New Insights into the Pathogenesis and Therapies of IgA Nephropathy

New Insights into the Pathogenesis and Therapies of IgA Nephropathy

Editors

Hitoshi Suzuki
Jan Novak

MDPI • Basel • Beijing • Wuhan • Barcelona • Belgrade • Manchester • Tokyo • Cluj • Tianjin

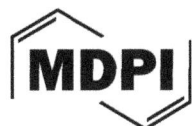

Editors

Hitoshi Suzuki
Department of Nephrology, Juntendo University Faculty of Medicine, Tokyo, Japan

Jan Novak
Department of Microbiology, University of Alabama at Birmingham, Birmingham, AL 35294, USA

Editorial Office
MDPI
St. Alban-Anlage 66
4052 Basel, Switzerland

This is a reprint of articles from the Special Issue published online in the open access journal *Journal of Clinical Medicine* (ISSN 2077-0383) (available at: https://www.mdpi.com/journal/jcm/special_issues/Nephropathy_Therapies).

For citation purposes, cite each article independently as indicated on the article page online and as indicated below:

LastName, A.A.; LastName, B.B.; LastName, C.C. Article Title. *Journal Name* **Year**, *Volume Number*, Page Range.

ISBN 978-3-0365-5041-1 (Hbk)
ISBN 978-3-0365-5042-8 (PDF)

© 2022 by the authors. Articles in this book are Open Access and distributed under the Creative Commons Attribution (CC BY) license, which allows users to download, copy and build upon published articles, as long as the author and publisher are properly credited, which ensures maximum dissemination and a wider impact of our publications.

The book as a whole is distributed by MDPI under the terms and conditions of the Creative Commons license CC BY-NC-ND.

Contents

About the Editors vii

Hitoshi Suzuki and Jan Novak
Special Issue: New Insights into the Pathogenesis and Therapies of IgA Nephropathy
Reprinted from: *J. Clin. Med.* **2022**, *11*, 4378, doi:10.3390/jcm11154378 1

Yukako Ohyama, Matthew B. Renfrow, Jan Novak and Kazuo Takahashi
Aberrantly Glycosylated IgA1 in IgA Nephropathy: What We Know and What We Don't Know
Reprinted from: *J. Clin. Med.* **2021**, *10*, 3467, doi:10.3390/jcm10163467 5

Yusuke Fukao, Hitoshi Suzuki, Jin Sug Kim, Kyung Hwan Jeong, Yuko Makita, Toshiki Kano, Yoshihito Nihei, Maiko Nakayama, Mingfeng Lee, Rina Kato, Jer-Ming Chang, Sang Ho Lee and Yusuke Suzuki
Galactose-Deficient IgA1 as a Candidate Urinary Marker of IgA Nephropathy
Reprinted from: *J. Clin. Med.* **2022**, *11*, 3173, doi:10.3390/jcm11113173 25

Barbora Knoppova, Colin Reily, R. Glenn King, Bruce A. Julian, Jan Novak and Todd J. Green
Pathogenesis of IgA Nephropathy: Current Understanding and Implications for Development of Disease-Specific Treatment
Reprinted from: *J. Clin. Med.* **2021**, *10*, 4501, doi:10.3390/jcm10194501 35

Felix Poppelaars, Bernardo Faria, Wilhelm Schwaeble and Mohamed R. Daha
The Contribution of Complement to the Pathogenesis of IgA Nephropathy: Are Complement-Targeted Therapies Moving from Rare Disorders to More Common Diseases?
Reprinted from: *J. Clin. Med.* **2021**, *10*, 4715, doi:10.3390/jcm10204715 57

Małgorzata Mizerska-Wasiak, Agnieszka Such-Gruchot, Karolina Cichoń-Kawa, Agnieszka Turczyn, Jadwiga Małdyk, Monika Miklaszewska, Dorota Drożdż, Agnieszka Firszt-Adamczyk, Roman Stankiewicz, Agnieszka Rybi-Szumińska, Anna Wasilewska, Maria Szczepańska, Beata Bieniaś, Przemysław Sikora, Agnieszka Pukajło-Marczyk, Danuta Zwolińska, Monika Pawlak-Bratkowska, Marcin Tkaczyk, Jacek Zachwieja, Magdalena Drożyńska-Duklas, Aleksandra Żurowska, Katarzyna Gadomska-Prokop, Ryszard Grenda and Małgorzata Pańczyk-Tomaszewska
The Role of Complement Component C3 Activation in the Clinical Presentation and Prognosis of IgA Nephropathy—A National Study in Children
Reprinted from: *J. Clin. Med.* **2021**, *10*, 4405, doi:10.3390/jcm10194405 79

Evangeline Pillebout
IgA Vasculitis and IgA Nephropathy: Same Disease?
Reprinted from: *J. Clin. Med.* **2021**, *10*, 2310, doi:10.3390/jcm10112310 91

Lingyun Lai, Shaojun Liu, Maria Azrad, Stacy Hall, Chuanming Hao, Jan Novak, Bruce A. Julian and Lea Novak
IgA Vasculitis with Nephritis in Adults: Histological and Clinical Assessment
Reprinted from: *J. Clin. Med.* **2021**, *10*, 4851, doi:10.3390/jcm10214851 105

Hernán Trimarchi, Mark Haas and Rosanna Coppo
Crescents and IgA Nephropathy: A Delicate Marriage
Reprinted from: *J. Clin. Med.* **2022**, *11*, 3569, doi:10.3390/jcm11133569 115

Yu Ah Hong, Ji Won Min, Myung Ah Ha, Eun Sil Koh, Hyung Duk Kim, Tae Hyun Ban, Young Soo Kim, Yong Kyun Kim, Dongryul Kim, Seok Joon Shin, Won Jung Choi, Yoon Kyung Chang, Suk Young Kim, Cheol Whee Park, Young Ok Kim, Chul Woo Yang and Hye Eun Yoon
The Impact of Obesity on the Severity of Clinicopathologic Parameters in Patients with IgA Nephropathy
Reprinted from: *J. Clin. Med.* **2020**, *10*, 2824, doi:10.3390/jcm10092824 . . . . **127**

Batoul Wehbi, Virginie Pascal, Lina Zawil, Michel Cogné and Jean-Claude Aldigier
History of IgA Nephropathy Mouse Models
Reprinted from: *J. Clin. Med.* **2021**, *10*, 3142, doi:10.3390/jcm10143142 . . . . **141**

Dita Maixnerova, Delphine El Mehdi, Dana V. Rizk, Hong Zhang and Vladimir Tesar
New Treatment Strategies for IgA Nephropathy: Targeting Plasma Cells as the Main Source of Pathogenic Antibodies
Reprinted from: *J. Clin. Med.* **2022**, *11*, 2810, doi:10.3390/jcm11102810 . . . . **153**

Chee Kay Cheung, Arun Rajasekaran, Jonathan Barratt and Dana V. Rizk
An Update on the Current State of Management and Clinical Trials for IgA Nephropathy
Reprinted from: *J. Clin. Med.* **2021**, *10*, 2493, doi:10.3390/jcm10112493 . . . . **165**

About the Editors

Hitoshi Suzuki

Hitoshi Suzuki, M.D., Ph.D., is a professor of the Department of Nephrology at Juntendo University Urayasu Hospital. He received his M.D. and Ph.D. from Juntendo University, Faculty of Medicine. He has investigated genetic factors, the role of bone-marrow-derived cells, and mucosal immunity involved in the pathogenesis of IgA nephropathy. After the postgraduate course, he studied abroad at the University of Alabama at Birmingham, USA to study molecular mechanisms of IgA nephropathy from 2005 to 2009 (mentor: Prof. Jan Novak). We have cloned IgA- and IgG-secreting cell lines from patients with IgA nephropathy and healthy controls and have analyzed molecular mechanisms and characteristics of aberrantly glycosylated IgA1 (galactose-deficient IgA1; Gd-IgA1) and the anti-Gd-IgA1 antibodies that formed the nephritogenic immune complexes. Furthermore, we have proposed 'A Multi-hit Mechanism', the widely accepted concept of pathogenesis of IgA nephropathy.

Jan Novak

Jan Novak is a Professor in the Department of Microbiology at the University of Alabama at Birmingham (UAB), Birmingham, AL, USA. He received his BS and MS in Biology from the Charles University, Prague, Czech Republic and PhD in Cell and Molecular Biology from the Czech Academy of Sciences. He has been at UAB since 1992. He was appointed to the rank of Distinguished Professor in 2022.

Dr. Novak's research interests include glycoimmunobiology and functional glycomics in health and disease, informing the emerging field of Glycomedicine. Major topics include renal and autoimmune diseases, cancer, mucosal infections, and biologically active compounds. Dr. Novak has been involved in many collaborative interdisciplinary studies, including those related to IgA nephropathy. These studies and related discoveries led to a multi-hit hypothesis for the pathogenesis of IgA nephropathy, a current "roadmap" for the development of disease-specific treatment and biomarkers.

Dr. Novak is an active member of the American Society of Nephrology (ASN) and a member of a steering committee of the International IgA Nephropathy Network. He is a member of the editorial board and an Associate Editor for the journal *Kidney Diseases*. In 2012, he co-organized an ASN early program, a 2-day conference on alloimmunity and autoimmunity. In 2013, he co-organized at UAB a mini-symposium "Glycoimmunobiology 2013", and in 2018 together with several colleagues at UAB established a new advanced course "Glycosylation in health and diseases". In 2021, he and his colleagues were invited by the NIH Glycobiology Scientific Interest Group to present a Special Topics Seminar Series on "Glycosylation in Human Health and Disease".

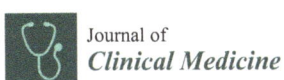

Editorial

Special Issue: New Insights into the Pathogenesis and Therapies of IgA Nephropathy

Hitoshi Suzuki [1,*] and Jan Novak [2,*]

1. Department of Nephrology, Juntendo University Urayasu Hospital, Chiba 279-0021, Japan
2. Department of Microbiology, University of Alabama at Birmingham, Birmingham, AL 35294, USA
* Correspondence: shitoshi@juntendo.ac.jp (H.S.); jannovak@uab.edu (J.N.)

IgA nephropathy (IgAN) is the most common form of primary glomerulonephritis worldwide [1]. Up to 40% of IgAN patients progress to kidney failure within 20 years following diagnosis [2]. Moreover, life expectancy is reduced by a decade in patients with IgAN [3]. IgA vasculitis with nephritis (IgAVN), formerly known as Henoch–Schönlein purpura nephritis, is a systemic form of vasculitis with renal manifestations similar to IgAN and with variable clinical outcome [4]. Thus, IgAN and IgAVN are significant public health problems.

The pathologic assessment of a renal biopsy specimen is the current "gold standard" for diagnosis of IgAN (for review, see [5–9]). Routine immunofluorescence reveals presence of glomerular immunodeposits consisting of IgA, with variable IgG and/or IgM. Complement C3 is present in most cases, but C1q is absent. Light microscopy provides an assessment of disease severity and prognosis based on the Oxford classification system. Its expanded version, termed MEST-C score, provides an evaluation of five different features: Mesangial cellularity, Endothelial hypercellularity, Segmental sclerosis, Tubular atrophy/interstitial fibrosis, and Crescents. IgAVN presents, in addition to kidney vasculitis features, with a greater frequency of severe lesions, such as glomerular necrosis and crescents. However, the pathologic findings for patients with IgAN as well as IgAVN may be impacted by the time between disease onset, diagnostic renal biopsy, and prior medications. Thus, a renal biopsy provides a snap shot in time since the inherent risks associated with renal biopsy hinder the use of a repeat biopsy. Minimally invasive approaches, such as those based on liquid biopsy biomarkers (e.g., blood, urine), are needed for monitoring disease progression, responses to treatments, and the identification of patients at risk of disease progression who may benefit from participation in new clinical trials.

In the last two decades, extensive studies, using genetic, cellular, biochemical, and immunologic approaches, have enabled the formulation of a multi-hit pathogenesis model for IgAN [10], which has been expanded to IgAVN [11]. This hypothesis postulates that glomerular immunodeposits originate from circulating immune complexes consisting of aberrantly glycosylated IgA1 bound by IgG autoantibodies. This IgA1 has some of the 3 to 6 clustered hinge-region O-glycans deficient in galactose (galactose-deficient IgA1). These IgA1-IgG circulating immune complexes have been found in patients with IgAN as well as IgAVN. Moreover, glomerular immunodeposits of patients with IgAN are enriched in galactose-deficient IgA1 glycoforms and the corresponding IgG autoantibodies [12–14]. Furthermore, the elevated serum levels of galactose-deficient IgA1 and corresponding IgG autoantibodies predict disease progression. The pathogenic role of immune complexes consisting of galactose-deficient IgA1 and IgG autoantibodies was recently confirmed in an experimental animal model [15,16]. Moreover, there are genetic elements involved in disease susceptibility and progression that can be associated with this multi-step mechanism [17–23].

Despite the progress since the disease was initially described in 1968 [24], disease-specific therapy to slow or prevent the progression of kidney injury is still not available. To

Citation: Suzuki, H.; Novak, J. Special Issue: New Insights into the Pathogenesis and Therapies of IgA Nephropathy. *J. Clin. Med.* 2022, *11*, 4378. https://doi.org/10.3390/jcm11154378

Received: 19 July 2022
Accepted: 24 July 2022
Published: 28 July 2022

Publisher's Note: MDPI stays neutral with regard to jurisdictional claims in published maps and institutional affiliations.

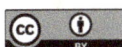

Copyright: © 2022 by the authors. Licensee MDPI, Basel, Switzerland. This article is an open access article distributed under the terms and conditions of the Creative Commons Attribution (CC BY) license (https://creativecommons.org/licenses/by/4.0/).

develop a curative treatment, new strategies for early diagnosis, disease-specific targets, and methods for the assessment of clinical responses in clinical trials need to be identified and developed.

This Special Issue presents a collection of reviews and clinical and experimental studies focused on specific aspects of the current research of the diagnosis, prognosis, disease pathogenesis, determination of disease activity, and emerging strategies for the treatment of IgAN and IgAVN. Of the twelve papers in this Special Issue, two are focused on IgAVN, nine on IgAN, and one makes a comparison between IgAN and IgAVN. Two papers are related to pathology, specifically, the prognostic significance of crescents in IgAN (Trimarch et al. [25]) and the light microscopic features observed at different times since disease onset in adult patients with IgAVN (Lai et al. [26]). Another paper compares features of IgAN and IgAVN (Pillebout et al. [27]). Two reviews focus on the two key factors in IgAN, the autoantigen (galactose-deficient IgA1) and the corresponding autoantibodies (Ohyama et al. and Knoppova et al. [28,29]), whereas an experimental study postulates that urinary galactose-deficient IgA1 may be a disease-specific biomarker useful for the assessment of disease activity in IgAN (Fukao et al. [30]). Two additional studies consider the role of complement in disease pathogenesis as it relates to therapeutic approaches or the diagnosis and prognosis of disease progression (Poppelaars et al. and Mizerska-Wasiak et al. [31,32]). Another study postulates that obesity may play a role in mesangial lesions in IgAN (Hong et al. [33]). In the last three papers, the authors review the characteristics of various murine models of IgAN (Wehbi et al. [34]) and provide updates on the current clinical trials in IgAN (Cheung et al. [35] and Maixnerova et al. [36]).

Although the papers in this Special Issue do not cover all current activities in the field, we found these publications to be inspirational and informative. We hope that the readers of this Special Issue will reach the same conclusion.

Author Contributions: H.S. and J.N. worked together on the initial draft and its further editing. All authors have read and agreed to the published version of the manuscript.

Funding: This research received no external funding.

Conflicts of Interest: H.S. and J.N. are co-inventors for a US patent application 14/318,082 (assigned to UAB Research Foundation). J.N. is a co-founder and co-owner of and consultant for Reliant Glycosciences, LLC.

References

1. Lai, K.N.; Tang, S.C.W.; Schena, F.P.; Novak, J.; Tomino, Y.; Fogo, A.B.; Glassock, R.J. IgA nephropathy. *Nat. Rev. Dis. Prim.* **2016**, *2*, 16001. [CrossRef]
2. Wyatt, R.J.; Julian, B.A. IgA nephropathy. *N. Engl. J. Med.* **2013**, *368*, 2402–2414. [CrossRef]
3. Hastings, M.C.; Bursac, Z.; Julian, B.A.; Baca, E.V.; Featherston, J.; Woodford, S.Y.; Bailey, L.; Wyatt, R.J. Life expectancy for patients from the southeastern United States with IgA nephropathy. *Kidney Int. Rep.* **2017**, *3*, 99–104. [CrossRef] [PubMed]
4. Davin, J.-C.; Ten Berge, I.J.; Weening, J.J. What is the difference between IgA nephropathy and Henoch-Schönlein purpura nephritis? *Kidney Int.* **2001**, *59*, 823–834. [CrossRef] [PubMed]
5. Clarkson, A.R.; Woodroffe, A.J.; Aarons, I.; Hiki, Y.; Hale, G. IgA nephropathy. *Annu. Rev. Med.* **1987**, *38*, 157–168. [CrossRef]
6. Jennette, J.C. The Immunohistology of IgA nephropathy. *Am. J. Kidney Dis.* **1988**, *12*, 348–352. [CrossRef]
7. Roberts, I.S.D. Pathology of IgA nephropathy. *Nat. Rev. Nephrol.* **2014**, *10*, 445–454. [CrossRef] [PubMed]
8. Rodrigues, J.C.; Haas, M.; Reich, H.N. IgA nephropathy. *Clin. J. Am. Soc. Nephrol.* **2017**, *12*, 677–686. [CrossRef] [PubMed]
9. Fogo, A.B.; Lusco, M.A.; Najafian, B.; Alpers, C.E. AJKD atlas of renal pathology: IgA nephropathy. *Am. J. Kidney Dis.* **2015**, *66*, e33–e34. [CrossRef] [PubMed]
10. Suzuki, H.; Kiryluk, K.; Novak, J.; Moldoveanu, Z.; Herr, A.B.; Renfrow, M.B.; Wyatt, R.J.; Scolari, F.; Mestecky, J.; Gharavi, A.G.; et al. The pathophysiology of IgA nephropathy. *J. Am. Soc. Nephrol.* **2011**, *22*, 1795–1803. [CrossRef]
11. Hastings, M.C.; Rizk, D.V.; Kiryluk, K.; Nelson, R.; Zahr, R.S.; Novak, J.; Wyatt, R.J. IgA vasculitis with nephritis: Update of pathogenesis with clinical implications. *Pediatr. Nephrol.* **2021**, *37*, 719–733. [CrossRef] [PubMed]
12. Hiki, Y.; Odani, H.; Takahashi, M.; Yasuda, Y.; Nishimoto, A.; Iwase, H.; Shinzato, T.; Kobayashi, Y.; Maeda, K. Mass spectrometry proves under-*O*-glycosylation of glomerular IgA1 in IgA nephropathy. *Kidney Int.* **2001**, *59*, 1077–1085. [CrossRef] [PubMed]
13. Allen, A.C.; Bailey, E.M.; Brenchley, P.E.; Buck, K.S.; Barratt, J.; Feehally, J. Mesangial IgA1 in IgA nephropathy exhibits aberrant *O*-glycosylation: Observations in three patients. *Kidney Int.* **2001**, *60*, 969–973. [CrossRef] [PubMed]

14. Rizk, D.V.; Saha, M.K.; Hall, S.; Novak, L.; Brown, R.; Huang, Z.-Q.; Fatima, H.; Julian, B.A.; Novak, J. Glomerular immunodeposits of patients with IgA nephropathy are enriched for IgG autoantibodies specific for galactose-deficient IgA1. *J. Am. Soc. Nephrol.* **2019**, *30*, 2017–2026. [CrossRef]
15. Moldoveanu, Z.; Suzuki, H.; Reily, C.; Satake, K.; Novak, L.; Xu, N.; Huang, Z.-Q.; Knoppova, B.; Khan, A.; Hall, S.; et al. Experimental evidence of pathogenic role of IgG autoantibodies in IgA nephropathy. *J. Autoimmun.* **2021**, *118*, 102593. [CrossRef] [PubMed]
16. Makita, Y.; Suzuki, H.; Nakano, D.; Yanagawa, H.; Kano, T.; Novak, J.; Nishiyama, A.; Suzuki, Y. Glomerular deposition of galactose-deficient IgA1-containing immune complexes via glomerular endothelial cell injuries. *Nephrol. Dial. Transplant.* **2022**; Online ahead of print. [CrossRef]
17. Julian, B.A.; Quiggins, P.A.; Thompson, J.S.; Woodford, S.Y.; Gleason, K.; Wyatt, R.J. Familial IgA nephropathy. *N. Engl. J. Med.* **1985**, *312*, 202–208. [CrossRef]
18. Gharavi, A.G.; Moldoveanu, Z.; Wyatt, R.; Barker, C.V.; Woodford, S.Y.; Lifton, R.P.; Mestecky, J.; Novak, J.; Julian, B.A. Aberrant IgA1 glycosylation is inherited in familial and sporadic IgA nephropathy. *J. Am. Soc. Nephrol.* **2008**, *19*, 1008–1014. [CrossRef] [PubMed]
19. Kiryluk, K.; Li, Y.; Sanna-Cherchi, S.; Rohanizadegan, M.; Suzuki, H.; Eitner, F.; Snyder, H.J.; Choi, M.; Hou, P.; Scolari, F.; et al. Geographic differences in genetic susceptibility to IgA nephropathy: GWAS replication study and geospatial risk analysis. *PLoS Genet.* **2012**, *8*, e1002765. [CrossRef]
20. Gharavi, A.G.; Kiryluk, K.; Choi, M.; Li, Y.; Hou, P.; Xie, J.; Sanna-Cherchi, S.; Men, C.J.; Julian, B.A.; Wyatt, R.; et al. Genome-wide association study identifies susceptibility loci for IgA nephropathy. *Nat. Genet.* **2011**, *43*, 321–327. [CrossRef]
21. Kiryluk, K.; Li, Y.; Scolari, F.; Sanna-Cherchi, S.; Choi, M.; Verbitsky, M.; Fasel, D.; Lata, S.; Prakash, S.; Shapiro, S.; et al. Discovery of new risk loci for IgA nephropathy implicates genes involved in immunity against intestinal pathogens. *Nat. Genet.* **2014**, *46*, 1187–1196. [CrossRef] [PubMed]
22. Kiryluk, K.; Li, Y.; Moldoveanu, Z.; Suzuki, H.; Reily, C.; Hou, P.; Xie, J.; Mladkova, N.; Prakash, S.; Fischman, C.; et al. GWAS for serum galactose-deficient IgA1 implicates critical genes of the O-glycosylation pathway. *PLoS Genet.* **2017**, *13*, e1006609. [CrossRef] [PubMed]
23. Gale, D.P.; Molyneux, K.; Wimbury, D.; Higgins, P.; Levine, A.P.; Caplin, B.; Ferlin, A.; Yin, P.; Nelson, C.P.; Stanescu, H.; et al. Galactosylation of IgA1 is associated with common variation in *C1GALT1*. *J. Am. Soc. Nephrol.* **2017**, *28*, 2158–2166. [CrossRef] [PubMed]
24. Berger, J.; Hinglais, N. Intercapillary deposits of IgA-IgG. *J. Urol. Nephrol.* **1968**, *74*, 694–695.
25. Trimarchi, H.; Haas, M.; Coppo, R. Crescents and IgA nephropathy: A delicate marriage. *J. Clin. Med.* **2022**, *11*, 3569. [CrossRef] [PubMed]
26. Lai, L.; Liu, S.; Azrad, M.; Hall, S.; Hao, C.; Novak, J.; Julian, B.A.; Novak, L. IgA vasculitis with nephritis in adults: Histological and clinical assessment. *J. Clin. Med.* **2021**, *10*, 4851. [CrossRef] [PubMed]
27. Pillebout, E. IgA vasculitis and IgA nephropathy: Same disease? *J. Clin. Med.* **2021**, *10*, 2310. [CrossRef]
28. Ohyama, Y.; Renfrow, M.B.; Novak, J.; Takahashi, K. Aberrantly glycosylated IgA1 in IgA nephropathy: What we know and what we don't know. *J. Clin. Med.* **2021**, *10*, 3467. [CrossRef]
29. Knoppova, B.; Reily, C.; King, R.G.; Julian, B.A.; Novak, J.; Green, T.J. Pathogenesis of IgA nephropathy: Current understanding and implications for development of disease-specific treatment. *J. Clin. Med.* **2021**, *10*, 4501. [CrossRef] [PubMed]
30. Fukao, Y.; Suzuki, H.; Kim, J.S.; Jeong, K.H.; Makita, Y.; Kano, T.; Nihei, Y.; Nakayama, M.; Lee, M.; Kato, R.; et al. Galactose-deficient IgA1 as a candidate urinary marker of IgA nephropathy. *J. Clin. Med.* **2022**, *11*, 3173. [CrossRef] [PubMed]
31. Poppelaars, F.; Faria, B.; Schwaeble, W.; Daha, M.R. The Contribution of complement to the pathogenesis of IgA nephropathy: Are complement-targeted therapies moving from rare disorders to more common diseases? *J. Clin. Med.* **2021**, *10*, 4715. [CrossRef] [PubMed]
32. Mizerska-Wasiak, M.; Such-Gruchot, A.; Cichoń-Kawa, K.; Turczyn, A.; Małdyk, J.; Miklaszewska, M.; Drożdż, D.; Firszt-Adamczyk, A.; Stankiewicz, R.; Rybi-Szumińska, A.; et al. The role of complement component C3 activation in the clinical presentation and prognosis of IgA nephropathy—A national study in children. *J. Clin. Med.* **2021**, *10*, 4405. [CrossRef] [PubMed]
33. Hong, Y.A.; Min, J.W.; Ha, M.A.; Koh, E.S.; Kim, H.D.; Ban, T.H.; Kim, Y.S.; Kim, Y.K.; Kim, D.; Shin, S.J.; et al. The impact of obesity on the severity of clinicopathologic parameters in patients with IgA nephropathy. *J. Clin. Med.* **2020**, *9*, 2824. [CrossRef] [PubMed]
34. Wehbi, B.; Pascal, V.; Zawil, L.; Cogné, M.; Aldigier, J.-C. History of IgA nephropathy mouse models. *J. Clin. Med.* **2021**, *10*, 3142. [CrossRef] [PubMed]
35. Cheung, C.K.; Rajasekaran, A.; Barratt, J.; Rizk, D.V. An update on the current state of management and clinical trials for IgA nephropathy. *J. Clin. Med.* **2021**, *10*, 2493. [CrossRef] [PubMed]
36. Maixnerova, D.; El Mehdi, D.; Rizk, D.V.; Zhang, H.; Tesar, V. New treatment strategies for IgA nephropathy: Targeting plasma cells as the main source of pathogenic antibodies. *J. Clin. Med.* **2022**, *11*, 2810. [CrossRef] [PubMed]

Review

Aberrantly Glycosylated IgA1 in IgA Nephropathy: What We Know and What We Don't Know

Yukako Ohyama [1], Matthew B. Renfrow [2], Jan Novak [2] and Kazuo Takahashi [1,*]

1 Department of Biomedical Molecular Sciences, Fujita Health University School of Medicine, Toyoake, Aichi 470-1192, Japan; yukako.oyama@fujita-hu.ac.jp
2 Departments of Biochemistry and Molecular Genetics and Microbiology, University of Alabama at Birmingham, Birmingham, AL 35294, USA; renfrow@uab.edu (M.B.R.); jannovak@uab.edu (J.N.)
* Correspondence: kazuot@fujita-hu.ac.jp; Tel.: +81-(562)-93-2430; Fax: +81-(562)-93-1830

Abstract: IgA nephropathy (IgAN), the most common primary glomerular disease worldwide, is characterized by glomerular deposition of IgA1-containing immune complexes. The IgA1 hinge region (HR) has up to six clustered *O*-glycans consisting of Ser/Thr-linked *N*-acetylgalactosamine usually with β1,3-linked galactose and variable sialylation. Circulating levels of IgA1 with abnormally *O*-glycosylated HR, termed galactose-deficient IgA1 (Gd-IgA1), are increased in patients with IgAN. Current evidence suggests that IgAN is induced by multiple sequential pathogenic steps, and production of aberrantly glycosylated IgA1 is considered the initial step. Thus, the mechanisms of biosynthesis of aberrantly glycosylated IgA1 and the involvement of aberrant glycoforms of IgA1 in disease development have been studied. Furthermore, Gd-IgA1 represents an attractive biomarker for IgAN, and its clinical significance is still being evaluated. To elucidate the pathogenesis of IgAN, it is important to deconvolute the biosynthetic origins of Gd-IgA1 and characterize the pathogenic IgA1 HR *O*-glycoform(s), including the glycan structures and their sites of attachment. These efforts will likely lead to development of new biomarkers. Here, we review the IgA1 HR *O*-glycosylation in general and the role of aberrantly glycosylated IgA1 in the pathogenesis of IgAN in particular.

Keywords: IgA nephropathy; aberrantly glycosylated IgA1; galactose-deficient IgA1; glycosylation of IgA1; biomarker

1. Introduction

IgA nephropathy (IgAN) is a mesangioproliferative glomerulonephritis associated with depositions of IgA-containing immune complexes [1]. These deposits are exclusively of IgA1 subclass [2]. Recurrence of IgAN is common in patients after transplantation [3–6]. Conversely, when kidneys with subclinical IgA deposits are transplanted into patients with end-stage renal disease other than IgAN, the deposited IgA in the donor kidney is cleared [7–9]. Furthermore, IgA deposits disappear when bone-marrow transplantations are performed for patients with IgAN [10]. Conversely, IgAN can develop after bone-marrow transplantation due to a non-graft-versus-host-disease-related multi-hit process associated with glomerular deposition of aberrantly glycosylated IgA1 (see for details below) [11]. Based on these observations, it is thought that the glomerular IgA deposits are derived from circulating IgA1-containing complexes. Elevated IgA serum levels alone are not sufficient to induce IgAN, as patients with IgA myeloma, who have abnormally increased serum IgA levels, rarely suffer from concomitant IgAN [12–14]. According to these observations, the pathogenetic mechanisms underlying IgAN appear to involve qualitative features of IgA1 rather than a mere elevation in blood levels of total IgA1.

Patients with IgAN present with a variety of clinical, laboratory, and histopathological findings. In addition to primary IgAN, many patients with liver disease, collagen disease, inflammatory bowel syndrome, malignant tumor, and infection exhibit IgA glomerular deposition, i.e., secondary IgAN [15,16]. Due to these many clinical features and types of secondary IgAN, it has been assumed that IgAN may represent a group of diseases rather than a single disease [17,18].

Most human circulatory IgA is derived from B cells in the bone marrow. Ninety-percent of IgA1 is mainly present as a monomeric form [19], whereas glomerular IgA deposits contain mainly polymeric IgA1, i.e., two or more monomers connected by joining chain (J chain) [20,21]. IgA deposition may not necessarily be associated with glomerular damage, unless it is accompanied by deposition of complement [22,23]. The development of IgAN likely involves several complex mechanisms, including (over)production and glomerular deposition of IgA1-containing immune complexes, activation of mesangial cells and subsequent glomerular injury [14,15,18,24–27]. As many patients with IgAN exhibit exacerbation concurrently with upper-respiratory-tract infections, the involvement of mucosal immunity in the disease pathogenesis is suspected [25,28].

IgA1 is a highly glycosylated molecule, carrying both N-linked and O-linked glycans. The importance of aberrant IgA1 O-glycosylation in the pathogenesis of IgAN has been first observed based on differences in lectin reactivities with serum IgA1 from patients with IgAN vs. healthy subjects [29]. This conclusion was further supported by the observed enrichment of aberrant IgA1 O-glycoforms in the glomerular immunodeposits of IgAN patients [30,31].

The circulating levels of polymeric IgA with aberrantly glycosylated IgA1, with some O-glycans in the hinge region (HR) galactose (Gal)-deficient, are elevated in most patients with IgAN [32,33]. Mesangial deposition of macromolecular IgA1 is thought to occur in patients with IgAN due to the formation of immune complexes. Particularly, autoantibodies specific for Gd-IgA1 bind Gd-IgA1 and form circulating immune complexes (CICs) [25]. Furthermore, IgA and aberrantly glycosylated IgA1 may bind to the soluble form of the Fcα receptor (sCD89) [34], and aberrantly glycosylated IgA1 may form protein aggregates [35]. IgA1-containing immune complexes activate the complement system, as evidenced by complement C3 in glomerular immunodeposits, leading to glomerular and renal tubular injury [36], as well as by the presence of C3 in the circulating IgA1-containing immune complexes (for review and details see [37–42]). Here, we review pathological and clinical significance of aberrant glycosylation of IgA1 in IgAN.

2. Structure of IgA

IgA production in humans is approximately 66 mg/kg/day, which is approximately twice that of IgG and 10 times that of IgM [43]. Two-thirds of IgA is secreted into the mucosal surfaces as the dominant isotype of secretory antibodies. Human IgA exists in two subclasses, IgA1 and IgA2; these two glycoproteins differ in number of N-glycans and the presence of O-glycans in IgA1. Compared with IgA2, IgA1 has clustered O-glycans in its HR, whereas IgA2 HR is short and without glycosylation sites. Figure 1a shows the glycan binding sites. The J chain, which is essential for the formation of polymeric IgA, has an N-glycan (Figure 1b). Most IgA in the mucosal tissues is produced by B cells as dimeric IgA with a disulfide-bond connected 16-kDa J chain. Polymeric IgA can bind to the polymeric immunoglobulin receptor (pIgR). Once polymeric IgA is bound to the pIgR at the basolateral side of the epithelium, it is transported to the luminal side through transcytosis, and a portion of pIgR is cleaved and remains attached to IgA to form secretory IgA (sIgA). This pIgR fragment, termed the secretory component (SC), has seven N-glycans (Figure 1c). Glycans on IgA and SC can bind or repel glycans on bacterial surfaces to prevent invasion into the blood/tissues [44].

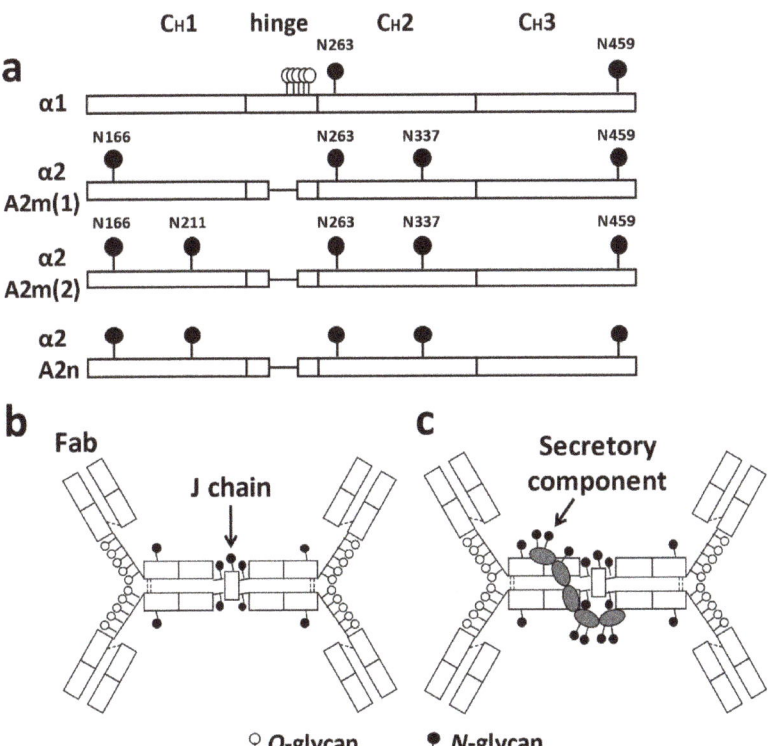

Figure 1. Molecular structure of IgA and its glycosylation sites. (**a**) Human IgA has two subclasses: IgA1 and IgA2. IgA1 harbors clustered O-glycans in its hinge region. IgA1 and IgA2 have several N-glycans in their constant region of heavy chains. IgA1 has two N-glycosylation sites at asparagine (Asn)^{263} and Asn^{459}. Three allotypes of IgA2 are known, designated A2m (1), A2m (2), and IgA2 (n). All allotypes have N-glycans at Asn^{166}, Asn^{263}, Asn^{337}, and Asn^{459}. A2m (2) and IgA2 (n) allotypes have a fifth N-glycan at Asn^{211} [45]. (**b**,**c**) Schematic representation of dimeric IgA1 and secretory IgA1. Both the joining chain (J chain) and the secretory component have N-glycan(s). Fab, antigen-binding fragment.

2.1. Glycosylation of IgA1

Figure 2 shows the structure of IgA1 [46]. Clustered O-glycans on IgA1 HR are present only in hominid primates [47–49]. Human IgA1 has two N-glycosylation sites in the CH2 region and in the tailpiece (asparagine (Asn)^{263} and Asn^{459}) (Figure 1a), and nine potential O-glycosylation sites (serine (Ser) and threonine (Thr)) in the proline (Pro)-rich HR (Figure 2a). Glycosylation in IgA1 HR occurs at specific sites [50–53]; usually three to six O-glycans are attached per HR [46,54], and the O-glycans of IgA1 are the core 1 glycans. Six different types of O-glycans can be found in IgA1 HR (Figure 2b). These features, number of attached O-glycans, glycan structures, and their attachment sites, contribute to the IgA1 HR O-glycoform diversity.

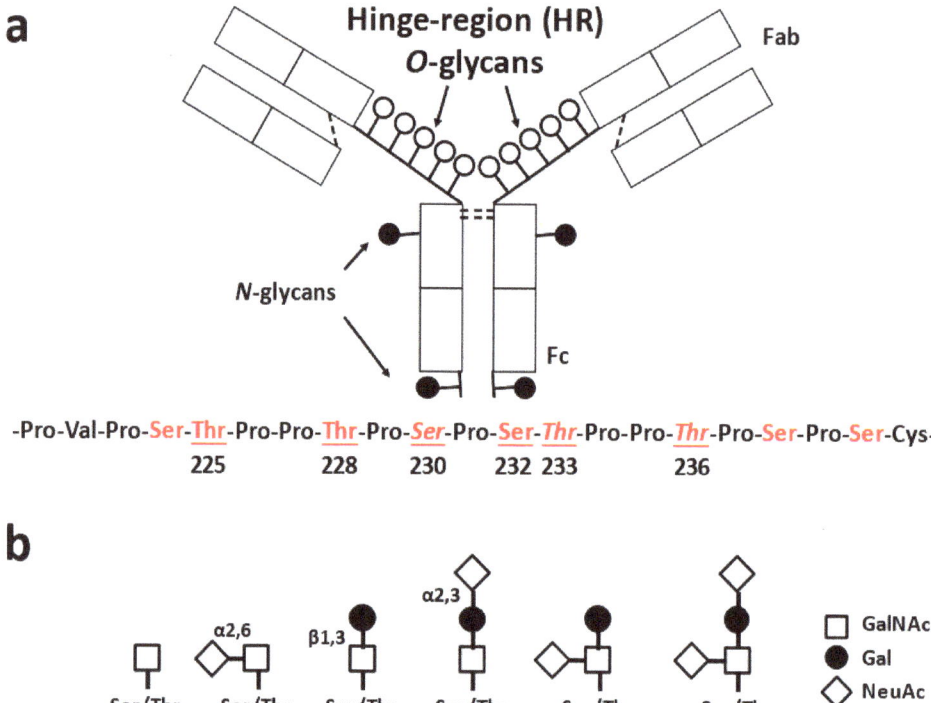

Figure 2. Schematic representation of human IgA1. The IgA1 heavy chain has three to six *O*-glycans in its hinge region (HR) and two *N*-glycosylation sites [46,54]. There are nine potential *O*-glycosylation sites, marked in red font, of which up to six sites can be *O*-glycosylated (underlined serine (Ser) and threonine (Thr)). Ser/Thr in italic (230, 233, 236) show the frequent sites with galactose (Gal)-deficient *O*-glycan (**a**) [50,52,53,55]. There are *O*-glycan variants of circulatory IgA1. *N*-acetylgalactosamine (GalNAc) is attached to Ser/Thr residues and can be extended by the attachment of Gal to GalNAc residues. GalNAc or Gal or both can be sialylated. Due of diversity of the glycan attachment sites, the number of *O*-glycans in HR, and variability of *O*-glycan structures, IgA1-HR *O*-glycoforms exhibit wide heterogeneity. Gd-IgA1-specific antibodies are considered to recognize Gal-deficient IgA1 glycoforms with terminal GalNAc (left structure). NeuAc, *N*-acetylneuraminic acid (**b**).

O-glycans of IgA1 are synthesized in a step-wise manner by glycosyltransferases in the Golgi apparatus of IgA1-secreting cells [56] (Figure 3). IgA1 HR *O*-glycosylation is initiated by the attachment of *N*-acetylgalactosamine (GalNAc) to Ser or Thr, catalyzed by UDP-*N*-acetylgalactosaminyltransferase 2 (GalNAc-T2) [51]. Other GalNAc-Ts can also participate in IgA1 HR glycosylation [57–60]. The addition of galactose (Gal) is mediated by the core 1 β1,3-galactosyltransferase (C1GalT1). The stability of C1GalT1 protein depends on its interaction with a specific molecular chaperone, Cosmc. In the absence of Cosmc, the C1GalT1 protein is rapidly degraded and, thus, Gal cannot be attached to GalNAc [61]. Furthermore, *N*-acetylneuraminic acid (NeuAc) is transferred to Gal and/or GalNAc by α2,3-sialyltransferase (ST3Gal1) and α2,6-sialyltransferase (ST6GalNAc2), respectively. If NeuAc is attached to GalNAc prior to the attachment of Gal, this premature sialylation precludes subsequent attachment of a Gal residue [62–64].

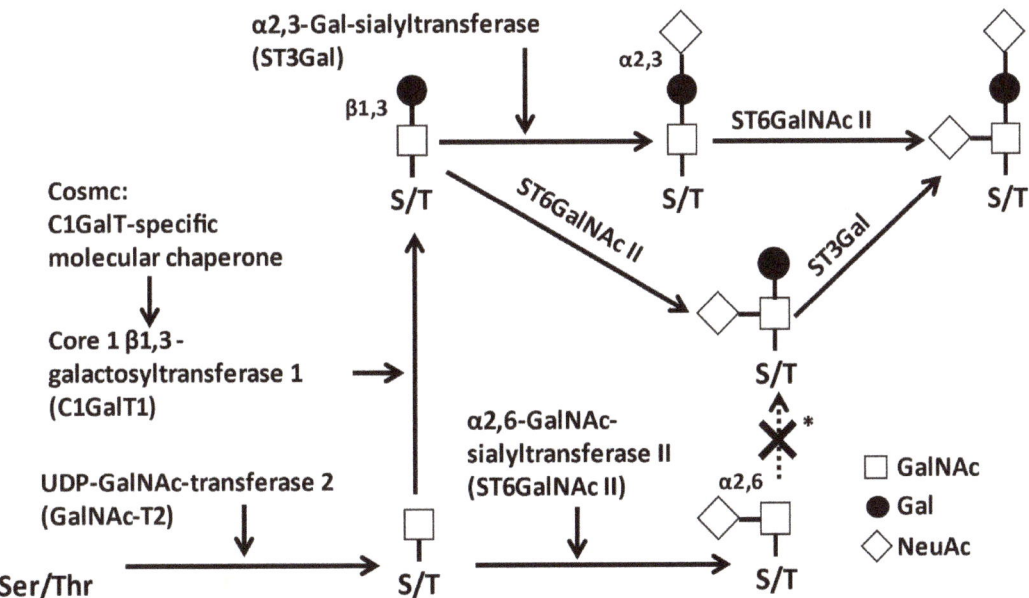

Figure 3. *O*-Glycosylation pathways of the human IgA1 hinge region (HR). The biosynthesis process starts with the attachment of *N*-acetylgalactosamine (GalNAc) to Ser/Thr residues in the HR by UDP-GalNAc-transferase 2 (GalNAc-T2). GalNAc residues are extended by galactose or *N*-acetylneuraminic acid (NeuAc) by core 1 β1,3-galactosyltransferase (C1GalT1) and its molecular chaperone Cosmc or α2,6 sialyltransferase (ST6GalNAc2), respectively. Finally, the *O*-glycan structure is completed by attachment of NeuAc to the galactose residue and/or GalNAc residues, each of which is mediated by α2,3-sialyltransferase (ST3Gal1) and ST6GalNAc2. The sialylation of GalNAc before the attachment of galactose prevents galactosylation of GalNAc (marked by *) [62].

2.2. Biological Roles of O-Glycosylation in IgA1 HR

Protein glycosylation impacts many biological functions [65], and *O*-glycosylation of IgA1 HR also influences the structural and functional characteristics of the IgA1 molecule. *O*-glycosylation in IgA1 HR probably imparts the T-shaped antigen-binding fragment (Fab) arms. The difference in the arrangement of Fab and Fc (fragment crystallizable) segments between IgA1 and IgA2 was previously demonstrated using X-ray and neutron scattering procedures [66]. The structural differences between IgA1 and IgA2 may be driven by the backbone amino-acid sequence and *O*-glycosylation of IgA HR; *O*-glycosylation of Ser/Thr residues affects *cis/trans* isomerization of Pro residues in HR [67]. Appropriate glycosylation of HR may decrease unfavorable relative orientations between Fab and Fc in IgA1 by stabilizing the conformation of HR. In addition, HR *O*-glycans add hydrophilic characteristics to IgA1 [55].

In addition to the structural influence on IgA1 molecules, IgA1 HR *O*-glycans mediate antigen-nonspecific binding to bacteria [58,68]. This function enables IgA to participate in innate immunity, in addition to adaptive immunity. It is possible that the *O*-glycans in IgA1 HR are related to enhanced innate immune functions of hominoid-primates IgA1 subclass.

2.3. Aberrantly Glycosylated IgA1

IgA1 with some HR *O*-glycan(s) Gal-deficient can be detected by lectins, such as *Helix aspersa* agglutinin (HAA), a lectin specific for terminal GalNAc [32,69–72]. HAA in enzyme-linked immunosorbent assay (ELISA) revealed elevated levels of Gal-deficient IgA1 (Gd-IgA1) in the circulation in patients with IgAN. The term "Gd-IgA1" is often used as a synonym for "aberrantly glycosylated IgA1", but it should be noted that not all

O-glycans in Gd-IgA1 HR have to be Gal-deficient. Other types of aberrant glycosylation of IgA1 may include underglycosylation, i.e., a lower number of O-glycans per HR compared to IgA1 from healthy subjects, or over-sialylation, elevated amount of NeuAc in IgA1 HR in patients with IgAN [73–76]. It is to be noted that IgA1 O-glycans are presented as a heterogeneous mixture of glycoforms in patients with IgAN as well as in healthy subjects. Thus, "aberrantly glycosylated IgA1" is also present in the circulation of healthy individuals [53,77] and often a cut-off point is used to define "normal" vs. "abnormal" glycoforms of IgA1. To identify IgA1 O-glycoforms that are elevated in the circulation of patients with IgAN, quantitative analyses are required, including site-specific attachment of Gal-deficient O-glycan. The detailed structures of aberrantly glycosylated IgA1 specific for IgAN have not been reported. The levels of Gd-IgA1 produced by cultured IgA1-producing cells from peripheral blood correlate with the donors' serum levels of Gd-IgA1 measured by lectin ELISA. This observation suggests that aberrantly glycosylated IgA1 originates due to the abnormal biosynthetic processes in IgA1-producing cells rather than a removal of Gal from circulatory IgA1 in the blood [76]. Reduced C1GalT1 activity and elevated ST6GalNAc2 activity in IgA1-producing cell lines are associated with production of Gd-IgA1 in IgAN [76].

3. Pathogenic Significance of Aberrantly Glycosylated IgA1

In IgAN, circulatory IgA1 with some glycans deficient in Gal is considered a disease-specific abnormality as this type of aberrant glycosylation is not observed for other glycoproteins with O-glycans, such as IgD or C1 inhibitor [78]. However, a high level of circulatory aberrantly glycosylated IgA1 alone does not induce glomerular injury [79]. Additional factors are thought to be involved in the development of IgAN, namely unique autoantibodies specific for Gd-IgA1 that enable formation of IgA1-containing immune complexes in the circulation, some of which deposit in the kidneys and induce glomerular injury [80,81]. Here, we discuss the factors related to the production of aberrantly glycosylated IgA1 (genetic factors, mucosal immunity) and Gd-IgA1 involvement in this postulated multi-hit mechanism.

3.1. Genetic Factors Associated to Gd-IgA1 Production

Increased serum levels of Gd-IgA1 are observed in 47% of first-degree relatives of patients with familial IgAN and 25% of first-degree relatives of patients with sporadic IgAN [79]. Furthermore, increased serum levels of aberrantly glycosylated IgA1 are observed in first-degree relatives of both pediatric and adult patients with IgAN [79,82–85], indicating a relationship between genetic background and aberrantly glycosylated IgA1. Regarding the production of aberrantly glycosylated IgA1, several single-nucleotide polymorphisms of *C1GALT1* [86–88] and *ST6GALNAC2* [88,89] genes represent IgAN-susceptibility alleles. However, no mutations were found in the exon of the gene encoding Cosmc, the molecular chaperone specific for C1GalT1 [90].

Genome-wide association studies of IgAN have identified many IgAN susceptibility loci, mainly in the MHC region at 6p21 [91,92], the *DEFA* locus at 8p23 [91–93], the *TNFSF13* locus at 17p13 [91], the *HORMAD2* locus at 22q12 [94], the *CFH/CFHR* locus at 1q32, the *ITGAM-ITGAX* locus at 16p11 [92], the *VAV3* locus at 1p13 [92] and the *CARD9* locus at 9q34 [92]. Except *C1GALT1*, genomic regions encoding other enzymes involved in IgA1 O-glycosylation have not been confirmed as IgAN susceptibility loci. Two genome-wide association studies confirmed that Gd-IgA1 serum levels are heritable and influenced by genetic variation at the *C1GALT1* gene [95,96]. Furthermore, two significant loci, in *C1GALT1* (rs13226913) and *C1GALT1C1* (rs5910940), which encode C1GalT1 and Cosmc, respectively, were identified in quantitative trait genome-wide association studies for serum levels of Gd-IgA1. In particular, the Gd-IgA1-increasing allele rs13226913 is rare or absent in some Asian populations and is the predominant allele in Europeans [96].

In addition, some microRNAs (miRNAs) are involved in regulating expression of some glycosyltransferases [97]. Relevant to IgAN, it was noted that expression of two miRNAs was associated with IgA1 O-glycosylation; expression of miR-148b targeting *C1GALT1* and miR-let-7b targeting *GALNT2* is elevated in peripheral blood mononuclear cells (PBMCs) of IgAN patients vs. healthy subjects [98,99]. These two miRNAs can be also detected in serum samples. A 2016 study found differences in the expression patterns between Caucasians and Asians, with significant upregulation in Caucasians [100]. From these reports, Gd-IgA1 levels are affected by the different alleles of the gene encoding *C1GALT1* and the different expression levels of miRNAs that control the expression of *C1GALT1* and *GALNT2*. Furthermore, the frequency of Gd-IgA1-increasing alleles and miR-148b that regulate *C1GALT1* expression are both higher in Caucasians than in Asians and may contribute to higher Gd-IgA1 levels in Caucasians than in Asians [95]. More recent studies identified additional mechanisms involving competing endogenous RNA molecules involved in regulation of IgA1 O-glycosylation, indicating that there is more to be discovered on the regulation of IgA1 O-glycosylation in general and in IgAN specifically [101–103]

3.2. Alteration of Mucosal Immunity Associated with Gd-IgA1 Production

Mucosal immunity is closely associated with IgAN. Patients with IgAN often present with an episode of macroscopic hematuria after upper-respiratory-tract or gastrointestinal tract infections. Furthermore, IgAN is associated with diseases involving mucosal abnormalities, such as ulcerative colitis, Crohn's disease, and coeliac disease [104–107].

Mesangial IgA1 deposits in IgAN resemble mucosal IgA, wherein they are both polymeric and relatively poorly O-galactosylated [30,31,108,109]. As the number of polymeric IgA-secreting plasma cells is increased in the bone marrow of IgAN patients [110], it has been speculated that mis-homing of mucosally imprinted B cells to the bone marrow may mediate production of "mucosal IgA1" into the circulation. IgD O-glycosylation is apparently normal in patients with IgAN [78] and, thus, factors specific for IgA1-producing cells are thought to affect O-glycosylation of IgA1 in IgAN, such as the microenvironment with antigen-mediated activation and class-switching signals [111].

The tonsils represent a mucosa-associated lymphoid tissue involved in IgA production, and tonsillectomy, often combined with steroid pulse, has been reported to be an effective treatment of IgAN in east Asia [112–114]. With regards to the expression of O-glycosyltransferases in tonsillar CD19$^+$ lymphocytes, *C1GALT1*, *C1GALT1C1*, and *GALNT2* have significantly reduced expression in IgAN patients compared to the subjects with chronic tonsillitis [115]. T-helper 2 (Th2)-cell polarity was observed in the tonsillar tissue of IgAN [116], and interleukin-4 (IL-4), a Th2 cytokine, reduced expression of C1GalT1 and Cosmc in a human B cell lines [117]. Studies using immortalized IgA1-secreting cell lines derived from peripheral blood of patients with IgAN and healthy controls provided additional insight into the regulation of glycogene expression by cytokines and Gd-IgA1 production [64,118]. IL-4 and, even more so, IL-6 enhance production of Gd-IgA1 due to further dysregulation of expression and activities of specific targets, including *C1GALT1*, *C1GALT1C1*, and *ST6GALNAC2* [64]. Leukemia inhibitory factor (LIF), an IL-6-related cytokine, also enhances Gd-IgA1 production [119]. Notably, both IL-6 and LIF enhance production of Gd-IgA1 in IgA1-secreting cell lines derived from IgAN patients due to abnormal signaling in JAK-STAT pathways that leads to further dysregulation of key glycosyltransferases [38,119–122]. Furthermore, a proliferation-inducing ligand (APRIL), known to play an important role in T cell-independent IgA class switching, is overproduced by CD19$^+$ B cells in tonsil germinal centers in IgAN [118]. In addition, in IgAN-prone ddY mice and in the human B cell line, APRIL and IL-6 expression is upregulated via activation by Toll-like receptor 9 (TLR9) by CpG-oligonucleotides (CpG-ODN) [123], resulting in increased Gd-IgA1 production. In summary, altered cytokine production and/or signaling responses in IgA1-producing cells in mucosal tissues may be one of the reasons for over-production of aberrantly glycosylated IgA1.

3.3. Antigenicity of Gd-IgA1 Related to Autoantibody Production

IgG or IgA1 autoantibodies targeting aberrantly glycosylated IgA1 have been identified in patients with IgAN [69,124,125]. IgG autoantibodies are predominant [126] and are found in the glomerular deposits of all patients [80]. Furthermore, a correlation between serum levels of Gd-IgA1 and the corresponding IgG autoantibodies was observed in sera of patients with IgAN, but not in sera of disease or healthy controls [126]. As described above, the alterations of *O*-glycosylation in IgA1 HR likely generate conformational changes in IgA1, contributing to the exposure of epitopes for anti-Gd-IgA1 autoantibodies, and driving the formation of IgA1-containing immune complexes (Figure 4c). IgG produced from IgG-producing cell lines derived from IgAN patients is highly reactive with desialylated and degalactosylated IgA1 and specific alterations of the amino acid sequence in the complementarity-determining region 3 (CDR3) in the variable region of the IgG heavy chains impacts the reactivity with Gd-IgA1 [125]. Notably, serum levels of IgG autoantibodies specific for Gd-IgA1 correlate with proteinuria [125]. Although the mechanism that leads to the formation of these autoantibodies has not been elucidated, these antibodies may be produced against some viruses and Gram-positive bacteria that express GalNAc-containing structures on their surfaces and they may acquire cross-reactivity with Gal-deficient IgA1 [25,56].

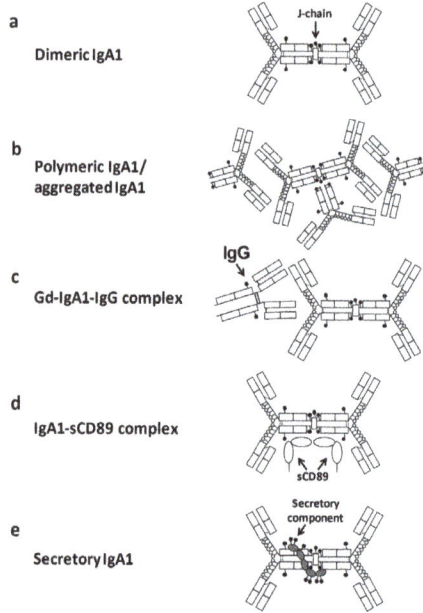

Figure 4. Macromolecular forms of IgA1. Although mesangially deposited IgA1 has not been fully characterized, Gd-IgA1-IgG (or IgA) immune complexes, IgA-IgA receptor complexes, self-aggregated IgA1 proteins, other serum protein complexes with IgA1, and secretory IgA1 are possible forms in the kidney deposits [23]. Dimeric IgA1 is composed of two monomeric IgA1 connected by joining chain (J chain) (**a**). Larger molecular forms of IgA1 may include complexes/aggregates of dimeric IgA1 and monomeric IgA1. Aberrantly glycosylated IgA1 may be prone to aggregation [127]. (**b**). Incomplete galactosylation of *O*-glycans in the IgA1 hinge region results in the exposure of terminal GalNAc and is recognized by autoantibodies (IgG of IgA), leading to the formation of IgA1-containing immune complexes (**c**). IgA1 complexes with soluble CD89 (sCD89) may be formed from CD89 cleaved from the surface of monocytes/macrophages (**d**). Secretory IgA1 consists of dimeric IgA1 with J chain and the secretory component (**e**). These macromolecular IgA1 forms (**a**–**e**) can form complexes with other serum proteins.

3.4. Impact of IgA1 O-Glycosylation of Interactions with IgA Receptors

There are five well-known IgA receptors: FcαR1 (CD89), asialoglycoprotein receptor (ASGPR), polymeric Ig receptor (pIgR), transferrin receptor (TfR; CD71), and Fc α/μ receptor. Some of these receptors are involved in IgA removal from the circulation, either for catabolism or transcytosis to mucosal surfaces.

ASGPR, which is expressed on the sinusoidal/lateral aspect of hepatocytes, is a receptor mediating endocytosis and catabolism of glycoproteins, including IgA [128]. In patients with secondary IgAN due to liver cirrhosis, reduced clearance of IgA-containing immune complexes (IgA-IC) has been reported, consistent with aberrant expression of hepatic ASGPR [16]. In primary IgAN, large size of IgA-IC is thought to limit access through the fenestration of endothelial cells to the space of Disse and, thus, to the ASGPR on hepatocytes, resulting in extended circulation time of IgA-IC [111].

CD89, a membrane glycoprotein expressed by cells of myeloid lineage, such as neutrophils, monocytes, macrophages, and eosinophils, binds to the constant region of the heavy chain of both the monomeric and dimeric forms of IgA1 and IgA2. It is thought that CD89 has a role in the removal of IgA-antigen complexes from the circulation [129]. In patients with IgAN, membrane expression of CD89 on circulating myeloid cells is decreased [129] and binding of monoclonal IgA to CD89 is impaired [130], which may contribute to a delayed IgA clearance. Notably, CD89 N-glycans significantly modulate binding affinity to IgA [131]. In addition, increased levels of soluble CD89 (sCD89) complexed with IgA are found in some patients with IgAN (Figure 4d) [132]. IgA-IC with sCD89 is possibly produced by shedding its extracellular portion after binding with IC containing polymeric Gd-IgA1. In mice generated by backcrossing between α1-knock-in mice and human CD89 transgenic mice, which spontaneously express human IgA1 and CD89, a complete human IgAN phenotype develops [133]. In addition, IgA-sCD89 complex levels are significantly higher in pre-transplantation patients with IgAN than in control groups and are also found in the mesangial deposition of IgAN [134].

Regarding IgA receptors expressed in human mesangial cells, Fcα/μR and CD71 receptors were detected [135,136], whereas CD89, ASGP-R, and pIgR were absent [137]. CD71 binds polymeric IgA1, but not monomeric IgA1 or IgA2, co-localizes with mesangial IgA1 deposits, and is overexpressed in patients with IgAN [136,138]. In addition, aberrantly glycosylated IgA1 and polymeric IgA1 show higher affinity for CD71, indicating that the formation of Gd-IgA1 immune complexes contributes to mesangial TfR-IgA1 interaction and glomerular deposition in IgAN [139].

Additional receptors able to bind IgA1 were identified in human mesangial cells: integrin α1/β1 and α2/β1 and β1,4-galactosyltransferase 1 [140,141]. Expression of the latter receptor in glomeruli is increased in IgAN, indicating that β1,4-galactosyltransferase 1 may play a role in IgA clearance and in the initial response to IgA deposition [140,142]. This observation on the role of β1,4-galactosyltransferase was reported earlier for binding of IgA1 to various cells [143].

3.5. Complement Activation

In IgAN, glomerular co-deposition of IgA and complement components of C3 are commonly observed, being present in at least 90% of renal biopsies [144]. As the membrane attack complex, the terminal product of the complement activation, is observed at high frequency, activation of the complement pathway has been considered to play a major role in glomerular injury in IgAN [145]. Although markers of the classical pathway, such as C1q and C4, are rarely observed, co-deposition of C3b, factor P, properdin, and factor H (FH) are observed in almost 100%, 75–100%, and 30–90% of cases, respectively [39,145]. In addition, cases with deposition of C4d, mannose-binding lectin (MBL), ficolin, and MBL-associated serine protease were observed, and associations of MBL and L-ficolin deposition with severity of renal histological damage have also been reported [146]. These aspects suggest that the alternative and lectin pathways are involved in IgAN pathophysiology [37].

Although the impact of aberrant IgA1 glycosylation on complement activation is not clearly understood, some reports suggest a relationship between complement activity and IgA1 glycosylation abnormalities. Polymeric IgA is more efficient in binding C3 and inducing glomerular injury compared to monomeric IgA in rats [147,148]. In humans, polymeric IgA1 is highly reactive with GalNAc-specific lectin HAA and shows a higher binding capacity for MBL via C-type lectin and higher C4 activation ability [149]. As recent studies showed that MBL binds to N-glycans of IgG and IgM [150,151], N-glycosylation of polymeric IgA may thus be associated with MBL binding and lectin pathway activation. In the comparison of N-glycosylation of IgA heavy chains between monomeric and polymeric IgA, oligomannose structure is elevated in polymeric IgA [149]. However, the N-glycans of the heavily glycosylated secretory component may also contribute to complement activation, as related to elevated concentration of secretory IgA in polymeric IgA is observed in IgAN [149]. Further investigations are required to determine which components and structures of N-glycans are involved in lectin-pathway activation and whether N- or O-glycosylation of IgA1 are involved in the alternative pathways of complement activation.

4. Clinical Significance of Aberrantly Glycosylated IgA1

In recent years, the validity of Gd-IgA1 and its associated molecules as diagnostic and prognostic markers has been assessed. Serum Gd-IgA1 levels can now be quantified using ELISA. Furthermore, detection and quantification of IgA1 HR O-glycosylation varieties and analysis of O-glycan attachment sites have been performed using high-resolution mass spectrometry.

4.1. Approaches for Detection of Aberrantly Glycosylated IgA1

For the detection of galactose-deficient O-glycan in IgA1 HR, some lectins that specifically bind to GalNAc residue have been used, such as *Helix aspersa* (HAA) or *H. pomatia* agglutinin (HPA) [70] and *Vicia villosa* lectin (VVL) [29]. A lectin-based assay for the detection of Gd-IgA1 was developed [70], and we confirmed that serum IgA1 in Japanese IgAN patients is also highly reactive with this lectin (Figure 5a) [32,33]. However, there are some limitations to the lectin-based assay. Lectin activity and stability may vary from lot to lot [152]. Additionally, lectin binding to GalNAc is affected by sialylation of GalNAc and Gal in the clustered IgA1 O-glycans [153].

For a lectin-independent detection of Gd-IgA1, monoclonal antibodies against human Gd-IgA1 HR peptides were developed, such as KM55 and 35A12, and ELISA methods using these monoclonal antibodies were established (Figure 5b) [152,154].

Although assays using lectin and monoclonal antibodies can detect Gd-IgA1, these methods cannot determine the number and the attachment site of O-glycans. The specific changes in IgA1 HR O-glycoforms in IgAN patients cannot be assessed by these analytical methods. For a detailed analysis of the O-glycoforms of IgA1 HR, which harbors clustered O-glycans, the HR glycopeptides need to be analyzed using high-resolution mass spectrometry combined with nanoflow liquid chromatography after digestion with endopeptidases, such as trypsin (Figure 5c). To identify the sites of O-glycan attachment, electron transfer dissociation (ETD) tandem MS has been used [52,53]. We previously developed an automated quantitative analytical workflow for profiling HR O-glycopeptide and for the detection and quantification of galactose-deficient glycan attachment sites [55]. Using this analytical method, the most frequently utilized Gal-deficient site in serum IgA1 in healthy subjects was T^{236}, followed by S^{230}, T^{233}, T^{228}, and S^{232} [55].

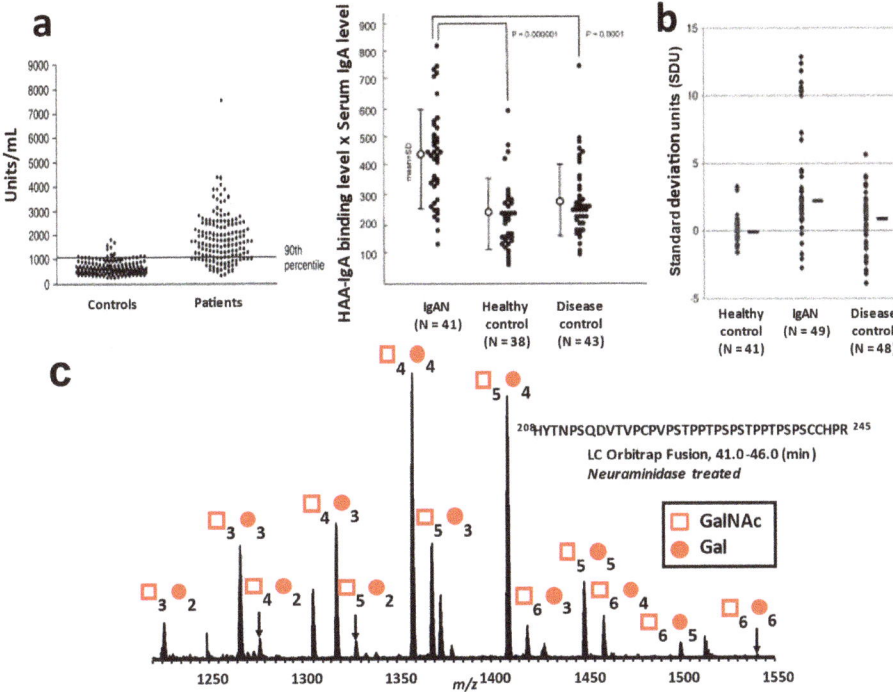

Figure 5. Detection of galactose-deficient IgA1 (Gd-IgA1). Serum Gd-IgA1 levels measured by *Helix aspersa* agglutinin (HAA)-based ELISA, due to HAA specificity for terminal GalNAc, is significantly higher in patients with IgAN than in healthy subjects (**a**) [32,33]. The left figure of (**a**) was published in *Kidney International* 2007, 71, 1148-54, Moldoveanu, Z. et al., Copyright 2007 Elsevier Inc and is republished with permission. The right figure of (**a**) is republished with permission of Oxford University Press, from *Nephrology Dialysis Transplantation* 2008, 23, 1931-9, Shimozato, S. et al., Copyright 2008 Oxford University Press. Detection of Gd-IgA1 using monoclonal antibody against human Gd-IgA1 hinge region (HR) peptide (**b**) [154]. The figure (**b**) was published in *Journal of Nephrology* 2015, 28, 181-6, Hiki, Y. et al., Copyright 2014, The Author(s). This article is under the terms of the Creative Commons CC BY license. A variety of IgA1 HR *O*-glycoforms can be detected by high-resolution mass spectrometry according to the difference in mass arising from the number of attached monosaccharides to the amino acid backbone of the IgA1 HR (His^{208}-Arg^{245}). The number of *N*-acetylgalactosamine (GalNAc; □) and galactose (Gal; •) are shown above the individual peaks (**c**).

4.2. Reliability of Gd-IgA1 as a Diagnostic and Prognostic Biomarker

Serum levels of Gd-IgA1 detected by lectin ELISA are significantly higher in patients with IgAN than in healthy controls or patients with other renal diseases [33,155]. However, it is still controversial whether higher levels of Gd-IgA1 recognized by HAA lectin are associated with clinical severity and outcome [32,33,155,156]. A couple of studies showed the predictive value of Gd-IgA1 serum levels [157,158]. Longitudinal changes in Gd-IgA1 serum levels before and after combination therapy, palatine tonsillectomy and steroid pulse therapy do not provide a clear picture [33,156]. Furthermore, rituximab therapy does not alter the Gd-IgA1 levels obtained by HAA ELISA [159].

Recently, several reports have been published on the validation of Gd-IgA1 measured using KM55. The serum level of Gd-IgA1 measured with KM55 is higher in patients with IgAN and HSPN than in patients with lupus nephritis (LN), ANCA-associated vasculitis (AAV), and minimal change disease in a Japanese cohort [160]. In addition, KM55 recognizes glomerular IgA1 in patients with IgAN and IgA vasculitis with nephritis (IgA-VN) [161]. Furthermore, elevation of serum KM55 Gd-IgA1 levels is associated with histopathologically advanced IgAN and predicts post-transplant recurrent IgAN [160,162]. KM55 recognizes GalNAc residues on Thr^{225} and Thr^{233} in synthetic glycopeptides in the PST(GalNAc)PP motif in IgA1 HR [163], but it is not known whether IgA1 with Gal-deficient O-glycan in these specific sites is associated with the pathogenesis of IgAN and IgA-VN.

However, the KM55-based method showed that serum Gd-IgA1 levels are elevated in patients with secondary IgAN to the same degree as in those with primary IgAN [164]. Immunostaining of Gd-IgA1 by KM55 was also observed in secondary IgAN and other IgA-depositing diseases, such as IgAN with hepatitis B virus, LN, cirrhosis, Crohn's disease, *Staphylococcus*-associated glomerulonephritis, and psoriasis [165,166]. Thus, the reliability of Gd-IgA1 measured by KM55 should be evaluated in a larger multicenter cohort.

5. Conclusions

The elevation in serum Gd-IgA1 levels and immunodeposits enriched for Gd-IgA1 glycoforms are characteristic features of IgAN. To clarify the characteristics of disease-specific IgA1, many studies have attempted to use lectin assays, monoclonal antibodies, mass spectrometry, and genetic and other types of analyses. However, the detailed characterization of O-glycoforms of IgA1 associated with IgAN is still to be performed. In addition, the effect of different O-glycoforms in IgA1 HR on the formation of immune complexes, mesangial deposition, and glomerular injury has not been fully elucidated. Table 1 summarizes what we know and what we do not know about glycosylation of IgA1 in IgAN.

Table 1. What we know and what we do not know about O-glycosylation of IgA1 in IgAN.

Characteristics of serum IgA1 in IgAN	
High reactivity with lectin from *Helix aspersa* (HAA)	Moldoveanu,2007 [32], Shimozato, 2008 [33]
High reactivity with monoclonal antibodies	Yasutake, 2015 [152], Hiki, 2015 [154]
IgA1 carbohydrates in IgAN assessed by mass spectrometry	
Decrease of galactose (Gal)	Hiki, 1998 [167], Inoue, 2012 [168], Nakazawa, 2019 [169]
Decrease of N-acetylgalactosamine (GalNAc)	Hiki,1998 [167], Odani, 2000 [170], Inoue, 2012 [168], Nakazawa, 2019 [169]
Decrease of sialic acid	Odani, 2000 [170]
Sites of glycan attachment	
Occur in specific sites	Renfrow, 2005 [50], Iwasaki, 2003 [51], Takahashi, 2010 [52], Takahashi, 2012 [53]
Disease in specific sites	Needs to be investigated
Expression of O-glycosyltransferases in B cells	
No decrease in the ratio of *C1GALT1: GALNT2* or *C1GALT1: C1GALT1C1*	Buck, 2008 [171]
Expression of *C1GALT1* and *ST6GALNAC2* altered in IgA1-producing cell lines from IgAN patients	Suzuki, 2008 [76]
Decreased *C1GALT1* expression in IgAN CD19+ B cells	Xing, 2020 [172]
O-Glycosylation characteristics of polymeric IgA1	
Polymeric IgA1 shows higher reactivity with HAA than in monomeric IgA1	Oortwijin, 2006 [149], Suzuki, 2008 [76], Novak, 2011 [173]
Polymeric IgA1 interacted with CD71 and its interaction is enhanced by sialidase and β-galactosidase	Moura, 2004 [139]

Table 1. *Cont.*

Epitopes recognized by IgG/A autoantibodies		
		Needs to be investigated
Clinical factors related to glycosylation of IgA1		
Genetic influences	Gd-IgA1 levels are highly inherited and affected by variants of glycosyltransferase	Tam,2009 [82], Kiryluk, 2011 [83], Gharavi, 2008 [79], Lin, 2009 [84], Hastings, 2010 [85], Gale, 2017 [95], Kiryluk, 2017 [96]
	Susceptibility to IgAN is affected by variants of glycosyltransferase	Li 2007 [86,89], Pirulli, 2009 [87], Zhu, 2009, [88]
Race differences	Gd-IgA1 levels elevated in Caucasian patients	Gale,2017 [95]
	Gd-IgA1-increasing allele is common in Europeans	Kiryluk, 2017 [96]
	MicroRNA regulating *C1GALT1* and *GALNT2* overexpressed in Caucasian patients	Serino, 2016 [100]
Age differences		Needs to be investigated
Disease activity	No association of Gd-IgA1 levels measured by HAA-based ELISA with disease activity	Moldoveanu, 2007 [32], Shimozato, 2008 [33]
	Positive association of Gd-IgA1 level measured by HAA-based ELISA with disease activity	Suzuki, 2014 [156], Sun, 2016 [155], Zhao, 2012 [157], Maixnerova, 2019 [158]
	Gd-IgA1 levels measured by KM55 associated with disease progression or recurrence	Wada, 2018 [160], Temurhan, 2017 [162]
Longitudinal changes	Longitudinal changes of Gd-IgA1 serum levels by HAA ELISA before and after therapy need additional studies	Shimozato, 2008 [33], Suzuki, 2014 [156], Lafayette, 2017 [159]
	O-Glycoform analyzed by MS changes between, before and after therapy	Iwatani, 2012 [174]

Recent genetic studies have shown that *O*-glycosylation of IgA1 is influenced by genetic variants of *O*-glycosyltransferase, and racial differences in variants have also been noted. Therefore, racial factors should be considered when investigating disease-specific *O*-glycoforms. By clarifying the disease-specific *O*-glycoform(s), the mechanism underlying aberrant glycosylation, and the effects of glycosylation changes, it is hoped that the elucidation of the etiology and development of diagnostic markers and new therapies for this disease will be advanced.

Author Contributions: Conceptualization, Y.O. and K.T.; validation, K.T.; writing—original draft preparation, Y.O. and K.T.; writing—review and editing, Y.O., M.B.R., J.N. and K.T.; visualization, Y.O. and K.T.; supervision, M.B.R. and J.N. All authors have read and agreed to the published version of the manuscript.

Funding: The work was funded by the JSPS KAKENHI (grant numbers 19K08691, 19K08715, 20K22915) and by Aichi Jinzou Foundation. J.N. and M.B.R. are supported in part by NIH grants DK078244, DK082753, AI149431, and GM098539.

Institutional Review Board Statement: Not applicable.

Informed Consent Statement: Not applicable.

Data Availability Statement: No new data were created or analyzed in this study. Data sharing is not applicable to this article.

Conflicts of Interest: M.B.R. and J.N. are co-founders and co-owners of and consultants for Reliant Glycosciences, LLC. M.B.R. and J.N. are co-inventors on US patent application 14/318,082 (assigned to UAB Research Foundation).

References

1. Berger, J.; Hinglais, N. Intercapillary deposits of IgA-IgG. *J. Urol. Nephrol.* **1968**, *74*, 694–695.
2. Conley, M.E.; Cooper, M.D.; Michael, A.F. Selective deposition of immunoglobulin A1 in immunoglobulin A nephropathy, anaphylactoid purpura nephritis, and systemic lupus erythematosus. *J. Clin. Investig.* **1980**, *66*, 1432–1436. [CrossRef] [PubMed]
3. Berger, J.; Yaneva, H.; Nabarra, B.; Barbanel, C. Recurrence of mesangial deposition of IgA after renal transplantation. *Kidney Int.* **1975**, *7*, 232–241. [CrossRef] [PubMed]
4. Ponticelli, C.; Traversi, L.; Feliciani, A.; Cesana, B.M.; Banfi, G.; Tarantino, A. Kidney transplantation in patients with IgA mesangial glomerulonephritis. *Kidney Int.* **2001**, *60*, 1948–1954. [CrossRef] [PubMed]
5. Berger, J. Recurrence of IgA nephropathy in renal allografts. *Am. J. Kidney Dis.* **1988**, *12*, 371–372. [CrossRef]
6. Floege, J. Recurrent IgA nephropathy after renal transplantation. *Semin. Nephrol.* **2004**, *24*, 287–291. [CrossRef] [PubMed]
7. Sanfilippo, F.; Croker, B.P.; Bollinger, R.R. Fate of four cadaveric donor renal allografts with mesangial IgA deposits. *Transplantation* **1982**, *33*, 370–376. [CrossRef] [PubMed]
8. Silva, F.G.; Chander, P.; Pirani, C.L.; Hardy, M.A. Disappearance of glomerular mesangial IgA deposits after renal allograft transplantation. *Transplantation* **1982**, *33*, 241–246.
9. Cuevas, X.; Lloveras, J.; Mir, M.; Aubia, J.; Masramon, J. Disappearance of mesangial IgA deposits from the kidneys of two donors after transplantation. *Transplant. Proc.* **1987**, *19*, 2208–2209.
10. Iwata, Y.; Wada, T.; Uchiyama, A.; Miwa, A.; Nakaya, I.; Tohyama, T.; Yamada, Y.; Kurokawa, T.; Yoshida, T.; Ohta, S.; et al. Remission of IgA nephropathy after allogeneic peripheral blood stem cell transplantation followed by immunosuppression for acute lymphocytic leukemia. *Intern. Med.* **2006**, *45*, 1291–1295. [CrossRef]
11. Hu, S.L.; Colvin, G.A.; Rifai, A.; Suzuki, H.; Novak, J.; Esparza, A.; Farooqi, S.; Julian, B.A. Glomerulonephritis after hematopoietic cell transplantation: IgA nephropathy with increased excretion of galactose-deficient IgA1. *Nephrol. Dial. Transplant.* **2010**, *25*, 1708–1713. [CrossRef] [PubMed]
12. Zickerman, A.M.; Allen, A.C.; Talwar, V.; Olczak, S.A.; Brownlee, A.; Holland, M.; Furness, P.N.; Brunskill, N.J.; Feehally, J. IgA myeloma presenting as Henoch-Schönlein purpura with nephritis. *Am. J. Kidney Dis.* **2000**, *36*, E19. [CrossRef] [PubMed]
13. Van Der Helm-Van Mil, A.H.; Smith, A.C.; Pouria, S.; Tarelli, E.; Brunskill, N.J.; Eikenboom, H.C. Immunoglobulin A multiple myeloma presenting with Henoch-Schönlein purpura associated with reduced sialylation of IgA1. *Br. J. Haematol.* **2003**, *122*, 915–917. [CrossRef] [PubMed]
14. Floege, J. The pathogenesis of IgA nephropathy: What is new and how does it change therapeutic approaches? *Am. J. Kidney Dis.* **2011**, *58*, 992–1004. [CrossRef] [PubMed]
15. Donadio, J.V.; Grande, J.P. IgA nephropathy. *N. Engl. J. Med.* **2002**, *347*, 738–748. [CrossRef]
16. Pouria, S.; Barratt, J. Secondary IgA nephropathy. *Semin. Nephrol.* **2008**, *28*, 27–37. [CrossRef] [PubMed]
17. Glassock, R.J. The pathogenesis of IgA nephropathy. *Curr. Opin. Nephrol. Hypertens.* **2011**, *20*, 153–160. [CrossRef]
18. Boyd, J.K.; Cheung, C.K.; Molyneux, K.; Feehally, J.; Barratt, J. An update on the pathogenesis and treatment of IgA nephropathy. *Kidney Int.* **2012**, *81*, 833–843. [CrossRef]
19. Mestecky, J. Immunobiology of IgA. *Am. J. Kidney Dis.* **1988**, *12*, 378–383. [CrossRef]
20. Tomino, Y.; Sakai, H.; Miura, M.; Endoh, M.; Nomoto, Y. Detection of polymeric IgA in glomeruli from patients with IgA nephropathy. *Clin. Exp. Immunol.* **1982**, *49*, 419–425.
21. Bene, M.C.; Faure, G.; Duheille, J. IgA nephropathy: Characterization of the polymeric nature of mesangial deposits by in vitro binding of free secretory component. *Clin. Exp. Immunol.* **1982**, *47*, 527–534. [PubMed]
22. Suzuki, K.; Honda, K.; Tanabe, K.; Toma, H.; Nihei, H.; Yamaguchi, Y. Incidence of latent mesangial IgA deposition in renal allograft donors in Japan. *Kidney Int.* **2003**, *63*, 2286–2294. [CrossRef] [PubMed]
23. Van Der Boog, P.J.M.; Van Kooten, C.; De Fijter, J.W.; Daha, M.R. Role of macromolecular IgA in IgA nephropathy. *Kidney Int.* **2005**, *67*, 813–821. [CrossRef]
24. Narita, I.; Gejyo, F. Pathogenetic significance of aberrant glycosylation of IgA1 in IgA nephropathy. *Clin. Exp. Immunol.* **2008**, *12*, 332–338. [CrossRef]
25. Suzuki, H.; Kiryluk, K.; Novak, J.; Moldoveanu, Z.; Herr, A.B.; Renfrow, M.B.; Wyatt, R.J.; Scolari, F.; Mestecky, J.; Gharavi, A.G.; et al. The pathophysiology of IgA nephropathy. *J. Am. Soc. Nephrol.* **2011**, *22*, 1795–1803. [CrossRef] [PubMed]
26. Mestecky, J.; Raska, M.; Julian, B.A.; Gharavi, A.G.; Renfrow, M.B.; Moldoveanu, Z.; Novak, L.; Matousovic, K.; Novak, J. IgA nephropathy: Molecular mechanisms of the disease. *Annu. Rev. Pathol.* **2013**, *8*, 217–240. [CrossRef]
27. Novak, J.; Julian, B.A.; Mestecky, J.; Renfrow, M.B. Glycosylation of IgA1 and pathogenesis of IgA nephropathy. *Semin. Immunopathol.* **2012**, *34*, 365–382. [CrossRef]
28. Coppo, R.; Amore, A.; Peruzzi, L.; Vergano, L.; Camilla, R. Innate immunity and IgA nephropathy. *J. Nephrol.* **2010**, *23*, 626–632.
29. Allen, A.C.; Harper, S.J.; Feehally, J. Galactosylation of N- and O-linked carbohydrate moieties of IgA1 and IgG in IgA nephropathy. *Clin. Exp. Immunol.* **1995**, *100*, 470–474. [CrossRef]
30. Allen, A.C.; Bailey, E.M.; Brenchley, P.E.; Buck, K.S.; Barratt, J.; Feehally, J. Mesangial IgA1 in IgA nephropathy exhibits aberrant O-glycosylation: Observations in three patients. *Kidney Int.* **2001**, *60*, 969–973. [CrossRef]
31. Hiki, Y.; Odani, H.; Takahashi, M.; Yasuda, Y.; Nishimoto, A.; Iwase, H.; Shinzato, T.; Kobayashi, Y.; Maeda, K. Mass spectrometry proves under-O-glycosylation of glomerular IgA1 in IgA nephropathy. *Kidney Int.* **2001**, *59*, 1077–1085. [CrossRef] [PubMed]

32. Moldoveanu, Z.; Wyatt, R.J.; Lee, J.Y.; Tomana, M.; Julian, B.A.; Mestecky, J.; Huang, W.Q.; Anreddy, S.R.; Hall, S.; Hastings, M.C.; et al. Patients with IgA nephropathy have increased serum galactose-deficient IgA1 levels. *Kidney Int.* **2007**, *71*, 1148–1154. [CrossRef] [PubMed]
33. Shimozato, S.; Hiki, Y.; Odani, H.; Takahashi, K.; Yamamoto, K.; Sugiyama, S. Serum under-galactosylated IgA1 is increased in Japanese patients with IgA nephropathy. *Nephrol. Dial. Transplant.* **2008**, *23*, 1931–1939. [CrossRef] [PubMed]
34. Moura, I.C.; Benhamou, M.; Launay, P.; Vrtovsnik, F.; Blank, U.; Monteiro, R.C. The glomerular response to IgA deposition in IgA nephropathy. *Semin. Nephrol.* **2008**, *28*, 88–95. [CrossRef]
35. Hiki, Y. O-linked oligosaccharides of the IgA1 hinge region: Roles of its aberrant structure in the occurrence and/or progression of IgA nephropathy. *Clin. Exp. Immunol.* **2009**, *13*, 415–423. [CrossRef]
36. Lai, K.N. Pathogenesis of IgA nephropathy. *Nat. Rev. Nephrol.* **2012**, *8*, 275–283. [CrossRef]
37. Rizk, D.V.; Maillard, N.; Julian, B.A.; Knoppova, B.; Green, T.J.; Novak, J.; Wyatt, R.J. The emerging role of complement proteins as a target for therapy of IgA nephropathy. *Front. Immunol.* **2019**, *10*, 504. [CrossRef]
38. Knoppova, B.; Reily, C.; Maillard, N.; Rizk, D.V.; Moldoveanu, Z.; Mestecky, J.; Raska, M.; Renfrow, M.B.; Julian, B.A.; Novak, J. The origin and activities of IgA1-containing immune complexes in IgA nephropathy. *Front. Immunol.* **2016**, *7*, 117. [CrossRef]
39. Maillard, N.; Wyatt, R.J.; Julian, B.A.; Kiryluk, K.; Gharavi, A.; Fremeaux-Bacchi, V.; Novak, J. Current understanding of the role of complement in IgA nephropathy. *J. Am. Soc. Nephrol.* **2015**, *26*, 1503–1512. [CrossRef]
40. Yagame, M.; Tomino, Y.; Miura, M.; Tanigaki, T.; Suga, T.; Nomoto, Y.; Sakai, H. Detection of IgA-class circulating immune complexes (CIC) in sera from patients with IgA nephropathy using a solid-phase anti-C3 Facb enzyme immunoassay (EIA). *Clin. Exp. Immunol.* **1987**, *67*, 270–276.
41. Valentijn, R.M.; van Es, L.A.; Daha, M.R. The specific detection of IgG, IgA and the complement components C3 and C4 in circulating immune complexes. *J. Clin. Lab. Immunol.* **1984**, *14*, 81–86. [PubMed]
42. Czerkinsky, C.; Koopman, W.J.; Jackson, S.; Collins, J.E.; Crago, S.S.; Schrohenloher, R.E.; Julian, B.A.; Galla, J.H.; Mestecky, J. Circulating immune complexes and immunoglobulin A rheumatoid factor in patients with mesangial immunoglobulin A nephropathies. *J. Clin. Investig.* **1986**, *77*, 1931–1938. [CrossRef] [PubMed]
43. Papista, C.; Berthelot, L.; Monteiro, R.C. Dysfunctions of the Iga system: A common link between intestinal and renal diseases. *Cell. Mol. Immunol.* **2011**, *8*, 126–134. [CrossRef]
44. Arnold, J.N.; Wormald, M.R.; Sim, R.B.; Rudd, P.M.; Dwek, R.A. The impact of glycosylation on the biological function and structure of human immunoglobulins. *Annu. Rev. Immunol.* **2007**, *25*, 21–50. [CrossRef] [PubMed]
45. Tsuzukida, Y.; Wang, C.C.; Putnam, F.W. Structure of the A2m(1) allotype of human IgA—A recombinant molecule. *Proc. Natl. Acad. Sci. USA* **1979**, *76*, 1104–1108. [CrossRef] [PubMed]
46. Mattu, T.S.; Pleass, R.J.; Willis, A.C.; Kilian, M.; Wormald, M.R.; Lellouch, A.C.; Rudd, P.M.; Woof, J.M.; Dwek, R.A. The glycosylation and structure of human serum IgA1, Fab, and Fc regions and the role of N-glycosylation on Fcα receptor interactions. *J. Biol. Chem.* **1998**, *273*, 2260–2272. [CrossRef] [PubMed]
47. Woof, J.M.; Mestecky, J. Mucosal immunoglobulins. *Immunol. Rev.* **2005**, *206*, 64–82. [CrossRef]
48. Woof, J.M.; Mestecky, J. Mucosal Immunoglobulins. In *Mucosal Immunology*, 3rd ed.; Academic Press: New York, NY, USA, 2005; Volume 1, pp. 153–181.
49. Peppard, J.V.; Kaetzel, C.S.; Russell, M.W. Phylogeny and Comparative Physiology of IgA. In *Mucosal Immunology*, 3rd ed.; Academic Press: New York, NY, USA, 2005; pp. 195–210.
50. Renfrow, M.B.; Cooper, H.J.; Tomana, M.; Kulhavy, R.; Hiki, Y.; Toma, K.; Emmett, M.R.; Mestecky, J.; Marshall, A.G.; Novak, J. Determination of aberrant O-glycosylation in the IgA1 hinge region by electron capture dissociation fourier transform-ion cyclotron resonance mass spectrometry. *J. Biol. Chem.* **2005**, *280*, 19136–19145. [CrossRef]
51. Iwasaki, H.; Zhang, Y.; Tachibana, K.; Gotoh, M.; Kikuchi, N.; Kwon, Y.D.; Togayachi, A.; Kudo, T.; Kubota, T.; Narimatsu, H. Initiation of O-glycan synthesis in IgA1 hinge region is determined by a single enzyme, UDP-N-acetyl-α-D-galactosamine:polypeptide N-acetylgalactosaminyltransferase 2. *J. Biol. Chem.* **2003**, *278*, 5613–5621. [CrossRef]
52. Takahashi, K.; Wall, S.B.; Suzuki, H.; Smith, A.D.t.; Hall, S.; Poulsen, K.; Kilian, M.; Mobley, J.A.; Julian, B.A.; Mestecky, J.; et al. Clustered O-glycans of IgA1: Defining macro- and microheterogeneity by use of electron capture/transfer dissociation. *Mol. Cell. Proteom.* **2010**, *9*, 2545–2557. [CrossRef]
53. Takahashi, K.; Smith, A.D.; Poulsen, K.; Kilian, M.; Julian, B.A.; Mestecky, J.; Novak, J.; Renfrow, M.B. Naturally occurring structural isomers in serum IgA1 O-glycosylation. *J. Proteome Res.* **2012**, *11*, 692–702. [CrossRef]
54. Tarelli, E.; Smith, A.C.; Hendry, B.M.; Challacombe, S.J.; Pouria, S. Human serum IgA1 is substituted with up to six O-glycans as shown by matrix assisted laser desorption ionisation time-of-flight mass spectrometry. *Carbohydr. Res.* **2004**, *339*, 2329–2335. [CrossRef]
55. Ohyama, Y.; Yamaguchi, H.; Nakajima, K.; Mizuno, T.; Fukamachi, Y.; Yokoi, Y.; Tsuboi, N.; Inaguma, D.; Hasegawa, M.; Renfrow, M.B.; et al. Analysis of O-glycoforms of the IgA1 hinge region by sequential deglycosylation. *Sci. Rep.* **2020**, *10*, 671. [CrossRef]
56. Novak, J.; Julian, B.A.; Tomana, M.; Mestecky, J. IgA glycosylation and IgA immune complexes in the pathogenesis of IgA nephropathy. *Semin. Nephrol.* **2008**, *28*, 78–87. [CrossRef]

57. Wandall, H.H.; Irazoqui, F.; Tarp, M.A.; Bennett, E.P.; Mandel, U.; Takeuchi, H.; Kato, K.; Irimura, T.; Suryanarayanan, G.; Hollingsworth, M.A.; et al. The lectin domains of polypeptide GalNAc-transferases exhibit carbohydrate-binding specificity for GalNAc: Lectin binding to GalNAc-glycopeptide substrates is required for high density GalNAc-O-glycosylation. *Glycobiology* **2007**, *17*, 374–387. [CrossRef]
58. Reily, C.; Stewart, T.J.; Renfrow, M.B.; Novak, J. Glycosylation in health and disease. *Nat. Rev. Nephrol.* **2019**, *15*, 346–366. [CrossRef] [PubMed]
59. Stewart, T.J.; Takahashi, K.; Whitaker, R.H.; Raska, M.; Placzek, W.J.; Novak, J.; Renfrow, M.B. IgA1 hinge-region clustered glycan fidelity is established early during semi-ordered glycosylation by GalNAc-T2. *Glycobiology* **2019**, *29*, 543–556. [CrossRef]
60. Stewart, T.J.; Takahashi, K.; Xu, N.; Prakash, A.; Brown, R.; Raska, M.; Renfrow, M.B.; Novak, J. Quantitative assessment of successive carbohydrate additions to the clustered O-glycosylation sites of IgA1 by glycosyltransferases. *Glycobiology* **2021**, *31*, 540–556. [CrossRef] [PubMed]
61. Ju, T.; Cummings, R.D. Protein glycosylation: Chaperone mutation in Tn syndrome. *Nature* **2005**, *437*, 1252. [CrossRef] [PubMed]
62. Schachter, H.; McGuire, E.J.; Roseman, S. Sialic acids. 13. A uridine diphosphate D-galactose: Mucin galactosyltransferase from porcine submaxillary gland. *J. Biol. Chem.* **1971**, *246*, 5321–5328. [CrossRef]
63. Novak, J.; Julian, B.A.; Tomana, M.; Mesteck, J. Progress in molecular and genetic studies of IgA nephropathy. *J. Clin. Immunol.* **2001**, *21*, 310–327. [CrossRef] [PubMed]
64. Suzuki, H.; Raska, M.; Yamada, K.; Moldoveanu, Z.; Julian, B.A.; Wyatt, R.J.; Tomino, Y.; Gharavi, A.G.; Novak, J. Cytokines alter IgA1 O-glycosylation by dysregulating C1GalT1 and ST6GalNAc-II enzymes. *J. Biol. Chem.* **2014**, *289*, 5330–5339. [CrossRef] [PubMed]
65. Varki, A. Biological roles of glycans. *Glycobiology* **2017**, *27*, 3–49. [CrossRef] [PubMed]
66. Furtado, P.B.; Whitty, P.W.; Robertson, A.; Eaton, J.T.; Almogren, A.; Kerr, M.A.; Woof, J.M.; Perkins, S.J. Solution structure determination of monomeric human IgA2 by X-ray and neutron scattering, analytical ultracentrifugation and constrained modelling: A comparison with monomeric human IgA1. *J. Mol. Biol.* **2004**, *338*, 921–941. [CrossRef] [PubMed]
67. Narimatsu, Y.; Joshi, H.J.; Schjoldager, K.T.; Hintze, J.; Halim, A.; Steentoft, C.; Nason, R.; Mandel, U.; Bennett, E.P.; Clausen, H.; et al. Exploring Regulation of Protein O-Glycosylation in Isogenic Human HEK293 Cells by Differential O-Glycoproteomics. *Mol. Cell. Proteom.* **2019**, *18*, 1396–1409. [CrossRef] [PubMed]
68. Royle, L.; Roos, A.; Harvey, D.J.; Wormald, M.R.; van Gijlswijk-Janssens, D.; Redwan, E.-R.M.; Wilson, I.A.; Daha, M.R.; Dwek, R.A.; Rudd, P.M. Secretory IgA N- and O-glycans provide a link between the innate and adaptive immune systems. *J. Biol. Chem.* **2003**, *278*, 20140–20153. [CrossRef]
69. Tomana, M.; Novak, J.; Julian, B.A.; Matousovic, K.; Konecny, K.; Mestecky, J. Circulating immune complexes in IgA nephropathy consist of IgA1 with galactose-deficient hinge region and antiglycan antibodies. *J. Clin. Investig.* **1999**, *104*, 73–81. [CrossRef]
70. Moore, J.S.; Kulhavy, R.; Tomana, M.; Moldoveanu, Z.; Suzuki, H.; Brown, R.; Hall, S.; Kilian, M.; Poulsen, K.; Mestecky, J.; et al. Reactivities of N-acetylgalactosamine-specific lectins with human IgA1 proteins. *Mol. Immunol.* **2007**, *44*, 2598–2604. [CrossRef]
71. Reily, C.; Rizk, D.V.; Julian, B.A.; Novak, J. Assay for galactose-deficient IgA1 enables mechanistic studies with primary cells from IgA nephropathy patients. *Biotechniques* **2018**, *65*, 71–77. [CrossRef] [PubMed]
72. Gomes, M.M.; Suzuki, H.; Brooks, M.T.; Tomana, M.; Moldoveanu, Z.; Mestecky, J.; Julian, B.A.; Novak, J.; Herr, A.B. Recognition of galactose-deficient O-glycans in the hinge region of IgA1 by N-acetylgalactosamine-specific snail lectins: A comparative binding study. *Biochemistry* **2010**, *49*, 5671–5682. [CrossRef]
73. Leung, J.C.; Poon, P.Y.; Lai, K.N. Increased sialylation of polymeric immunoglobulin A1: Mechanism of selective glomerular deposition in immunoglobulin A nephropathy? *J. Lab. Clin. Med.* **1999**, *133*, 152–160. [CrossRef]
74. Amore, A.; Cirina, P.; Conti, G.; Brusa, P.; Peruzzi, L.; Coppo, R. Glycosylation of circulating IgA in patients with IgA nephropathy modulates proliferation and apoptosis of mesangial cells. *J. Am. Soc. Nephrol.* **2001**, *12*, 1862–1871. [CrossRef] [PubMed]
75. Leung, J.C.; Tang, S.C.; Chan, D.T.; Lui, S.L.; Lai, K.N. Increased sialylation of polymeric lambda-IgA1 in patients with IgA nephropathy. *J. Clin. Lab. Anal.* **2002**, *16*, 11–19. [CrossRef] [PubMed]
76. Suzuki, H.; Moldoveanu, Z.; Hall, S.; Brown, R.; Vu, H.L.; Novak, L.; Julian, B.A.; Tomana, M.; Wyatt, R.J.; Edberg, J.C.; et al. IgA1-secreting cell lines from patients with IgA nephropathy produce aberrantly glycosylated IgA1. *J. Clin. Investig.* **2008**, *118*, 629–639. [CrossRef] [PubMed]
77. Wada, Y.; Tajiri, M.; Ohshima, S. Quantitation of saccharide compositions of O-glycans by mass spectrometry of glycopeptides and its application to rheumatoid arthritis. *J. Proteome Res.* **2010**, *9*, 1367–1373. [CrossRef]
78. Smith, A.C.; de Wolff, J.F.; Molyneux, K.; Feehally, J.; Barratt, J. O-glycosylation of serum IgD in IgA nephropathy. *J. Am. Soc. Nephrol.* **2006**, *17*, 1192–1199. [CrossRef]
79. Gharavi, A.G.; Moldoveanu, Z.; Wyatt, R.J.; Barker, C.V.; Woodford, S.Y.; Lifton, R.P.; Mestecky, J.; Novak, J.; Julian, B.A. Aberrant IgA1 glycosylation is inherited in familial and sporadic IgA nephropathy. *J. Am. Soc. Nephrol.* **2008**, *19*, 1008–1014. [CrossRef]
80. Rizk, D.V.; Saha, M.K.; Hall, S.; Novak, L.; Brown, R.; Huang, Z.Q.; Fatima, H.; Julian, B.A.; Novak, J. Glomerular immunodeposits of patients with IgA nephropathy are enriched for IgG autoantibodies specific for galactose-deficient IgA1. *J. Am. Soc. Nephrol.* **2019**, *30*, 2017–2026. [CrossRef]
81. Moldoveanu, Z.; Suzuki, H.; Reily, C.; Satake, K.; Novak, L.; Xu, N.; Huang, Z.Q.; Knoppova, B.; Khan, A.; Hall, S.; et al. Experimental evidence of pathogenic role of IgG autoantibodies in IgA nephropathy. *J. Autoimmun.* **2021**, *118*, 102593. [CrossRef]

82. Tam, K.Y.; Leung, J.C.K.; Chan, L.Y.Y.; Lam, M.F.; Tang, S.C.W.; Lai, K.N. Macromolecular IgA1 taken from patients with familial IgA nephropathy or their asymptomatic relatives have higher reactivity to mesangial cells in vitro. *Kidney Int.* **2009**, *75*, 1330–1339. [CrossRef] [PubMed]
83. Kiryluk, K.; Moldoveanu, Z.; Sanders, J.T.; Eison, T.M.; Suzuki, H.; Julian, B.A.; Novak, J.; Gharavi, A.G.; Wyatt, R.J. Aberrant glycosylation of IgA1 is inherited in both pediatric IgA nephropathy and Henoch-Schönlein purpura nephritis. *Kidney Int.* **2011**, *80*, 79–87. [CrossRef]
84. Lin, X.; Ding, J.; Zhu, L.; Shi, S.; Jiang, L.; Zhao, M.; Zhang, H. Aberrant galactosylation of IgA1 is involved in the genetic susceptibility of Chinese patients with IgA nephropathy. *Nephrol. Dial. Transplant.* **2009**, *24*, 3372–3375. [CrossRef] [PubMed]
85. Hastings, M.C.; Moldoveanu, Z.; Julian, B.A.; Novak, J.; Sanders, J.T.; McGlothan, K.R.; Gharavi, A.G.; Wyatt, R.J. Galactose-deficient IgA1 in African Americans with IgA nephropathy: Serum levels and heritability. *Clin. J. Am. Soc. Nephrol.* **2010**, *5*, 2069–2074. [CrossRef] [PubMed]
86. Li, G.S.; Zhang, H.; Lv, J.C.; Shen, Y.; Wang, H.Y. Variants of C1GALT1 gene are associated with the genetic susceptibility to IgA nephropathy. *Kidney Int.* **2007**, *71*, 448–453. [CrossRef]
87. Pirulli, D.; Crovella, S.; Ulivi, S.; Zadro, C.; Bertok, S.; Rendine, S.; Scolari, F.; Foramitti, M.; Ravani, P.; Roccatello, D.; et al. Genetic variant of C1GalT1 contributes to the susceptibility to IgA nephropathy. *J. Nephrol.* **2009**, *22*, 152–159.
88. Zhu, L.; Tang, W.; Li, G.; Lv, J.; Ding, J.; Yu, L.; Zhao, M.; Li, Y.; Zhang, X.; Shen, Y.; et al. Interaction between variants of two glycosyltransferase genes in IgA nephropathy. *Kidney Int.* **2009**, *76*, 190–198. [CrossRef] [PubMed]
89. Li, G.S.; Zhu, L.; Zhang, H.; Lv, J.C.; Ding, J.X.; Zhao, M.H.; Shen, Y.; Wang, H.Y. Variants of the ST6GALNAC2 promoter influence transcriptional activity and contribute to genetic susceptibility to IgA nephropathy. *Hum. Mutat.* **2007**, *28*, 950–957. [CrossRef] [PubMed]
90. Malycha, F.; Eggermann, T.; Hristov, M.; Schena, F.P.; Mertens, P.R.; Zerres, K.; Floege, J.; Eitner, F. No evidence for a role of *cosmc*-chaperone mutations in European IgA nephropathy patients. *Nephrol. Dial. Transplant.* **2009**, *24*, 321–324. [CrossRef] [PubMed]
91. Yu, X.Q.; Li, M.; Zhang, H.; Low, H.Q.; Wei, X.; Wang, J.Q.; Sun, L.D.; Sim, K.S.; Li, Y.; Foo, J.N.; et al. A genome-wide association study in Han Chinese identifies multiple susceptibility loci for IgA nephropathy. *Nat. Genet.* **2011**, *44*, 178–182. [CrossRef] [PubMed]
92. Kiryluk, K.; Li, Y.; Scolari, F.; Sanna-Cherchi, S.; Choi, M.; Verbitsky, M.; Fasel, D.; Lata, S.; Prakash, S.; Shapiro, S.; et al. Discovery of new risk loci for IgA nephropathy implicates genes involved in immunity against intestinal pathogens. *Nat. Genet.* **2014**, *46*, 1187–1196. [CrossRef]
93. Qi, Y.Y.; Zhou, X.J.; Cheng, F.J.; Hou, P.; Zhu, L.; Shi, S.F.; Liu, L.J.; Lv, J.C.; Zhang, H. DEFA gene variants associated with IgA nephropathy in a Chinese population. *Genes Immun.* **2015**, *16*, 231–237. [CrossRef]
94. Gharavi, A.G.; Kiryluk, K.; Choi, M.; Li, Y.; Hou, P.; Xie, J.; Sanna-Cherchi, S.; Men, C.J.; Julian, B.A.; Wyatt, R.J.; et al. Genome-wide association study identifies susceptibility loci for IgA nephropathy. *Nat. Genet.* **2011**, *43*, 321–327. [CrossRef] [PubMed]
95. Gale, D.P.; Molyneux, K.; Wimbury, D.; Higgins, P.; Levine, A.P.; Caplin, B.; Ferlin, A.; Yin, P.; Nelson, C.P.; Stanescu, H.; et al. Galactosylation of IgA1 Is Associated with Common Variation in C1GALT1. *J. Am. Soc. Nephrol.* **2017**, *28*, 2158–2166. [CrossRef]
96. Kiryluk, K.; Li, Y.; Moldoveanu, Z.; Suzuki, H.; Reily, C.; Hou, P.; Xie, J.; Mladkova, N.; Prakash, S.; Fischman, C.; et al. GWAS for serum galactose-deficient IgA1 implicates critical genes of the O-glycosylation pathway. *PLoS Genet.* **2017**, *13*, e1006609. [CrossRef]
97. Thu, C.T.; Mahal, L.K. Sweet Control: MicroRNA regulation of the glycome. *Biochemistry* **2020**, *59*, 3098–3110. [CrossRef] [PubMed]
98. Serino, G.; Sallustio, F.; Cox, S.N.; Pesce, F.; Schena, F.P. Abnormal miR-148b expression promotes aberrant glycosylation of IgA1 in IgA nephropathy. *J. Am. Soc. Nephrol.* **2012**, *23*, 814–824. [CrossRef] [PubMed]
99. Serino, G.; Sallustio, F.; Curci, C.; Cox, S.N.; Pesce, F.; De Palma, G.; Schena, F.P. Role of let-7b in the regulation of N-acetylgalactosaminyltransferase 2 in IgA nephropathy. *Nephrol. Dial. Transplant.* **2015**, *30*, 1132–1139. [CrossRef] [PubMed]
100. Serino, G.; Pesce, F.; Sallustio, F.; De Palma, G.; Cox, S.N.; Curci, C.; Zaza, G.; Lai, K.N.; Leung, J.C.; Tang, S.C.; et al. In a retrospective international study, circulating miR-148b and let-7b were found to be serum markers for detecting primary IgA nephropathy. *Kidney Int.* **2016**, *89*, 683–692. [CrossRef] [PubMed]
101. Liu, H.; Liu, D.; Liu, Y.; Xia, M.; Li, Y.; Li, M.; Liu, H. Comprehensive analysis of circRNA expression profiles and circRNA-associated competing endogenous RNA networks in IgA nephropathy. *PeerJ* **2020**, *8*, e10395. [CrossRef]
102. Liu, C.; Ye, M.Y.; Yan, W.Z.; Peng, X.F.; He, L.Y.; Peng, Y.M. microRNA-630 regulates underglycosylated IgA1 production in the tonsils by targeting TLR4 in IgA nephropathy. *Front. Immunol.* **2020**, *11*, 563699. [CrossRef] [PubMed]
103. Wang, Z.; Liao, Y.; Wang, L.; Lin, Y.; Ye, Z.; Zeng, X.; Liu, X.; Wei, F.; Yang, N. Small RNA deep sequencing reveals novel miRNAs in peripheral blood mononuclear cells from patients with IgA nephropathy. *Mol. Med. Rep.* **2020**, *22*, 3378–3386. [CrossRef]
104. Trimarchi, H.M.; Iotti, A.; Iotti, R.; Freixas, E.A.; Peters, R. Immunoglobulin A nephropathy and ulcerative colitis. A focus on their pathogenesis. *Am. J. Nephrol.* **2001**, *21*, 400–405. [CrossRef]
105. Forshaw, M.J.; Guirguis, O.; Hennigan, T.W. IgA nephropathy in association with Crohn's disease. *Int. J. Colorectal. Dis.* **2005**, *20*, 463–465. [CrossRef]

106. de Moura, C.G.; de Moura, T.G.; de Souza, S.P.; Testagrossa, L. Inflammatory bowel disease, ankylosing spondylitis, and IgA nephropathy. *J. Clin. Rheumatol.* **2006**, *12*, 106–107. [CrossRef] [PubMed]
107. Smerud, H.K.; Fellstrom, B.; Hallgren, R.; Osagie, S.; Venge, P.; Kristjansson, G. Gluten sensitivity in patients with IgA nephropathy. *Nephrol. Dial. Transplant.* **2009**, *24*, 2476–2481. [CrossRef] [PubMed]
108. Zhang, J.J.; Xu, L.X.; Liu, G.; Zhao, M.H.; Wang, H.Y. The level of serum secretory IgA of patients with IgA nephropathy is elevated and associated with pathological phenotypes. *Nephrol. Dial. Transplant.* **2008**, *23*, 207–212. [CrossRef] [PubMed]
109. Oortwijn, B.D.; Rastaldi, M.P.; Roos, A.; Mattinzoli, D.; Daha, M.R.; van Kooten, C. Demonstration of secretory IgA in kidneys of patients with IgA nephropathy. *Nephrol. Dial. Transplant.* **2007**, *22*, 3191–3195. [CrossRef] [PubMed]
110. Harper, S.J.; Allen, A.C.; Pringle, J.H.; Feehally, J. Increased dimeric IgA producing B cells in the bone marrow in IgA nephropathy determined by in situ hybridisation for J chain mRNA. *J. Clin. Pathol.* **1996**, *49*, 38–42. [CrossRef]
111. Novak, J.; Barratt, J.; Julian, B.A.; Renfrow, M.B. Aberrant glycosylation of the IgA1 molecule in IgA nephropathy. *Semin. Nephrol.* **2018**, *38*, 461–476. [CrossRef]
112. Hirano, K.; Matsuzaki, K.; Yasuda, T.; Nishikawa, M.; Yasuda, Y.; Koike, K.; Maruyama, S.; Yokoo, T.; Matsuo, S.; Kawamura, T.; et al. Association between tonsillectomy and outcomes in patients with immunoglobulin A nephropathy. *JAMA Netw Open* **2019**, *2*, e194772. [CrossRef] [PubMed]
113. Xie, Y.; Chen, X.; Nishi, S.; Narita, I.; Gejyo, F. Relationship between tonsils and IgA nephropathy as well as indications of tonsillectomy. *Kidney Int.* **2004**, *65*, 1135–1144. [CrossRef] [PubMed]
114. Xie, Y.; Nishi, S.; Ueno, M.; Imai, N.; Sakatsume, M.; Narita, I.; Suzuki, Y.; Akazawa, K.; Shimada, H.; Arakawa, M.; et al. The efficacy of tonsillectomy on long-term renal survival in patients with IgA nephropathy. *Kidney Int.* **2003**, *63*, 1861–1867. [CrossRef]
115. Inoue, T.; Sugiyama, H.; Hiki, Y.; Takiue, K.; Morinaga, H.; Kitagawa, M.; Maeshima, Y.; Fukushima, K.; Nishizaki, K.; Akagi, H.; et al. Differential expression of glycogenes in tonsillar B lymphocytes in association with proteinuria and renal dysfunction in IgA nephropathy. *Clin. Immunol.* **2010**, *136*, 447–455. [CrossRef]
116. He, L.; Peng, Y.; Liu, H.; Yin, W.; Chen, X.; Peng, X.; Shao, J.; Liu, Y.; Liu, F. Th1/Th2 polarization in tonsillar lymphocyte form patients with IgA nephropathy. *Ren. Fail.* **2014**, *36*, 407–412. [CrossRef]
117. Yamada, K.; Kobayashi, N.; Ikeda, T.; Suzuki, Y.; Tsuge, T.; Horikoshi, S.; Emancipator, S.N.; Tomino, Y. Down-regulation of core 1 beta1,3-galactosyltransferase and Cosmc by Th2 cytokine alters O-glycosylation of IgA1. *Nephrol. Dial. Transplant.* **2010**, *25*, 3890–3897. [CrossRef] [PubMed]
118. Muto, M.; Manfroi, B.; Suzuki, H.; Joh, K.; Nagai, M.; Wakai, S.; Righini, C.; Maiguma, M.; Izui, S.; Tomino, Y.; et al. Toll-Like Receptor 9 stimulation induces aberrant expression of a proliferation-inducing ligand by tonsillar germinal center B cells in IgA nephropathy. *J. Am. Soc. Nephrol.* **2017**, *28*, 1227–1238. [CrossRef] [PubMed]
119. Yamada, K.; Huang, Z.Q.; Raska, M.; Reily, C.; Anderson, J.C.; Suzuki, H.; Kiryluk, K.; Gharavi, A.G.; Julian, B.A.; Willey, C.D.; et al. Leukemia inhibitory factor signaling enhances production of galactose-deficient IgA1 in IgA nephropathy. *Kidney Dis.* **2020**, *6*, 168–180. [CrossRef]
120. Yamada, K.; Huang, Z.Q.; Raska, M.; Reily, C.; Anderson, J.C.; Suzuki, H.; Ueda, H.; Moldoveanu, Z.; Kiryluk, K.; Suzuki, Y.; et al. Inhibition of STAT3 signaling reduces IgA1 autoantigen production in IgA nephropathy. *Kidney Int. Rep.* **2017**, *2*, 1194–1207. [CrossRef]
121. Novak, J.; Rizk, D.; Takahashi, K.; Zhang, X.; Bian, Q.; Ueda, H.; Ueda, Y.; Reily, C.; Lai, L.Y.; Hao, C.; et al. New insights into the pathogenesis of IgA nephropathy. *Kidney Dis.* **2015**, *1*, 8–18. [CrossRef] [PubMed]
122. Reily, C.; Ueda, H.; Huang, Z.Q.; Mestecky, J.; Julian, B.A.; Willey, C.D.; Novak, J. Cellular signaling and production of galactose-deficient IgA1 in IgA nephropathy, an autoimmune disease. *J. Immunol. Res.* **2014**, *2014*, 197548. [CrossRef] [PubMed]
123. Makita, Y.; Suzuki, H.; Kano, T.; Takahata, A.; Julian, B.A.; Novak, J.; Suzuki, Y. TLR9 activation induces aberrant IgA glycosylation via APRIL- and IL-6-mediated pathways in IgA nephropathy. *Kidney Int.* **2019**, *97*, 340–349. [CrossRef] [PubMed]
124. Tomana, M.; Matousovic, K.; Julian, B.A.; Radl, J.; Konecny, K.; Mestecky, J. Galactose-deficient IgA1 in sera of IgA nephropathy patients is present in complexes with IgG. *Kidney Int.* **1997**, *52*, 509–516. [CrossRef]
125. Suzuki, H.; Fan, R.; Zhang, Z.; Brown, R.; Hall, S.; Julian, B.A.; Chatham, W.W.; Suzuki, Y.; Wyatt, R.J.; Moldoveanu, Z.; et al. Aberrantly glycosylated IgA1 in IgA nephropathy patients is recognized by IgG antibodies with restricted heterogeneity. *J. Clin. Investig.* **2009**, *119*, 1668–1677. [CrossRef] [PubMed]
126. Placzek, W.J.; Yanagawa, H.; Makita, Y.; Renfrow, M.B.; Julian, B.A.; Rizk, D.V.; Suzuki, Y.; Novak, J.; Suzuki, H. Serum galactose-deficient-IgA1 and IgG autoantibodies correlate in patients with IgA nephropathy. *PLoS ONE* **2018**, *13*, e0190967. [CrossRef] [PubMed]
127. Kokubo, T.; Hiki, Y.; Iwase, H.; Tanaka, A.; Toma, K.; Hotta, K.; Kobayashi, Y. Protective role of IgA1 glycans against IgA1 self-aggregation and adhesion to extracellular matrix proteins. *J. Am. Soc. Nephrol.* **1998**, *9*, 2048–2054. [CrossRef] [PubMed]
128. Schwartz, A.L.; Fridovich, S.E.; Knowles, B.B.; Lodish, H.F. Characterization of the asialoglycoprotein receptor in a continuous hepatoma line. *J. Biol. Chem.* **1981**, *256*, 8878–8881. [CrossRef]
129. Grossetete, B.; Launay, P.; Lehuen, A.; Jungers, P.; Bach, J.F.; Monteiro, R.C. Down-regulation of Fc alpha receptors on blood cells of IgA nephropathy patients: Evidence for a negative regulatory role of serum IgA. *Kidney Int.* **1998**, *53*, 1321–1335. [CrossRef] [PubMed]

130. van Zandbergen, G.; van Kooten, C.; Mohamad, N.K.; Reterink, T.J.; de Fijter, J.W.; van de Winkel, J.G.; Daha, M.R. Reduced binding of immunoglobulin A (IgA) from patients with primary IgA nephropathy to the myeloid IgA Fc-receptor, CD89. *Nephrol. Dial. Transplant.* **1998**, *13*, 3058–3064. [CrossRef]
131. Goritzer, K.; Turupcu, A.; Maresch, D.; Novak, J.; Altmann, F.; Oostenbrink, C.; Obinger, C.; Strasser, R. Distinct Fc α receptor N-glycans modulate the binding affinity to immunoglobulin A (IgA) antibodies. *J. Biol. Chem.* **2019**, *294*, 13995–14008. [CrossRef]
132. Launay, P.; Grossetete, B.; Arcos-Fajardo, M.; Gaudin, E.; Torres, S.P.; Beaudoin, L.; Patey-Mariaud de Serre, N.; Lehuen, A.; Monteiro, R.C. Fcα receptor (CD89) mediates the development of immunoglobulin A (IgA) nephropathy (Berger's disease). Evidence for pathogenic soluble receptor-IgA complexes in patients and CD89 transgenic mice. *J. Exp. Med.* **2000**, *191*, 1999–2009. [CrossRef] [PubMed]
133. Berthelot, L.; Papista, C.; Maciel, T.T.; Biarnes-Pelicot, M.; Tissandie, E.; Wang, P.H.; Tamouza, H.; Jamin, A.; Bex-Coudrat, J.; Gestin, A.; et al. Transglutaminase is essential for IgA nephropathy development acting through IgA receptors. *J. Exp. Med.* **2012**, *209*, 793–806. [CrossRef]
134. Berthelot, L.; Robert, T.; Vuiblet, V.; Tabary, T.; Braconnier, A.; Drame, M.; Toupance, O.; Rieu, P.; Monteiro, R.C.; Toure, F. Recurrent IgA nephropathy is predicted by altered glycosylated IgA, autoantibodies and soluble CD89 complexes. *Kidney Int.* **2015**, *88*, 815–822. [CrossRef]
135. McDonald, K.J.; Cameron, A.J.; Allen, J.M.; Jardine, A.G. Expression of Fc alpha/mu receptor by human mesangial cells: A candidate receptor for immune complex deposition in IgA nephropathy. *Biochem. Biophys. Res. Commun.* **2002**, *290*, 438–442. [CrossRef]
136. Moura, I.C.; Centelles, M.N.; Arcos-Fajardo, M.; Malheiros, D.M.; Collawn, J.F.; Cooper, M.D.; Monteiro, R.C. Identification of the transferrin receptor as a novel immunoglobulin (Ig)A1 receptor and its enhanced expression on mesangial cells in IgA nephropathy. *J. Exp. Med.* **2001**, *194*, 417–425. [CrossRef]
137. Leung, J.C.; Tsang, A.W.; Chan, D.T.; Lai, K.N. Absence of CD89, polymeric immunoglobulin receptor, and asialoglycoprotein receptor on human mesangial cells. *J. Am. Soc. Nephrol.* **2000**, *11*, 241–249. [CrossRef]
138. Haddad, E. Enhanced expression of the CD71 mesangial IgA1 receptor in Berger Disease and Henoch-Schönlein Nephritis: Association between CD71 expression and IgA deposits. *J. Am. Soc. Nephrol.* **2003**, *14*, 327–337. [CrossRef] [PubMed]
139. Moura, I.C. Glycosylation and size of IgA1 are essential for interaction with mesangial transferrin receptor in IgA nephropathy. *J. Am. Soc. Nephrol.* **2004**, *15*, 622–634. [CrossRef] [PubMed]
140. Molyneux, K.; Wimbury, D.; Pawluczyk, I.; Muto, M.; Bhachu, J.; Mertens, P.R.; Feehally, J.; Barratt, J. β1,4-galactosyltransferase 1 is a novel receptor for IgA in human mesangial cells. *Kidney Int.* **2017**, *92*, 1458–1468. [CrossRef] [PubMed]
141. Kaneko, Y.; Otsuka, T.; Tsuchida, Y.; Gejyo, F.; Narita, I. Integrin α1/β1 and α2/β1 as a receptor for IgA1 in human glomerular mesangial cells in IgA nephropathy. *Int. Immunol.* **2012**, *24*, 219–232. [CrossRef]
142. Monteiro, R.C. Recent advances in the physiopathology of IgA nephropathy. *Nephrol. Ther.* **2018**, *14* (Suppl. 1), S1–S8. [CrossRef] [PubMed]
143. Tomana, M.; Zikan, J.; Moldoveanu, Z.; Kulhavy, R.; Bennett, J.C.; Mestecky, J. Interactions of cell-surface galactosyltransferase with immunoglobulins. *Mol. Immunol.* **1993**, *30*, 265–275. [CrossRef]
144. Tortajada, A.; Gutierrez, E.; Pickering, M.C.; Praga Terente, M.; Medjeral-Thomas, N. The role of complement in IgA nephropathy. *Mol. Immunol.* **2019**, *114*, 123–132. [CrossRef] [PubMed]
145. Rauterberg, E.W.; Lieberknecht, H.M.; Wingen, A.M.; Ritz, E. Complement membrane attack (MAC) in idiopathic IgA-glomerulonephritis. *Kidney Int.* **1987**, *31*, 820–829. [CrossRef]
146. Roos, A.; Rastaldi, M.P.; Calvaresi, N.; Oortwijn, B.D.; Schlagwein, N.; van Gijlswijk-Janssen, D.J.; Stahl, G.L.; Matsushita, M.; Fujita, T.; van Kooten, C.; et al. Glomerular activation of the lectin pathway of complement in IgA nephropathy is associated with more severe renal disease. *J. Am. Soc. Nephrol.* **2006**, *17*, 1724–1734. [CrossRef] [PubMed]
147. Stad, R.K.; Bogers, W.M.; Thoomes-van der Sluys, M.E.; Van Es, L.A.; Daha, M.R. In vivo activation of complement by IgA in a rat model. *Clin. Exp. Immunol.* **1992**, *87*, 138–143. [CrossRef]
148. Stad, R.K.; Bruijn, J.A.; van Gijlswijk-Janssen, D.J.; van Es, L.A.; Daha, M.R. An acute model for IgA-mediated glomerular inflammation in rats induced by monoclonal polymeric rat IgA antibodies. *Clin. Exp. Immunol.* **1993**, *92*, 514–521. [CrossRef]
149. Oortwijn, B.D.; Roos, A.; Royle, L.; van Gijlswijk-Janssen, D.J.; Faber-Krol, M.C.; Eijgenraam, J.W.; Dwek, R.A.; Daha, M.R.; Rudd, P.M.; van Kooten, C. Differential glycosylation of polymeric and monomeric IgA: A possible role in glomerular inflammation in IgA nephropathy. *J. Am. Soc. Nephrol.* **2006**, *17*, 3529–3539. [CrossRef]
150. Arnold, J.N.; Wormald, M.R.; Suter, D.M.; Radcliffe, C.M.; Harvey, D.J.; Dwek, R.A.; Rudd, P.M.; Sim, R.B. Human serum IgM glycosylation: Identification of glycoforms that can bind to mannan-binding lectin. *J. Biol. Chem.* **2005**, *280*, 29080–29087. [CrossRef]
151. Malhotra, R.; Wormald, M.R.; Rudd, P.M.; Fischer, P.B.; Dwek, R.A.; Sim, R.B. Glycosylation changes of IgG associated with rheumatoid arthritis can activate complement via the mannose-binding protein. *Nat. Med.* **1995**, *1*, 237–243. [CrossRef]
152. Yasutake, J.; Suzuki, Y.; Suzuki, H.; Hiura, N.; Yanagawa, H.; Makita, Y.; Kaneko, E.; Tomino, Y. Novel lectin-independent approach to detect galactose-deficient IgA1 in IgA nephropathy. *Nephrol. Dial. Transplant.* **2015**, *30*, 1315–1321. [CrossRef]
153. Takahashi, K.; Raska, M.; Stuchlova Horynova, M.; Hall, S.D.; Poulsen, K.; Kilian, M.; Hiki, Y.; Yuzawa, Y.; Moldoveanu, Z.; Julian, B.A.; et al. Enzymatic sialylation of IgA1 O-glycans: Implications for studies of IgA nephropathy. *PLoS ONE* **2014**, *9*, e99026. [CrossRef]

154. Hiki, Y.; Hori, H.; Yamamoto, K.; Yamamoto, Y.; Yuzawa, Y.; Kitaguchi, N.; Takahashi, K. Specificity of two monoclonal antibodies against a synthetic glycopeptide, an analogue to the hypo-galactosylated IgA1 hinge region. *J. Nephrol.* **2015**, *28*, 181–186. [CrossRef] [PubMed]
155. Sun, Q.; Zhang, Z.; Zhang, H.; Liu, X. Aberrant IgA1 glycosylation in IgA nephropathy: A Systematic Review. *PLoS ONE* **2016**, *11*, e0166700. [CrossRef]
156. Suzuki, Y.; Matsuzaki, K.; Suzuki, H.; Okazaki, K.; Yanagawa, H.; Ieiri, N.; Sato, M.; Sato, T.; Taguma, Y.; Matsuoka, J.; et al. Serum levels of galactose-deficient immunoglobulin (Ig) A1 and related immune complex are associated with disease activity of IgA nephropathy. *Clin. Exp. Immunol.* **2014**, *18*, 770–777. [CrossRef] [PubMed]
157. Zhao, N.; Hou, P.; Lv, J.; Moldoveanu, Z.; Li, Y.; Kiryluk, K.; Gharavi, A.G.; Novak, J.; Zhang, H. The level of galactose-deficient IgA1 in the sera of patients with IgA nephropathy is associated with disease progression. *Kidney Int.* **2012**, *82*, 790–796. [CrossRef] [PubMed]
158. Maixnerova, D.; Ling, C.; Hall, S.; Reily, C.; Brown, R.; Neprasova, M.; Suchanek, M.; Honsova, E.; Zima, T.; Novak, J.; et al. Galactose-deficient IgA1 and the corresponding IgG autoantibodies predict IgA nephropathy progression. *PLoS ONE* **2019**, *14*, e0212254. [CrossRef]
159. Lafayette, R.A.; Canetta, P.A.; Rovin, B.H.; Appel, G.B.; Novak, J.; Nath, K.A.; Sethi, S.; Tumlin, J.A.; Mehta, K.; Hogan, M.; et al. A Randomized, controlled trial of Rituximab in IgA nephropathy with proteinuria and renal dysfunction. *J. Am. Soc. Nephrol.* **2017**, *28*, 1306–1313. [CrossRef]
160. Wada, Y.; Matsumoto, K.; Suzuki, T.; Saito, T.; Kanazawa, N.; Tachibana, S.; Iseri, K.; Sugiyama, M.; Iyoda, M.; Shibata, T. Clinical significance of serum and mesangial galactose-deficient IgA1 in patients with IgA nephropathy. *PLoS ONE* **2018**, *13*, e0206865. [CrossRef] [PubMed]
161. Suzuki, H.; Yasutake, J.; Makita, Y.; Tanbo, Y.; Yamasaki, K.; Sofue, T.; Kano, T.; Suzuki, Y. IgA nephropathy and IgA vasculitis with nephritis have a shared feature involving galactose-deficient IgA1-oriented pathogenesis. *Kidney Int.* **2018**, *93*, 700–705. [CrossRef]
162. Temurhan, S.; Akgul, S.U.; Caliskan, Y.; Artan, A.S.; Kekik, C.; Yazici, H.; Demir, E.; Caliskan, B.; Turkmen, A.; Oguz, F.S.; et al. A Novel biomarker for post-transplant recurrent IgA nephropathy. *Transplant. Proc.* **2017**, *49*, 541–545. [CrossRef]
163. Yamasaki, K.; Suzuki, H.; Yasutake, J.; Yamazaki, Y.; Suzuki, Y. Galactose-Deficient IgA1-Specific Antibody Recognizes GalNAc-Modified Unique Epitope on Hinge Region of IgA1. *Monoclon. Antib. Immunodiagn. Immunother.* **2018**, *37*, 252–256. [CrossRef] [PubMed]
164. Wang, M.; Lv, J.; Zhang, X.; Chen, P.; Zhao, M.; Zhang, H. Secondary IgA Nephropathy shares the same immune features with primary IgA nephropathy. *Kidney Int. Rep.* **2020**, *5*, 165–172. [CrossRef]
165. Zhao, L.; Peng, L.; Yang, D.; Chen, S.; Lan, Z.; Zhu, X.; Yuan, S.; Chen, G.; Liu, Y.; Liu, H. Immunostaining of galactose-deficient IgA1 by KM55 is not specific for immunoglobulin A nephropathy. *Clin. Immunol.* **2020**, *217*, 108483. [CrossRef]
166. Cassol, C.A.; Bott, C.; Nadasdy, G.M.; Alberton, V.; Malvar, A.; Nagaraja, H.N.; Nadasdy, T.; Rovin, B.H.; Satoskar, A.A. Immunostaining for galactose-deficient immunoglobulin A is not specific for primary immunoglobulin A nephropathy. *Nephrol. Dial. Transplant.* **2020**, *35*, 2123–2129. [CrossRef]
167. Hiki, Y.; Tanaka, A.; Kokubo, T.; Iwase, H.; Nishikido, J.; Hotta, K.; Kobayashi, Y. Analyses of IgA1 hinge glycopeptides in IgA nephropathy by matrix-assisted laser desorption/ionization time-of-flight mass spectrometry. *J. Am. Soc. Nephrol.* **1998**, *9*, 577–582. [CrossRef] [PubMed]
168. Inoue, T.; Iijima, H.; Tajiri, M.; Shinzaki, S.; Shiraishi, E.; Hiyama, S.; Mukai, A.; Nakajima, S.; Iwatani, H.; Nishida, T.; et al. Deficiency of N-acetylgalactosamine in O-linked oligosaccharides of IgA is a novel biologic marker for Crohn's disease. *Inflamm. Bowel Dis.* **2012**, *18*, 1723–1734. [CrossRef]
169. Nakazawa, S.; Imamura, R.; Kawamura, M.; Kato, T.; Abe, T.; Namba, T.; Iwatani, H.; Yamanaka, K.; Uemura, M.; Kishikawa, H.; et al. Difference in IgA1 O-glycosylation between IgA deposition donors and IgA nephropathy recipients. *Biochem. Biophys. Res. Commun.* **2019**, *508*, 1106–1112. [CrossRef] [PubMed]
170. Odani, H.; Hiki, Y.; Takahashi, M.; Nishimoto, A.; Yasuda, Y.; Iwase, H.; Shinzato, T.; Maeda, K. Direct evidence for decreased sialylation and galactosylation of human serum IgA1 Fc O-glycosylated hinge peptides in IgA nephropathy by mass spectrometry. *Biochem. Biophys. Res. Commun.* **2000**, *271*, 268–274. [CrossRef]
171. Buck, K.S.; Smith, A.C.; Molyneux, K.; El-Barbary, H.; Feehally, J.; Barratt, J. B-cell O-galactosyltransferase activity, and expression of O-glycosylation genes in bone marrow in IgA nephropathy. *Kidney Int.* **2008**, *73*, 1128–1136. [CrossRef]
172. Xing, Y.; Li, L.; Zhang, Y.; Wang, F.; He, D.; Liu, Y.; Jia, J.; Yan, T.; Lin, S. C1GALT1 expression is associated with galactosylation of IgA1 in peripheral B lymphocyte in immunoglobulin a nephropathy. *BMC Nephrol.* **2020**, *21*, 18. [CrossRef]
173. Novak, J.; Raskova Kafkova, L.; Suzuki, H.; Tomana, M.; Matousovic, K.; Brown, R.; Hall, S.; Sanders, J.T.; Eison, T.M.; Moldoveanu, Z.; et al. IgA1 immune complexes from pediatric patients with IgA nephropathy activate cultured human mesangial cells. *Nephrol. Dial. Transplant.* **2011**, *26*, 3451–3457. [CrossRef] [PubMed]
174. Iwatani, H.; Inoue, T.; Wada, Y.; Nagasawa, Y.; Yamamoto, R.; Iijima, H.; Takehara, T.; Imai, E.; Rakugi, H.; Isaka, Y. Quantitative change of IgA hinge O-glycan composition is a novel marker of therapeutic responses of IgA nephropathy. *Biochem. Biophys. Res. Commun.* **2012**, *428*, 339–342. [CrossRef] [PubMed]

Journal of
Clinical Medicine

Article

Galactose-Deficient IgA1 as a Candidate Urinary Marker of IgA Nephropathy

Yusuke Fukao [1], Hitoshi Suzuki [1,2,*], Jin Sug Kim [3], Kyung Hwan Jeong [3], Yuko Makita [1], Toshiki Kano [1], Yoshihito Nihei [1], Maiko Nakayama [1], Mingfeng Lee [1], Rina Kato [1], Jer-Ming Chang [4], Sang Ho Lee [3] and Yusuke Suzuki [1,*]

1. Department of Nephrology, Faculty of Medicine, Juntendo University, Tokyo 113-8421, Japan; y-fukao@juntendo.ac.jp (Y.F.); ymakita@juntendo.ac.jp (Y.M.); tkano@juntendo.ac.jp (T.K.); y-nihei@juntendo.ac.jp (Y.N.); m-nakayama@juntendo.ac.jp (M.N.); m-ri@juntendo.ac.jp (M.L.); r-fujikawa@juntendo.ac.jp (R.K.)
2. Department of Nephrology, Juntendo University Urayasu Hospital, Chiba 279-0021, Japan
3. Division of Nephrology, Department of Internal Medicine, College of Medicine, Kyung Hee University, Seoul 130-701, Korea; jinsuk0902@naver.com (J.S.K.); kyunghwan@naver.com (K.H.J.); lshkidney@khu.ac.kr (S.H.L.)
4. Division of Nephrology, Kaohsiung Medical University Hospital, Kaohsiung 80756, Taiwan; jemich@cc.kmu.edu.tw
* Correspondence: shitoshi@juntendo.ac.jp (H.S.); yusuke@juntendo.ac.jp (Y.S.)

Abstract: In patients with IgA nephropathy (IgAN), circulatory IgA1 and IgA1 in the mesangial deposits contain galactose-deficient IgA1 (Gd-IgA1). Some of the Gd-IgA1 from the glomerular deposits is excreted in the urine and thus urinary Gd-IgA1 may represent a disease-specific marker. We recruited 338 Japanese biopsy-proven IgAN patients and 120 patients with other renal diseases (disease controls). Urine samples collected at the time of renal biopsy were used to measure Gd-IgA1 levels using a specific monoclonal antibody (KM55 mAb). Urinary Gd-IgA1 levels were significantly higher in patients with IgAN than in disease controls. Moreover, urinary Gd-IgA1 was significantly correlated with the severity of the histopathological parameters in IgAN patients. Next, we validated the use of urinary Gd-IgA1 levels in the other Asian cohorts. In the Korean cohort, urinary Gd-IgA1 levels were also higher in patients with IgAN than in disease controls. Even in Japanese patients with IgAN and trace proteinuria (less than 0.3 g/gCr), urinary Gd-IgA1 was detected. Thus, urinary Gd-IgA1 may be an early disease-specific biomarker useful for determining the disease activity of IgAN.

Keywords: urinary galactose-deficient IgA1; KM55; IgA nephropathy

1. Introduction

Immunoglobulin A nephropathy (IgAN) is the most common primary glomerulonephritis [1]. According to a systematic review of 40 worldwide studies, the incidence of IgAN is reportedly 2.5/100,000/year [2]. If left untreated, IgAN has a poor prognosis, developing into end-stage renal failure in approximately 20% to 40% of cases within 20 years after onset [3].

There are two IgA isotypes in humans, IgA1 and IgA2 [4]. Galactose-deficient IgA1 (Gd-IgA1), which lacks galactose (Gal) in the O-glycan side chains in the hinge region and exposes N-acetylgalactosamine (GalNAc), has been identified as one of the key molecules in the pathogenesis of IgAN and is increased in the sera of patients with IgAN [5]. According to the multi-hit hypothesis [6], Gd-IgA1 is recognized by anti-glycan autoantibodies, resulting in the formation of pathogenic immune complexes. These immune complexes are deposited in the kidneys, activate mesangial cells, and induce glomerular injury.

Serum Gd-IgA1 levels can predict IgAN progression [7,8]. In contrast, most relatives of IgAN patients with abnormal IgA1 glycoforms do not develop IgAN [9], and serum

Gd-IgA1 levels do not correlate with proteinuria [5], suggesting that serum Gd-IgA1 may not be a useful biomarker.

We previously developed a monoclonal antibody (KM55 mAb) that specifically recognizes Gd-IgA1, and demonstrated that glomerular Gd-IgA1 was specifically detected in IgAN and IgA vasculitis by immunohistochemical analysis using KM55 mAb [10,11].

In a mouse model, injection of purified nephritogenic IgA from IgAN-prone mice led to deposition in the glomeruli in nude mice. Parts of the injected IgA passed through into the bladder, suggesting that some parts of such glomerular IgA were cleared into the urine. In addition, the nephritogenic IgA had strong affinity not only to the glomerular mesangium, but also to the subepithelium [12]. On the other hand, several studies have supported that epithelial cells have the potential to clear matrix material and epithelial deposits into the cavity of Bowman's capsule [13]. Therefore, we hypothesized that urinary Gd-IgA1 could be a disease-specific marker. Indeed, an enzyme-linked immunosorbent assay (ELISA) using Helix aspersa agglutinin (HAA), a GalNAc-specific lectin, could detect urinary Gd-IgA1 and differentiate patients with IgAN from patients with other renal diseases [14]. However, lectin-dependent assays are not suitable for large-scale, multi-specimen testing because of the instability of glycan recognition. Thus, a novel and stable assay is required for the early detection of IgAN.

Many studies have shown that the degree of proteinuria is an outcome predictor in IgAN [15,16]. However, it is difficult to determine whether urinary protein excretion is due to active lesions triggered by glomerular immune deposition or chronic lesions represented by glomerulosclerosis and nephron reduction [17]. Therefore, proteinuria may not always reflect the disease activity, and its assessment is insufficient to determine the indications for treatment.

Several reports have indicated a high remission rate of tonsillectomy combined with steroid pulse therapy in the early stages of IgAN [18,19]. In addition, the renal biopsy findings of 56 patients with hematuria without overt proteinuria revealed that IgAN was common in their pathological diagnoses, and 31% of the patients with IgAN had crescentic lesions [20]. Thus, early diagnosis and treatment of IgAN are important for remission, and a useful biomarker for the indication of renal biopsy is desired.

There are no established disease-specific biomarkers for IgAN. Furthermore, repeated renal biopsies are difficult because of the invasiveness. We established a stable and simple ELISA for Gd-IgA1 using the KM55 mAb in 2015 [11]. In this study, we investigated the usefulness of urinary Gd-IgA1 as a disease-specific marker for IgAN from Japanese cohorts and further verified this using non-Japanese Asian cohorts.

2. Materials and Methods

2.1. Patients and Samples

We recruited 338 Japanese adults ($\geq$18 years old) with biopsy-proven IgAN and 120 patients with other renal diseases (disease controls) diagnosed at Juntendo University Hospital, Tokyo, Japan from 2015 to 2018. In addition, to validate the use of the urinary Gd-IgA1 level, we recruited 69 Korean and 35 Taiwanese biopsy-proven IgAN patients, as well as 39 Korean disease control patients.

Clinical and laboratory data were collected at the time of the renal biopsy. The laboratory parameters included serum creatinine (Cr) levels, serum Gd-IgA1 levels, urinary protein-to-creatinine ratios (UPCR), and urinary Gd-IgA1 levels.

2.2. Pathological Parameters

The histological samples were classified according to the clinical guidelines for IgAN from the Japanese Society of Nephrology (JSN) [21] or the Oxford classification [22,23]. Briefly, the histological grade (H-grade) of the JSN criteria was defined as 1 (0–24.9%), 2 (25–49.9%), 3 (50–74.9%), and 4 (75–100%) based on the percentage of glomeruli with pathological features, such as crescents, global sclerosis, and segmental sclerosis, which predict the progression to end-stage renal disease.

2.3. Measurement of Gd-IgA1

Serum and urinary Gd-IgA1 levels were determined using the KM55 mAb according to the manufacturer's instructions (Immuno-Biological Laboratories, Fujioka, Japan), and logarithmically transformed (log10 basis).

2.4. Statistical Analyses

Data are expressed as mean ± standard error. Comparisons between groups were performed using the Mann–Whitney U test. Spearman's correlation analysis was used to analyze the correlation between two variables. Statistical significance was defined as $p < 0.05$. Statistical analyses were performed using GraphPad Prism software ver.8.0 (GraphPad Software, San Diego, CA, USA).

3. Results

3.1. Demographic, Clinical, and Laboratory Findings

The clinical characteristics of the cohorts from each country at the time of renal biopsy are presented in Table 1. In the Japanese and Korean cohorts, there were no significant differences in age or sex between patients with IgAN and the disease controls. Compared to Japanese patients with IgAN, Korean patients showed higher levels of proteinuria and lower kidney function at the time of renal biopsy.

Table 1. Clinical characteristics of patients with IgAN and disease controls at the time of renal biopsy.

	Patients (n)	Age (year)	Sex	sCr (mg/dL)	eGFR (mL/min/1.73 m^2)	UPCR (g/gCr)
Japanese						data
IgAN	338	38.1	M177/F161	0.8	83.1	0.9
DC	120	49.2	M53/F67	1.0	79.9	2.4
Korean						
IgAN	69	40.5	M28/F41	1.3	76.5	1.5
DC	39	44.4	M16/F20	1.9	69.4	4.6

IgAN, IgA nephropathy; DC, disease control; M, male; F, female; sCr, serum creatinine; eGFR, estimated glomerular filtration rate; UPCR, urinary protein-to-creatinine ratio.

Other renal diseases included lupus nephritis, anti-neutrophil cytoplasmic antibody (ANCA)-associated glomerulonephritis, membranous nephropathy, focal segmental glomerulosclerosis, minimal change disease, membranoproliferative glomerulonephritis, non-IgA mesangial proliferative glomerulonephritis, tubulointerstitial nephritis, diabetic kidney disease, renal amyloidosis, nephrosclerosis, and thin basement membrane disease (Table 2).

Table 2. Clinical characteristics of disease control patients from the Japanese and Korean cohorts.

Disease Controls	Patients (n)	sCr (mg/dL)	eGFR (mL/min/1.73 m^2)	UPCR (g/gCr)
Japanese cohort				
ANCA-associated glomerulonephritis	15	1.7	37.1	2.0
Lupus nephritis	26	0.7	95.7	1.7
Minimal change disease	12	0.8	87.1	5.6
Membranous nephropathy	16	0.7	90.0	3.8
Membranoproliferative glomerulonephritis	4	0.9	103.9	1.6
Non-IgA mesangial proliferative glomerulonephritis	10	0.7	101.7	0.3
Focal segmental glomerulosclerosis	5	0.9	62.3	3.2
Tubulointerstitial nephritis	10	2.0	37.2	1.7
Renal amyloidosis	6	1.0	72.1	5.1

Table 2. Cont.

Disease Controls	Patients (n)	sCr (mg/dL)	eGFR (mL/min/1.73 m^2)	UPCR (g/gCr)
Diabetic kidney disease	5	1.3	56.1	1.8
Nephrosclerosis	4	0.7	77.4	0.3
Thin basement membrane disease	7	0.6	119.0	0.9
Korean cohort				
ANCA-associated glomerulonephritis	12	3.9	24.9	2.3
Lupus nephritis	7	0.9	85.8	4.2
Minimal change disease	16	1.2	85.7	7.6
Thin basement membrane disease	4	0.6	108.8	0.5

sCr, serum creatinine; eGFR, estimated glomerular filtration rate; UPCR, urinary protein-to-creatinine ratio; ANCA, anti-neutrophil cytoplasmic antibody.

3.2. Urinary Levels of Gd-IgA1 in the Japanese Cohort

In the Japanese cohort, urinary Gd-IgA1 levels were significantly elevated in patients with IgAN compared to those in disease controls ($p < 0.0001$) (Figure 1a). The levels of urinary Gd-IgA1 in each disease control group are shown in Figure 1b. Overall, urinary Gd-IgA1 levels were lower in the disease controls than in IgAN patients.

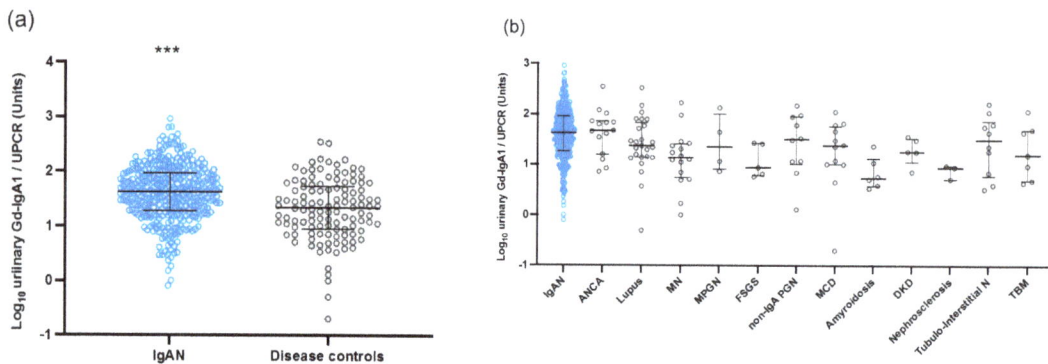

Figure 1. Urinary levels of Gd-IgA1 in Japanese cohort. (**a**) Urinary Gd-IgA1 levels were significantly elevated in patients with IgAN compared to those in disease controls. (**b**) Urinary Gd-IgA1 levels were lower in the disease controls than in IgAN patients. *** $p < 0.0001$.

3.3. Correlation between Urinary Gd-IgA1 and Laboratory and Pathological Findings in IgAN Patients from the Japanese Cohort

We assessed the association between urinary Gd-IgA1 levels and the clinical data and pathological parameters in patients with IgAN from the Japanese cohort. The levels of urinary Gd-IgA1 were associated with the levels of serum Gd-IgA1 ($p < 0.0001$) (Figure 2a), but not with proteinuria, in patients with IgAN (Figure 2b). As shown in Figure 2c, urinary Gd-IgA1 levels were positively correlated with the histological grade ($R = 0.4108$, $p < 0.0001$). Meanwhile, there were no significant correlations between the urinary Gd-IgA1 levels and the MEST-C scores of the Oxford classification. Then, we placed a threshold on the urinary Gd-IgA1 levels, i.e., >50 ng/mL, and analyzed the association between urinary Gd-IgA1 levels and MEST-C Oxford classification. As shown in Figure 2d, there were significant correlations between the urinary Gd-IgA1 levels and the T score of the Oxford classification in cases with urinary Gd-IgA1 greater than 50 ng/mL ($p < 0.01$).

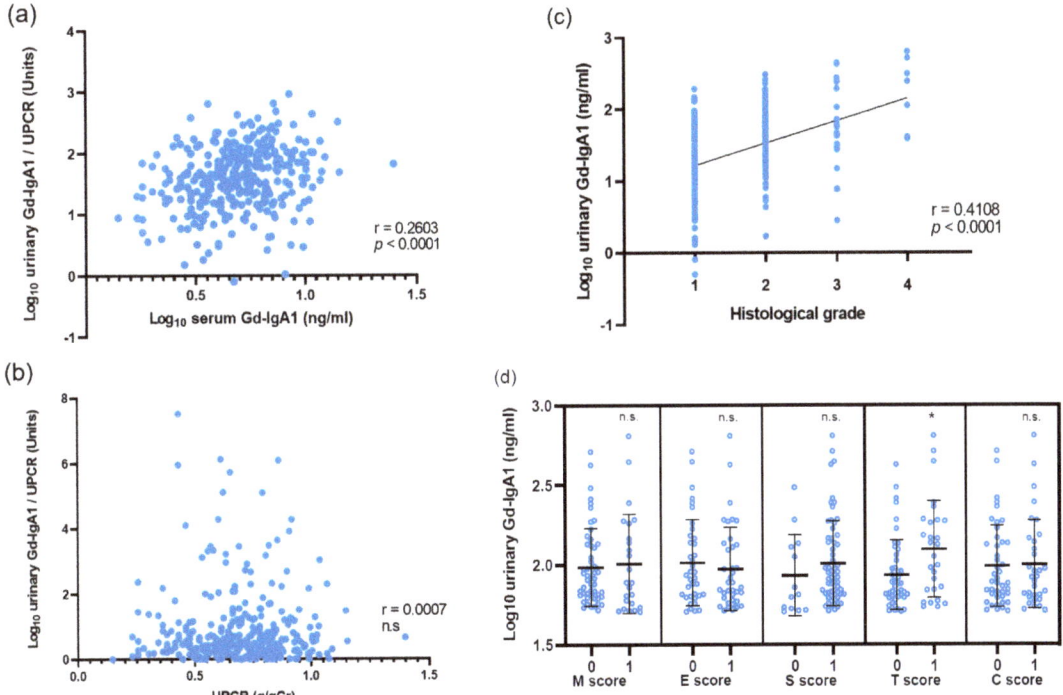

Figure 2. Correlation between urinary Gd-IgA1 and laboratory and pathological findings in IgAN patients from the Japanese cohort. (**a**) The levels of urinary Gd-IgA1 associated with the levels of serum Gd-IgA1. (**b**) The levels of urinary Gd-IgA1 did not correlate with the levels of proteinuria. (**c**) Urinary Gd-IgA1 levels were positively correlated with the histological grade. (**d**) Urinary Gd-IgA1 levels were positively correlated with the T score of the Oxford classification in cases with urinary Gd-IgA1 greater than 50 ng/mL. * $p < 0.01$, n.s.: not significant, Abbreviations: M (mesangial hypercellularity); E (endocapillary hypercellularity); S (segmental glomerulosclerosis); T (tubular atrophy/interstitial fibrosis); and C (cellular/fibrocellular crescents).

3.4. Validation in Korean Cohort

Next, we validated the use of urinary Gd-IgA1 levels for the diagnosis of IgAN using the Korean cohort. In the Korean cohort, the levels of urinary Gd-IgA1 in patients with IgAN were significantly higher compared with those in disease controls ($p < 0.0001$) (Figure 3a). Moreover, the levels of urinary Gd-IgA1 in patients with IgAN were higher than those in any of the disease controls (Figure 3b).

3.5. Difference in Clinical Features at the Time of Renal Biopsy in Patients with IgAN

Compared with the Japanese cohort, Korean and Taiwanese patients showed greater levels of proteinuria and lower kidney function at the time of renal biopsy (Table 3). In addition, levels of urinary Gd-IgA1 in the Korean and Taiwanese patients with IgAN were higher than those in the Japanese patients (Supplementary Figure S1).

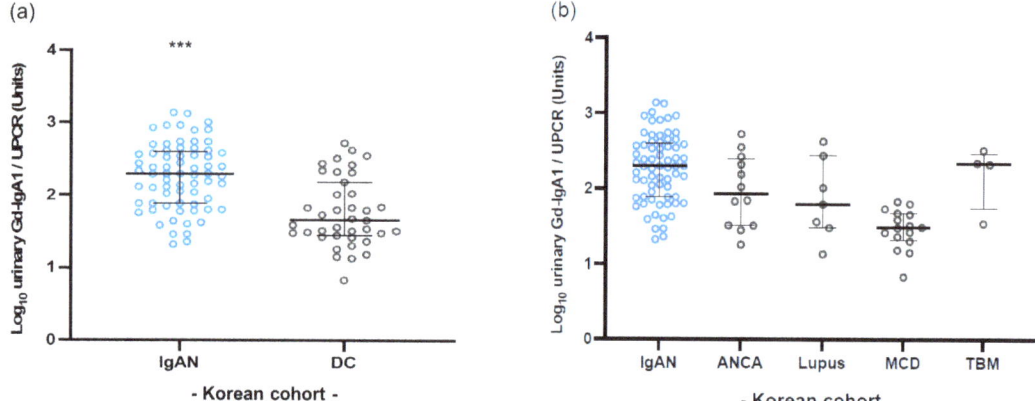

Figure 3. Urinary levels of Gd-IgA1 in Korean and Taiwanese cohorts. (**a**) The levels of urinary Gd-IgA1 in Korean patients with IgAN were significantly higher compared with those in disease controls. (**b**) The levels of urinary Gd-IgA1 in Korean patients with IgAN were higher than those in the any other disease controls. *** $p < 0.0001$.

Table 3. Clinical features of patients with IgAN at the time of renal biopsy.

	Patients (n)	Age (year)	Sex	sCr (mg/dL)	eGFR (mL/min/1.73 m^2)	UPCR (g/gCr)
Japanese IgAN	338	38.1	M177/F161	0.8	83.1	data 0.9
Korean IgAN	69	40.5	M28/F41	1.3	76.5	1.5
Taiwanese IgAN	35	36.6	M21/F14	1.9	51.9	1.4

IgAN, IgA nephropathy; M, male; F, female; sCr, serum creatinine; eGFR, estimated glomerular filtration rate; UPCR, urinary protein-to-creatinine ratio.

3.6. Urinary Gd-IgA1 Excretion with Trace Proteinuria

We assessed the urinary Gd-IgA1 excretion in cases with trace proteinuria (less than 0.3 g/gCr) using the Japanese cohort. Even in cases with trace proteinuria, urinary Gd-IgA1 was detected, and the levels of urinary Gd-IgA1 were higher in patients with IgAN than in disease controls (Figure 4).

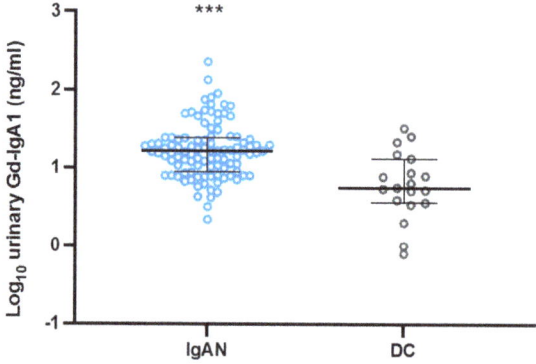

Figure 4. Urinary Gd-IgA1 excretion in cases with trace amounts of proteinuria (less than 0.3 g/gCr). *** $p < 0.0001$.

4. Discussion

A definitive diagnosis of IgAN requires a pathological diagnosis via renal biopsy. In Japan, an annual screening for urinary abnormalities is performed in school-aged children, and asymptomatic patients with microscopic hematuria or mild proteinuria are more likely to undergo renal biopsy than are patients in other countries [24,25]. Indications for renal biopsy vary in each country due to medical insurance. Clinical remission can be achieved with an early diagnosis and treatment [26]. Therefore, a useful biomarker for early detection is required.

Gd-IgA1 is a critical effector molecule in the pathogenesis of IgAN. Glomerular Gd-IgA1 has been specifically detected in patients with IgAN but not in those with other renal diseases [10]. A previous experiment using real-time imaging revealed that injected IgA from the serum of IgAN-prone mice bound to the glomeruli in normal mice, and these IgA deposits cleared over time [12]. Thus, we hypothesized that a fraction of the Gd-IgA1 in glomerular deposits may be excreted into the urine. Previous reports using HAA lectins supported this hypothesis [14]. In this study, we used a stable lectin-independent method with the KM55 mAb to measure the urinary levels of Gd-IgA1. Indeed, the urinary excretion of Gd-IgA1 was elevated in patients with IgAN compared with that in disease controls. This may be due to a mechanism in IgAN in which the greater the amount of Gd-IgA1 deposited, the more glomerular injury occurs, resulting in the increased excretion of urinary Gd-IgA1. As reported in a systematic review [27], the usefulness of serum Gd-IgA1 levels as a tool for assessing disease severity is controversial. In the present study, we found a correlation between urinary Gd-IgA1 levels and the histological severity in IgAN patients. Moreover, the T score of the Oxford classification was associated with urinary Gd-IgA1 levels. Previous reports indicated that the T score is associated with a poor renal outcome [28,29]. Of note, the T score was significantly associated with the renal outcome, independently of clinical data [30]. This suggests that urinary Gd-IgA1 may be useful in determining the disease activity of IgAN.

IgAN is a multifactorial disease with a complex pathogenesis involving genetic and environmental factors. Therefore, we validated the urinary Gd-IgA1 assay in different cohorts of IgAN patients. The levels of urinary Gd-IgA1 were also significantly higher in patients with IgAN than in disease controls in the Korean cohort. Of note, in the Taiwanese and Korean cohorts, urinary Gd-IgA1 levels were much higher than those in the Japanese cohort, which may be due to differences in indications for renal biopsy in these countries, resulting in a higher proportion of advanced-stage cases with a higher urinary protein level and lower eGFR at the time of the renal biopsy.

Clinically, a renal biopsy is rarely performed if proteinuria is negative, even in patients with hematuria. A single-center study in Japan reported that as many as 31% of IgAN patients with hematuria without overt proteinuria (less than 0.3 g/gCr) showed crescents in the renal biopsy findings [20]. Moreover, even in the early stages of IgAN, with normal kidney function and trace proteinuria, long-term renal survival is not always favorable [31]. As early identification and treatment can lead to clinical remission of IgAN [18], biomarkers that can be used for early diagnosis and enable determination of the timing of therapeutic interventions are needed. In the present study, even in patients with IgAN and trace proteinuria (less than 0.3 g/gCr), urinary Gd-IgA1 was detected. Importantly, this suggests that urinary Gd-IgA1 is an early biomarker compared to proteinuria in patients with IgAN.

There are several limitations in the present study. First, we only included Asian patients with IgAN. Large-scale, worldwide studies are needed to elucidate the underlying mechanisms of urinary Gd-IgA1 excretion. Moreover, longitudinal analysis during course of treatment is desired to elucidate disease activity.

In summary, we found higher urinary levels of Gd-IgA1 in patients with IgAN than in patients with other renal diseases. Urinary Gd-IgA1 may be a highly disease-specific marker in several Asian countries. Furthermore, urinary Gd-IgA1 can be detected in patients with trace proteinuria. The present study suggests that urinary Gd-IgA1 is useful not only for the early screening and diagnosis of IgAN but also for determining the disease severity.

Supplementary Materials: The following supporting information can be downloaded at: https://www.mdpi.com/article/10.3390/jcm11113173/s1, Supplementary Figure S1: Levels of urinary Gd-IgA1 in Japanese, Korean and Taiwanese patients with IgAN. Levels of urinary Gd-IgA1 in Korean and Taiwanese patients with IgAN were higher than those in the Japanese patients.

Author Contributions: Conceptualization, Y.F. and H.S.; writing, Y.F. and J.S.K.; review and editing, H.S., K.H.J., Y.M., T.K., Y.N., M.N., M.L., R.K., J.-M.C., S.H.L. and Y.S. All authors have read and agreed to the published version of the manuscript.

Funding: This study was supported, in part, by the JSPS KAKENHI, Grant Numbers 15K09274 and 18K08252, and the Practical Research Project for Renal Diseases from the Japan Agency for Medical Research and Development, AMED.

Institutional Review Board Statement: The study was conducted in accordance with the Declaration of Helsinki and approved by the ethics committee of Juntendo University Hospital (protocol code 2013058 and 858 and dates of approval 6 October 2013 and 19 June 2015), Kyung Hee University (protocol code 2009-06-301 and date of approval 15 February 2022) and Kaohsiung Medical University (protocol code KMUHIRB-G(I)-20180012 and date of approval 13 July 2018).

Informed Consent Statement: Informed consent was obtained from all subjects involved in the study.

Data Availability Statement: Not applicable.

Conflicts of Interest: The authors declare no conflict of interest.

References

1. Levy, M.; Berger, J. Worldwide perspective of IgA nephropathy. *Am. J. Kidney Dis.* **1988**, *12*, 340–347. [CrossRef]
2. McGrogan, A.; Franssen, C.F.; de Vries, C.S. The incidence of primary glomerulonephritis worldwide: A systematic review of the literature. *Nephrol. Dial. Transpl.* **2011**, *26*, 414–430. [CrossRef] [PubMed]
3. D'Amico, G. The commonest glomerulonephritis in the world: IgA nephropathy. *Q. J. Med.* **1987**, *64*, 709–727. [PubMed]
4. Brandtzaeg, P.; Johansen, F.E. Mucosal B cells: Phenotypic characteristics, transcriptional regulation, and homing properties. *Immunol. Rev.* **2005**, *206*, 32–63. [CrossRef] [PubMed]
5. Moldoveanu, Z.; Wyatt, R.J.; Lee, J.Y.; Tomana, M.; Julian, B.A.; Mestecky, J.; Huang, W.Q.; Anreddy, S.R.; Hall, S.; Hastings, M.C.; et al. Patients with IgA nephropathy have increased serum galactose-deficient IgA1 levels. *Kidney Int.* **2007**, *71*, 1148–1154. [CrossRef] [PubMed]
6. Suzuki, H.; Kiryluk, K.; Novak, J.; Moldoveanu, Z.; Herr, A.B.; Renfrow, M.B.; Wyatt, R.J.; Scolari, F.; Mestecky, J.; Gharavi, A.G.; et al. The pathophysiology of IgA nephropathy. *J. Am. Soc. Nephrol.* **2011**, *22*, 1795–1803. [CrossRef]
7. Maixnerova, D.; Ling, C.; Hall, S.; Reily, C.; Brown, R.; Neprasova, M.; Suchanek, M.; Honsova, E.; Zima, T.; Novak, J.; et al. Galactose-deficient IgA1 and the corresponding IgG autoantibodies predict IgA nephropathy progression. *PLoS ONE* **2019**, *14*, e0212254. [CrossRef]
8. Zhao, N.; Hou, P.; Lv, J.; Moldoveanu, Z.; Li, Y.; Kiryluk, K.; Gharavi, A.G.; Novak, J.; Zhang, H. The level of galactose-deficient IgA1 in the sera of patients with IgA nephropathy is associated with disease progression. *Kidney Int.* **2012**, *82*, 790–796. [CrossRef]
9. Gharavi, A.G.; Moldoveanu, Z.; Wyatt, R.J.; Barker, C.V.; Woodford, S.Y.; Lifton, R.P.; Mestecky, J.; Novak, J.; Julian, B.A. Aberrant IgA1 glycosylation is inherited in familial and sporadic IgA nephropathy. *J. Am. Soc. Nephrol.* **2008**, *19*, 1008–1014. [CrossRef]
10. Suzuki, H.; Yasutake, J.; Makita, Y.; Tanbo, Y.; Yamasaki, K.; Sofue, T.; Kano, T.; Suzuki, Y. IgA nephropathy and IgA vasculitis with nephritis have a shared feature involving galactose-deficient IgA1-oriented pathogenesis. *Kidney Int.* **2018**, *93*, 700–705. [CrossRef]
11. Yasutake, J.; Suzuki, Y.; Suzuki, H.; Hiura, N.; Yanagawa, H.; Makita, Y.; Kaneko, E.; Tomino, Y. Novel lectin-independent approach to detect galactose-deficient IgA1 in IgA nephropathy. *Nephrol. Dial. Transpl.* **2015**, *30*, 1315–1321. [CrossRef]
12. Yamaji, K.; Suzuki, Y.; Suzuki, H.; Satake, K.; Horikoshi, S.; Novak, J.; Tomino, Y. The kinetics of glomerular deposition of nephritogenic IgA. *PLoS ONE* **2014**, *9*, e113005. [CrossRef]
13. Li, C.; Ruotsalainen, V.; Tryggvason, K.; Shaw, A.S.; Miner, J.H. CD2AP is expressed with nephrin in developing podocytes and is found widely in mature kidney and elsewhere. *Am. J. Physiol. Renal. Physiol.* **2000**, *279*, F785–F792. [CrossRef] [PubMed]
14. Suzuki, H.; Allegri, L.; Suzuki, Y.; Hall, S.; Moldoveanu, Z.; Wyatt, R.J.; Novak, J.; Julian, B.A. Galactose-Deficient IgA1 as a Candidate Urinary Polypeptide Marker of IgA Nephropathy? *Dis. Markers* **2016**, *2016*, 7806438. [CrossRef] [PubMed]
15. Bartosik, L.P.; Lajoie, G.; Sugar, L.; Cattran, D.C. Predicting progression in IgA nephropathy. *Am. J. Kidney Dis.* **2001**, *38*, 728–735. [CrossRef] [PubMed]
16. Donadio, J.V.; Bergstralh, E.J.; Grande, J.P.; Rademcher, D.M. Proteinuria patterns and their association with subsequent end-stage renal disease in IgA nephropathy. *Nephrol. Dial. Transpl.* **2002**, *17*, 1197–1203. [CrossRef]
17. Suzuki, Y.; Matsuzaki, K.; Suzuki, H.; Sakamoto, N.; Joh, K.; Kawamura, T.; Tomino, Y.; Matsuo, S. Proposal of remission criteria for IgA nephropathy. *Clin. Exp. Nephrol.* **2014**, *18*, 481–486. [CrossRef]

18. Kawaguchi, T.; Ieiri, N.; Yamazaki, S.; Hayashino, Y.; Gillespie, B.; Miyazaki, M.; Taguma, Y.; Fukuhara, S.; Hotta, O. Clinical effectiveness of steroid pulse therapy combined with tonsillectomy in patients with immunoglobulin A nephropathy presenting glomerular haematuria and minimal proteinuria. *Nephrology* **2010**, *15*, 116–123. [CrossRef]
19. Komatsu, H.; Sato, Y.; Miyamoto, T.; Tamura, M.; Nakata, T.; Tomo, T.; Nishino, T.; Miyazaki, M.; Fujimoto, S. Significance of tonsillectomy combined with steroid pulse therapy for IgA nephropathy with mild proteinuria. *Clin. Exp. Nephrol.* **2016**, *20*, 94–102. [CrossRef]
20. Hoshino, Y.; Kaga, T.; Abe, Y.; Endo, M.; Wakai, S.; Tsuchiya, K.; Nitta, K. Renal biopsy findings and clinical indicators of patients with hematuria without overt proteinuria. *Clin. Exp. Nephrol.* **2015**, *19*, 918–924. [CrossRef]
21. Matsuo, S.; Kawamura, T.; Joh, K.; Utsunomiya, Y.; Okonogi, H.; Miyazaki, Y.; Koike, K.; Yokoo, T.; Matsushima, M.; Yoshimura, M.; et al. Clinical guides for immunoglobulin A (IgA) nephropathy in Japan, third version. *Jpn. J. Nephrol.* **2011**, *53*, 123–135.
22. Cattran, D.C.; Coppo, R.; Cook, H.T.; Feehally, J.; Roberts, I.S.; Troyanov, S.; Alpers, C.E.; Amore, A.; Barratt, J.; Berthoux, F.; et al. The Oxford classification of IgA nephropathy: Rationale, clinicopathological correlations, and classification. *Kidney Int.* **2009**, *76*, 534–545. [CrossRef] [PubMed]
23. Roberts, I.S.; Cook, H.T.; Troyanov, S.; Alpers, C.E.; Amore, A.; Barratt, J.; Berthoux, F.; Bonsib, S.; Bruijn, J.A.; Cattran, D.C.; et al. The Oxford classification of IgA nephropathy: Pathology definitions, correlations, and reproducibility. *Kidney Int.* **2009**, *76*, 546–556. [CrossRef]
24. Yap, H.K.; Quek, C.M.; Shen, Q.; Joshi, V.; Chia, K.S. Role of urinary screening programmes in children in the prevention of chronic kidney disease. *Ann. Acad. Med. Singap.* **2005**, *34*, 3–7.
25. Donadio, J.V.; Grande, J.P. IgA nephropathy. *N. Engl. J. Med.* **2002**, *347*, 738–748. [CrossRef] [PubMed]
26. Shoji, T.; Nakanishi, I.; Suzuki, A.; Hayashi, T.; Togawa, M.; Okada, N.; Imai, E.; Hori, M.; Tsubakihara, Y. Early treatment with corticosteroids ameliorates proteinuria, proliferative lesions, and mesangial phenotypic modulation in adult diffuse proliferative IgA nephropathy. *Am. J. Kidney Dis.* **2000**, *35*, 194–201. [CrossRef]
27. Sun, Q.; Zhang, Z.; Zhang, H.; Liu, X. Aberrant IgA1 Glycosylation in IgA Nephropathy: A Systematic Review. *PLoS ONE* **2016**, *11*, e0166700. [CrossRef]
28. Kaihan, A.B.; Yasuda, Y.; Katsuno, T.; Kato, S.; Imaizumi, T.; Ozeki, T.; Hishida, M.; Nagata, T.; Ando, M.; Tsuboi, N.; et al. The Japanese Histologic Classification and T-score in the Oxford Classification system could predict renal outcome in Japanese IgA nephropathy patients. *Clin. Exp. Nephrol.* **2017**, *21*, 986–994. [CrossRef]
29. Haaskjold, Y.L.; Bjørneklett, R.; Bostad, L.; Bostad, L.S.; Lura, N.G.; Knoop, T. Utilizing the MEST score for prognostic staging in IgA nephropathy. *BMC Nephrol.* **2022**, *23*, 26. [CrossRef] [PubMed]
30. Barbour, S.J.; Espino-Hernandez, G.; Reich, H.N.; Coppo, R.; Roberts, I.S.; Feehally, J.; Herzenberg, A.M.; Cattran, D.C.; Bavbek, N.; Cook, T.; et al. The MEST score provides earlier risk prediction in lgA nephropathy. *Kidney Int.* **2016**, *89*, 167–175. [CrossRef]
31. Lee, H.; Hwang, J.H.; Paik, J.H.; Ryu, H.J.; Kim, D.K.; Chin, H.J.; Oh, Y.K.; Joo, K.W.; Lim, C.S.; Kim, Y.S.; et al. Long-term prognosis of clinically early IgA nephropathy is not always favorable. *BMC Nephrol.* **2014**, *15*, 94. [CrossRef] [PubMed]

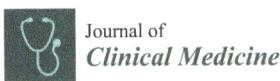

Review

Pathogenesis of IgA Nephropathy: Current Understanding and Implications for Development of Disease-Specific Treatment

Barbora Knoppova [1], Colin Reily [2], R. Glenn King [1], Bruce A. Julian [1,2], Jan Novak [1,*] and Todd J. Green [1,*]

[1] Department of Microbiology, University of Alabama at Birmingham, Birmingham, AL 35294, USA; barcak@uab.edu (B.K.); rgking@uab.edu (R.G.K.); bjulian@uabmc.edu (B.A.J.)

[2] Department of Medicine, University of Alabama at Birmingham, Birmingham, AL 35294, USA; creily@uab.edu

* Correspondence: jannovak@uab.edu (J.N.); tgreen@uab.edu (T.J.G.)

Abstract: IgA nephropathy, initially described in 1968 as a kidney disease with glomerular "intercapillary deposits of IgA-IgG", has no disease-specific treatment and is a common cause of kidney failure. Clinical observations and laboratory analyses suggest that IgA nephropathy is an autoimmune disease wherein the kidneys are damaged as innocent bystanders due to deposition of IgA1-IgG immune complexes from the circulation. A multi-hit hypothesis for the pathogenesis of IgA nephropathy describes four sequential steps in disease development. Specifically, patients with IgA nephropathy have elevated circulating levels of IgA1 with some *O*-glycans deficient in galactose (galactose-deficient IgA1) and these IgA1 glycoforms are recognized as autoantigens by unique IgG autoantibodies, resulting in formation of circulating immune complexes, some of which deposit in glomeruli and activate mesangial cells to induce kidney injury. This proposed mechanism is supported by observations that (i) glomerular immunodeposits in patients with IgA nephropathy are enriched for galactose-deficient IgA1 glycoforms and the corresponding IgG autoantibodies; (ii) circulatory levels of galactose-deficient IgA1 and IgG autoantibodies predict disease progression; and

(iii) pathogenic potential of galactose-deficient IgA1 and IgG autoantibodies was demonstrated in vivo. Thus, a better understanding of the structure–function of these immunoglobulins as autoantibodies and autoantigens will enable development of disease-specific treatments.

Keywords: IgA nephropathy; *O*-glycosylation; IgA1; autoantibody; immune complex

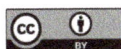

1. Introduction

IgA nephropathy (IgAN) is the most common form of primary glomerulonephritis in many countries [1]. It was initially described in 1968 by Drs. Jean Berger and Nicole Hinglais as a kidney disease with glomerular "intercapillary deposits of IgA-IgG" [2]. Five decades later, the diagnosis still requires examination of kidney tissue. Routine immunofluorescence microscopy reveals IgA as the predominant or co-dominant immunoglobulin in the glomerular immune deposits. This IgA has distinctive characteristics: it is restricted to the IgA1 subclass [3] and has less galactose in its *O*-glycans than does circulating IgA1 in healthy persons (galactose-deficient IgA1; Gd-IgA1) [4,5]. The immune proteins in the glomeruli of patients with IgAN generally include complement C3; IgG, IgM, or both, are often present [6,7]. Light microscopy typically shows glomerular injury as mesangial hypercellularity and increased mesangial matrix [8].

IgAN may affect individuals of nearly all ages, although the diagnosis is rare in children younger than five years of age. The incidence of IgAN peaks in the second and third decades of life [1,7]. In children and adolescents, painless visible hematuria, often concurrent with an infection of the upper respiratory or gastrointestinal tract, frequently heralds the onset of clinical disease. This manifestation may also accompany intense physical activity. Most patients with macroscopic (visible) hematuria have additional episodes over several years [9]. Visible hematuria due to IgAN rarely begins after age 40 years. For patients in their 30s and 40s, microscopic hematuria, with or without, proteinuria may be discovered at the time of routine health screenings. The magnitude of proteinuria varies widely between patients, although proteinuria without microscopic hematuria is uncommon. IgAN is a common cause of chronic kidney disease, particularly for patients with proteinuria persistently more than 1 g/day [10–12]. There is currently no disease-specific therapy and 30–40% of patients progress to kidney failure that reduces life expectancy by about 10 years [13].

The incidence of IgAN varies substantially between ethnic/racial groups, being highest in East Asians; the disease accounts for about 40% of all native-kidney biopsies in Japan, 25% in Europe, 12% in the United States, and less than 5% in central Africa [14]. Some of this variability can be explained by differences in health screening policies and biopsy practices between these regions, but genetic factors also likely contribute [15]. The incidence in the United States has been estimated at 1 per 100,000 person-years [16]. Distribution between the sexes varies by region for reasons not yet defined; the male:female ratio is 2–3:1 in North America [16–18] and Europe [19], but about 1:1 in East Asia [20]. The frequency of the disease may be underestimated. Autopsy studies found IgA glomerular deposits accompanied by glomerular pathology in 1.3% of victims of trauma in Finland [21] and 4% of victims in Singapore [22]. A Japanese study showed that 16% of kidney allografts (from living and deceased donors) had glomerular IgA deposits in biopsy specimens at the time of engraftment of which 10% exhibited histological features typical of IgAN [23]. A recent study confirmed these findings, with 13% of kidneys donated for transplantation exhibiting asymptomatic IgA deposition [24].

In IgAN, kidneys are injured innocently, as indicated by two key findings in kidney transplantation. IgAN often develops in allografts [25–27]; in contrast, IgA deposits disappear from allografts from donors with subclinical IgAN shortly after engraftment into non-IgAN recipients [28]. These observations suggest that the glomerular IgA is deposited from the circulation. While serum Gd-IgA1 levels are elevated in most patients with IgAN, such levels are not sufficient to induce the disease. Many first-degree relatives of patients with IgAN have comparably high levels for years without exhibiting any clinical feature of kidney disease [29]. Most of the circulating Gd-IgA1 is within immune complexes bound by IgG that recognizes galactose-deficient hinge-region (HR) O-glycans on the IgA1 heavy chain [30]. We have postulated that IgAN is an autoimmune disease with a multi-hit mechanism [31] (Figure 1): Gd-IgA1 is produced in greater quantities in IgAN patients compared with that in healthy individuals whereby circulating Gd-IgA1 levels are elevated (hit #1). These Gd-IgA1 molecules are recognized by IgG autoantibodies (hit #2), leading to formation of immune complexes in the blood (hit #3). Some of these circulating immune complexes accumulate in the glomerular mesangium and activate resident mesangial cells to induce kidney injury (hit #4). This proposed sequence is in agreement with the observations that serum levels of Gd-IgA1 (autoantigen) and the corresponding autoantibodies each correlate with disease severity and progression [30,32–34]. Furthermore, the IgG co-deposits in glomeruli are of the IgG1 and IgG3 subclasses [35] as are the IgG autoantibodies in the circulation [30]. IgG is the main autoantibody isotype; the levels of serum IgG autoantibodies in patients with IgAN correlate with those of the autoantigen, Gd-IgA1 [36], and predict disease progression and disease recurrence after transplantation [32,34,37–39]. Other studies revealed that IgG glomerular deposits were associated with a worse long-term outcome [40–42]. These studies together indicate the major role of IgG autoantibodies in IgAN pathogenesis [43].

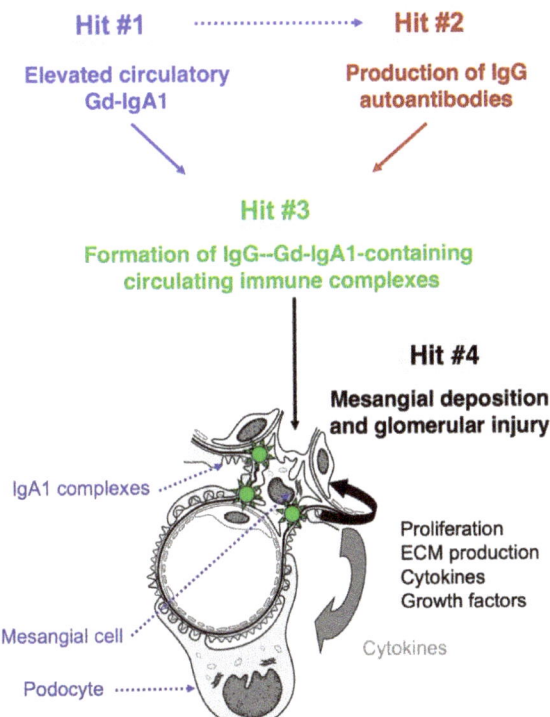

Figure 1. Model of pathogenesis of IgA nephropathy. IgA nephropathy (IgAN) is an autoimmune disease with a genetically and environmentally co-determined multi-hit process [31]. IgA1 with some O-glycans deficient in galactose (galactose-deficient IgA1; Gd-IgA1), in levels often elevated in the circulation of patients with IgAN (Hit #1), is recognized by IgG autoantibodies specific for Gd-IgA1 (Hit #2), and form pathogenic immune complexes, with other serum proteins being added (e.g., complement) (Hit #3). Blood levels of the autoantigen (Gd-IgA1) and the corresponding IgG autoantibodies correlate in IgAN patients, suggesting that elevated circulating levels of Gd-IgA1 are associated with the production of IgG autoantibodies specific for Gd-IgA1 (dashed arrow). Some of the immune complexes formed in the circulation deposit in the kidneys, activate mesangial cells, and induce glomerular injury (Hit #4). Figure modified with permission [44].

Routine immunofluorescence microscopy fails to reveal IgG in many kidney biopsies of patients with IgAN [41,45]. To address this apparent discrepancy with the proposed multi-hit mechanism of disease, we characterized the IgG extracted from glomeruli of remnant renal-biopsy specimens of patients with IgAN to test its antigenic specificity [46]. IgG was detected in glomerular immunodeposits of all IgAN patients, including those without IgG on routine immunofluorescence microscopy. Furthermore, this IgG, but not that in kidney biopsies from patients with membranous nephropathy and lupus nephritis, was enriched for autoantibodies specific for Gd-IgA1. Confocal microscopy using an IgG-specific nanobody confirmed that IgG was present in all IgAN biopsies, irrespective of whether IgG was detected by routine immunofluorescence microscopy. The IgA and IgG co-localized in the glomeruli, indicating that these immunoglobulins comprised immune complexes [46]. These findings strengthen the postulated multi-hit mechanism for the development of IgAN and the central role of IgG autoantibodies in the process, as confirmed recently in an experimental animal model [47].

Most cases of IgAN appear to be sporadic, although kindreds with familial IgAN are well described [48,49]. Genetically determined factors contribute to the pathogenesis of

IgAN, even in patients with apparently sporadic disease [50–54]. Genome-wide association studies of predominantly European and East Asian cohorts have identified at least 21 risk variants for IgAN [55]. Some variants affect the enzymes controlling the glycosylation of IgA1 [56–58] while others alter innate immunity or modulate the activity of the complement system [54,59]. The genetic variants identified so far account for about 7% of the disease risk. Moreover, the cumulative number of the risk variants is strongly associated with age at disease onset, increasing progressively with younger age at diagnosis [50–54].

2. Galactose-Deficient IgA1 (Hit #1)

In humans and higher primates, IgA exists in two isoforms (also called subclasses), IgA1 and IgA2 (~84% and ~16% of total circulatory IgA, respectively). Both isoforms can be in the monomeric and polymeric forms, mIgA, and pIgA. pIgA has a joining chain (J chain), a ~17-kDa protein that forms disulfide bridges with Cys residues at the tail piece of the α heavy chain on the Fc region, to join two IgA monomers [60]. Most pIgA1 and pIgA2 is produced in the mucosal tissues, where pIgA molecules are moved by transcytosis onto the mucosal surfaces. For mucosal secretions, pIgA is produced by IgA-secreting plasma cells in mucosal tissues, such as those in gut-associated lymphoid tissues (GALT) [61,62]. pIgA is bound at the basolateral face of the intestinal epithelial cells by the pIg-receptor (pIgR), which is responsible for transcytosis of pIgA or pIgM. Once the pIgR-IgA complex reaches the apical membrane, pIgR is cleaved to produce the secretory component (SC), and the protein complex containing pIgA and SC is secreted onto the mucosal surfaces as secretory IgA [63,64].

IgA1 has a unique HR between the first and second constant domains (CH1 and CH2) of the heavy chain, connecting the antigen-binding fragment (Fab, heavy-chain domains VH and CH1, and the entire light chain) with the Fc region. Each IgA1 HR contains 3–6 O-glycans, attached to some of the nine serine and threonine residues [65–69]. The O-glycans of the HR of circulatory IgA1 are core 1 O-glycans. The biosynthesis is initiated by addition of an N-acetylgalactosamine (GalNAc) residue by a GalNAc-transferase (GalNAc-T), such as GalNAc-T2. This initial step may be followed by addition of galactose to GalNAc in a β1–3 glycosidic bond by the enzyme core 1 β1,3-galactosyltransferase (C1GalT1). Proper folding of the C1GalT1 protein is facilitated by its chaperone, C1GalT1C1 (COSMC), without which C1GalT1 protein integrity and, thus, function is compromised [70,71]. Additional modifications of GalNAc-galactose disaccharide can then occur on circulatory IgA1: GalNAc can then be sialylated via an α2–6 linkage and/or galactose sialylated via an α2–3 linkage (Figure 2) [72–75]. O-glycans of the HR consisting of GalNAc alone or sialylated GalNAc are galactose-deficient. The serum IgA1 in patients with IgAN has more galactose-deficient HR glycans (Gd-IgA1) than in healthy persons [76–78]. Furthermore, the glomerular IgA deposits are enriched for Gd-IgA1 glycoforms, most likely due to deposition of some of the circulating Gd-IgA1 [46]. The serum Gd-IgA1 level predicts progression to end-stage kidney disease (ESKD) [33]. For patients with ESKD who undergo transplantation, recurrent disease in the allograft is predicted by elevated Gd-IgA1 levels, supporting the hypothesis on the extra-renal origin of IgAN [24,37].

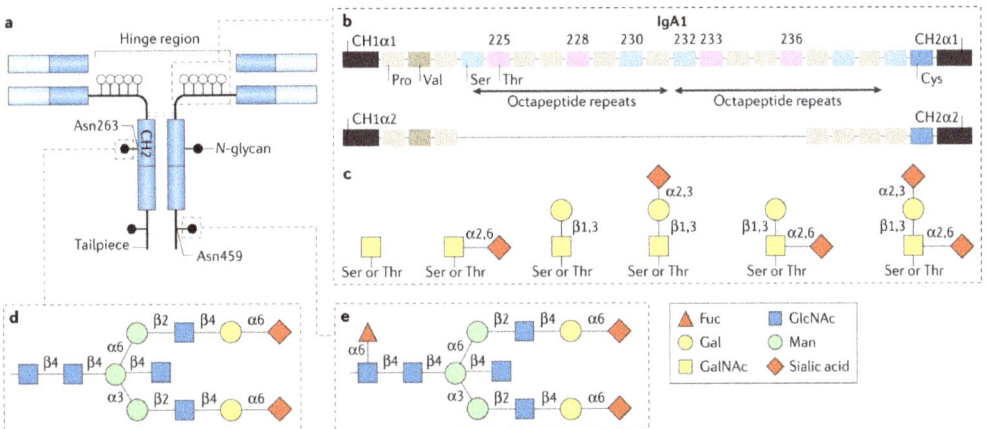

Figure 2. Structure and glycosylation of human IgA1. (**a**) Each heavy chain of IgA1 contains two N-glycans, one in the CH2 domain (Asn263) and the other in the tailpiece (Asn459). (**b**) The hinge-region (HR) of IgA1, unlike that of IgA2, contains nine Ser and Thr residues that are potential O-glycosylation sites. Only 3–6 of these residues are O-glycosylated and the most common IgA1 glycoforms have 4 or 5 O-glycans in the HR. (**c**) The O-glycan composition of normal circulatory IgA1 is variable but usually consists of a core 1 disaccharide structure with N-acetylgalactosamine (GalNAc) in β1,3-linkage with galactose (Gal); each of these monosaccharides can be sialylated. (**d**) The CH2 site of N-glycosylation contains digalactosylated biantennary glycans with or without a bisecting N-acetylglucosamine (GlcNAc), but it is not usually fucosylated. (**e**) The tailpiece N-glycosylation site contains fucosylated glycans. Figure reproduced with permission [43].

The mechanism(s) of Gd-IgA1 production in patients with IgAN is still under investigation. Gd-IgA1 in the circulation of patients with IgAN is predominantly polymeric [79] in contrast to the monomeric form for most of the circulatory IgA1. This fact raises questions about a potential mucosal origin of the Gd-IgA1-secreting cells and their localization (mucosal tissue vs. subsequent errant homing to bone marrow) [80,81]. Alteration in activity of several glycosylation enzymes has been associated with increased Gd-IgA1 production, including decreased expression and activity of C1GalT1 and increased expression and activity of ST6GalNAc2 [31,75,79,82]. The chaperone protein for C1GalT1, C1GalT1C1, is downregulated in B cells from IgAN patients compared to healthy controls and its activity inversely correlated with serum Gd-IgA1 levels [71]. Mechanistic studies found that some cytokines (e.g., leukemia inhibitory factor (LIF) and IL-6) increase Gd-IgA1 production in cultured IgA1-producing cell lines from IgAN patients but not in those from healthy controls. Specifically, supplementation of IL-6 and IL-4 in the media of cultured IgA1-producing cells from IgAN patients decreased expression and activity of C1GalT1 and increased expression of sialyltransferase ST6GalNAc2 [75]. IL-6-mediated activation increased and prolonged activation of the JAK-STAT pathway (detected as phospho-STAT3) was found in IgA1-secreting cells from IgAN patients compared to those from healthy controls [83]. Leukemia inhibitory factor (LIF) exhibits similar effects as IL-6 on IgA1-producing cells from IgAN patients, except that the signaling is mediated by STAT1. These cytokine effects underscore the role of aberrant signaling and cellular activation in Gd-IgA1 production in IgAN [84].

The synthesis of Gd-IgA1 is genetically co-determined. In patients with familial and sporadic IgAN, the serum level of Gd-IgA1 is a heritable trait; many blood relatives have higher levels than genetically distinct married-in relatives, but without any clinical manifestation of IgAN [29,85]. Genome-wide association studies (GWAS) of serum levels of Gd-IgA1 have identified single-nucleotide polymorphisms (SNPs) in the *C1GALT1* and *C1GALT1C1* loci that are related to the expression of specific genes. Reduced expression of *C1GALT1* and *C1GALT1C1* would be manifested by addition of less galactose to GalNAc of the IgA1 HR glycans. GWAS also revealed variants in several genes that influence the synthesis Gd-IgA1, including LIF [53,54].

Treatment of patients with IgAN has included several approaches that reduce circulating levels of Gd-IgA1. Tonsillectomy has been widely accepted in Japan [86–90]. Gd-IgA1 production by IgA1-secreting cells in tonsils is related to abnormalities in the expression of glycosyltransferase genes associated with core 1 O-glycosylation [91]. However, tonsillectomy has not improved kidney outcomes of IgAN patients in western Europeans, suggesting that the underlying mechanisms of Gd-IgA1 production may be distinct in different populations [92,93]. Although oral administration of corticosteroids may reduce Gd-IgA1 synthesis and, consequently, circulating levels of Gd-IgA1-IgG immune complexes [91,94,95], such therapy is not standard of care for most patients due to significant toxicity [96]. In the recent NEFIGAN trial, oral administration of a slow-release corticosteroid (TRF-budesonide) designed to reach the mucosal surface of the ileum significantly reduced proteinuria, slowed decline in kidney clearance function, and lowered serum levels of Gd-IgA1 and Gd-IgA1-IgG immune complexes [97–99].

Catabolism of circulatory polymeric and monomeric IgA occurs in the liver and depends on the asialoglycoprotein receptor (ASGPR) on hepatocytes [100,101]. The binding to ASGPR is dependent on the glycosylation status of IgA, in line with the well-known specificity of this hepatocyte lectin for glycans [102–106]. Circulating IgA1-IgG complexes may not be cleared as quickly in IgAN patients as in healthy controls. Clearance of an IgA1-IgG complexes-mimicking probe was delayed in IgAN patients compared with healthy controls) [107]. However, clearance of another protein probe (asialo α1 acid glycoprotein) was equivalent in the two cohorts, indicating that the liver clearance function is not generally impaired in IgAN patients.

The origins of Gd-IgA1 production have not been defined, despite many studies designed to evaluate the mechanisms of the synthesis of the immunoglobulin. There persists substantial technical difficulty in evaluating whether mucosal tissues are the site of Gd-IgA1-producing cells that secrete the galactose-deficient pIgA1 that enters the circulation. Additionally, as not all IgA1-secreting cells produce Gd-IgA1, many questions remain about how cytokines may control differential regulation of glycosylation in Gd-IgA1-producing cells. Future innovative single-cell analytics that identify signaling and transcriptional mechanisms in IgA1-secreting cells that produce Gd-IgA1 should find potential targets for novel, effective disease-specific therapy.

3. Autoantibodies (Hit #2)

Autoantibodies in patients with IgAN recognize the aberrantly glycosylated HR of IgA1 [30,108]. The specificity of serum IgG autoantibodies was assessed using a panel of well-defined glycoforms of potential antigens. Serum IgG of patients with IgAN exhibited significantly higher binding to enzymatically desialylated and degalactosylated IgA1, Fab fragment of Gd-IgA1 with O-glycosylated HR, and albumin-linked HR glycopeptide with three GalNAc residues compared to enzymatically galactosylated or sialylated Gd-IgA1 and albumin-linked HR peptide without any glycan. These experiments confirmed the specificity of autoantibodies for IgA1 with its HR containing terminal GalNAc [30,109]. Serum Gd-IgA1-specific antibodies can be of IgG, IgM, or IgA isotype, and it is thought that at least some of them can be induced by microbiota with GalNAc-containing epitopes [110–113]. Follow-up studies with serum specimens from IgAN patients revealed that IgG is the predominant autoantibody isotype specific for Gd-IgA1 [36,114].

IgG autoantibodies specific for Gd-IgA1 in patients with IgAN have a distinctive sequence signature. IgG autoantibodies were cloned from immortalized IgG-producing cells derived from peripheral blood of several patients with IgAN using single-cell RT-PCR [30]. Sequence analysis of variable regions of the heavy chains (VH) of these IgG autoantibodies revealed serine in the junction of framework 3 and the complementarity determining region 3 (CDR3). Follow-up studies confirmed that serine residue in this region was important for binding to Gd-IgA1. When the recombinant IgG autoantibody from an

IgAN patient was modified to replace serine with alanine in this position, the resultant IgG proteins exhibited reduced binding to Gd-IgA1. Conversely, IgG from a healthy control that weakly bound Gd-IgA1 had alanine in that amino-acid position; replacing it with serine significantly improved the binding, further confirming the importance of serine in this position for binding of IgG to Gd-IgA1 [30].

A follow-up study was performed to assess whether this single amino-acid alteration originates from a rare allele of a VH gene or somatic hypermutations, such as those occurring during antibody-maturation processes [115]. Germline genomic DNA from seven IgAN patients and six healthy controls was sequenced for the specific VH gene of each autoantibody. These genomic sequences were then compared with the sequences of the cloned VH regions of autoantibodies. Germline genomic VH genes of IgAN patients had nucleotide sequences encoding alanine or valine, but not serine. These findings identified several nucleotide mutations that resulted in a codon switch to serine. No such codon change was observed in sequences originating from healthy controls. These data indicate that serine in the framework 3-CDR3 region of these autoantibodies likely originates from somatic hypermutations that enhance the affinity for IgG autoantibodies in patients with IgAN [116].

It is not known what triggers the production of autoantibodies targeting IgA1 with terminal GalNAc residue(s) in the hinge-region. One hypothesis proposes that an infection by microorganisms carrying GalNAc on their outer surfaces elicits production of GalNAc-recognizing antibodies that cross-react with Gd-IgA1. Infection by Epstein–Barr virus, respiratory syncytial virus, herpes simplex virus, and streptococci may induce production of such antibodies [110–113,117]. Tn-antigen-specific antibodies (i.e., recognizing GalNAc-containing glycoconjugates) have been induced by ingestion or inhalation of live or killed *Escherichia coli* (O86) [118,119]. Upon infection of mucosal surfaces and gastrointestinal tract, susceptible individuals could react by producing hypermutated IgG against mucosal pathogens [120]. A recent study proposed an association between infection by *Streptococcus mutans* and severe outcome of IgAN [121]. Moreover, a study with *Bacteroidetes* bacteria found aberrant mucosal immune responses to tonsillar anaerobic microbiota and production of IgA specific for these bacteria may be involved in the pathophysiology of IgAN [122].

Regardless of the origin of Gd-IgA1-specific autoantibodies, their serum levels correlate with disease severity [30] and predict disease progression [32,34]. Therefore, measurement of serum levels of these autoantibodies may be a prognostic biomarker of IgAN. Furthermore, serum levels of Gd-IgA1-specific IgG autoantibodies correlate with the levels of serum Gd-IgA1 in IgAN patients [36], indicating potential utility of both biomarkers.

4. Other Types of Autoantibodies Targeting Aberrantly Glycosylated Proteins

Although the involvement of glycan-dependent Gd-IgA1-specific antibodies in IgAN is clear, the origin of these autoantibodies is currently unknown. Glycan-reactive antibodies are abundant in the circulation of healthy individuals and many specificities of these antibodies have been described. For example, antibodies against xenoantigens, such as α-galactose as well as allo- or auto-antigens, including blood groups which display potential self-reactivity, are all readily detectable [123]. Although high levels of self-reactive antibodies recognizing mature post-translational glycosylation are rare, antibodies that react with immature or truncated glycosylation precursors are abundant in humans. Many of these structures are also antigenic determinants of non-mammalian glycans, including commensal and pathogenic bacteria, which likely promote the production of most, if not all, natural glycan-reactive antibodies. Indeed, antibodies reactive with chitooligosaccharides, short polymers of *N*-acetylglucosamine (GlcNAc) residues that are structurally similar to the *N*-glycans, are among the most abundant glycan-specific antibodies in humans [124,125]. In rodents, the synthesis of these glycan-specific antibodies is driven by the commensal flora [124,125]. Whether Gd-IgA1-reactive antibodies are derived from naturally occurring precursors generated by microbial exposure or are the products of de novo responses against neoepitopes in Gd-IgA1 is unknown. These two possibilities are not mutually exclusive; a comparable scenario may be the antigenicity of tumor-associated antigen Tn-MUC1, i.e., MUC1 with terminal GalNAc residues (for review, see [126]).

Cellular transformation in cancer frequently alters glycosylation profiles. A similar process applies to the production of Gd-IgA1: the loss of function of the T-synthase (C1GalT1) or its molecular chaperone Cosmc (C1GalTC1) truncates the synthesis of the HR O-glycans after attachment of GalNAcα to serine or threonine [43]. The result is expression of tumor-associated antigen termed Tn antigen along with its sialylated form (sTn antigen). Similar to the glycan-reactive epitopes described above, the Tn and sTn antigens are among the epitopes covered by the natural antibody repertoire [127]. Moreover, like other glycan-specific antibodies, the anti-Tn reactivity in human serum antibodies is polyclonal in nature, exhibiting binding to an array of structurally similar glycans. In fact, human anti-Tn antibodies, including IgG and IgM isotypes, affinity-purified using terminal GalNAcα-containing matrix, demonstrate higher affinity for other glycan structures compared to terminal GalNAcα, including bacteria-derived products and cell-wall structures [128]. At least some of these antibodies clearly recognize tumor-associated Tn antigens [129]. MUC1 is a glycoprotein constitutively expressed by epithelial cells in many organs, including the lungs and gastrointestinal tract. Extensively glycosylated, 50% of the mass of MUC1 in normal healthy tissue is contributed by O-glycans [130]. Likely, because of its size, density of O-linked glycosylation, and high-expression levels in many tumors, aberrantly glycosylated MUC1 is an attractive tumor-associated antigen for immunotherapy. Considerable efforts have been devoted to harnessing antibodies toward aberrantly glycosylated MUC1 as cancer immunotherapy, through vaccination with glyco-MUC1 peptides or passive immunization [126].

As is the case with the other glycan epitopes described above, the fine-specificities of antibodies that recognize tumor-derived MUC1 are diverse, as are their antigenic targets. Immunization with MUC1 glycopeptides displaying aberrant glycan profiles generates antibodies that differ from the natural Tn-reactive antibodies [131]. Although direct binding to the Tn antigen has not been observed for most MUC1 antibodies generated in the efforts to develop anti-tumor therapeutics, Tn glycans appear to play a role in antigen binding. The affinity of many antibodies toward MUC1 peptides is increased in the presence of the Tn antigen, in some cases correlating with the number of Tn modifications on MUC1 peptides [132].

Several anti-MUC1 recombinant antibodies have been investigated as therapeutic reagents targeting breast, colon, and pancreatic cancers [133,134]. The mechanisms of action of the reagents vary, ranging from antibody-dependent cellular cytotoxicity to polarization of cell-associated MUC-1 promoting increased cell-mediated immunity [135,136]. For one such antibody, mAb-AR20.5 (BrevaRex), cellular and humoral immunity recognizing MUC1 were observed after its administration [137]. Initially, it was proposed that this mouse IgG1 antibody was activating the idiotypic network, resulting in the derivation of MUC1-reactive antibodies. It was subsequently determined, however, that the increase in anti-MUC1 serum antibody reactivity in patients receiving BrevaRex therapy was the result of the formation of immune complexes with BrevaRex and soluble MUC1 shed from tumors. These immune complexes promoted T cell-mediated and humoral immune activation directed toward the endogenous MUC1, resulting in elevated levels of antibody reactive with MUC1. Interestingly, a similar phenomenon has been observed for two other therapeutic antibodies targeting another mucin antigen (CA125) aberrantly glycosylated and shed from tumor cells [138,139]. Although there is much work to be done to determine the antigenic glycoforms of Gd-IgA1 contributing to IgAN and the autoantibodies that complex with Gd-IgA1 driving this disease, these examples offer a plausible mechanism by which the auto-immune responses to Gd-IgA1 could be initiated. Low affinity anti-Tn antibodies, which are universally present in human sera, may recognize Gd-IgA1 to form immune complexes, which, in turn, direct the activation of adaptive immunity, ultimately promoting epitope spreading and the generation of high-affinity pathogenic antibodies.

5. Circulating Immune Complexes (Hit #3)

Circulating immune complexes (CICs) in IgAN patients consist of IgG autoantibodies bound to polymeric IgA1 with galactose-deficient HR O-glycans [117,140,141]. Aggregates of Gd-IgA1 and fibronectin and extracellular matrix proteins have also been found in the circulation [142,143]. The latter study showed that besides IgG, CICs are composed of IgA, IgM, and complement C3 [144]. The biological activity of the CICs is determined by composition and size. The CICs containing high content of Gd-IgA1 induce proliferation of mesangial cells in culture, which was not observed for Gd-IgA1 alone or Gd-IgA1-lacking immune complexes [145]. Large-molecular-weight CICs (800–900 kDa) are biologically active. Cellular proliferation and overproduction of cytokines and components of extracellular matrix are observed in cultured primary mesangial cells stimulated with the large-molecular-weight CICs, whereas smaller complexes are inhibitory [145,146]. Experiments with in vitro produced immune complexes using Gd-IgA1 myeloma protein and anti-glycan IgG from cord blood of healthy women confirmed the stimulatory effects of IgA1-IgG immune complexes on mesangial cells [147].

Complement component C3 [148] and its fragments (iC3b, C3c, and C3dg) are also in the Gd-IgA1-IgG immune complexes, confirming the biologic capability of these complexes to activate the alternative complement pathway [149]. In a study of 81 IgAN patients, C3 activation was demonstrated in 75% of the adult and 57% of the pediatric patients. Involvement of the classical complement pathway, assessed by C4 activation, was detected in plasma of 20% of the adult and 5% of the pediatric patients [150]. Analysis of kidney biopsy specimens reveals C3 in most cases, indicating involvement of alternative complement pathway, whereas C1 is usually absent. Complement activation pathways are described in Figure 3 (for review, see [151,152]). Recent proteomics analysis of CICs identified association of Gd-IgA1 with α1-microglobulin. Elevated blood levels of Gd-IgA1-α1-microglobulin correlated with hypertension, eGFR levels, and extent of scarring in the kidney biopsy sections [153].

The levels of CICs in IgAN patients correlate with clinical and histological activity such as microscopic hematuria, episodes of macroscopic hematuria, and severity of glomerular injury [154]. At the time of macroscopic hematuria, the blood level of immune complexes of IgA1-IgG may significantly increase, although IgA1-IgM complexes may also be present [155].

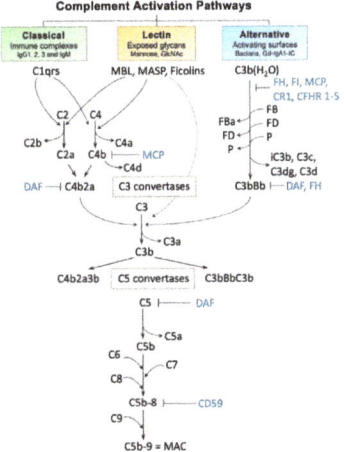

Figure 3. Complement activation pathways and selected regulatory proteins. The three pathways of complement activation, classical, lectin, and alternative, are initiated by interactions of complement proteins with distinct structures. The common activators for each pathway are described in the respective boxes. Complexes of antigen and antibody can activate the classical pathway.

Mannan-binding lectin recognizes carbohydrate structures and, upon association with serine proteases (MASP, mannose-associated serine proteases), can activate the lectin pathway. Complement C3 that is covalently bound to microorganism surfaces as C3b initiates the cascade of the alternative pathway. Each pathway can ultimately generate an active C3 convertase, resulting in cleavage of C3 component into C3a and C3b fragments. C3b can interact with C4b2b or C3bBb to produce C5 convertase that cleaves C5 into C5a and C5b fragments. C5b binds to the cell membrane and serves as a platform for assembly of the membrane attack complex (MAC) [156,157]. The formation of MAC can be inhibited by membrane-bound CD59 that binds to C8 and/or C9. Selected regulatory proteins are shown in light blue. CR1, complement receptor 1; CFHR 1–5, complement factor H-related proteins 1–5; DAF, decay-accelerating factor; FB, factor B; FD, factor D; FI, factor I; Gd-IgA1, galactose-deficient IgA1; Gd-IgA1-IC, galactose-deficient IgA1-containing immune complexes; MCP, membrane cofactor protein; P, properdin. Figure modified with permission [151].

6. Deposition of Circulating Immune Complexes and Renal Injury (Hit #4)

As detailed above, IgAN is an autoimmune disease characterized by the glomerular deposition of immune complexes containing Gd-IgA1 and IgG autoantibodies specific for Gd-IgA1 [46,158,159]. These IgA1-containing glomerular immunodeposits usually contain also complement C3. As IgAN patients often have elevated levels of circulatory Gd-IgA1 and IgG autoantibodies, and the Gd-IgA1-IgG immune complexes also contain C3 and the same subclasses of IgG (IgG1 and 3), it is thought that the glomerular immunodeposits originate from the circulation [31].

In vitro experiments using cultured primary human mesangial cells [160] have shown that IgA1-containing immune complexes in the sera of patients with IgAN can activate mesangial cells [44,145,161–171]. In contrast, free (uncomplexed) Gd-IgA1 did not stimulate proliferation of cultured mesangial cells [31,145–147,164,171,172]. Moreover, immune complexes formed in vitro from Gd-IgA1 and IgG autoantibody mimicked the stimulatory effect of Gd-IgA1-IgG-containing immune complexes in sera of IgAN patients [147,159,173].

It is not fully understood what types of receptors on mesangial cells are engaged by the pathogenic complexes. Mesangial cells express several receptors that can bind IgA1: transferrin receptor (CD71) [166,174–176], integrin β1 [177], and cell surface galactosyltransferase (e.g., β1,4-galactosyltransferase) [178]. The transferrin receptor (CD71) binds IgA1, but not IgA2, and the IgA1 binding is inhibitable by transferrin [175]. CD71 binds polymeric, but not monomeric IgA1, and the binding is dependent on glycosylation, namely O-glycosylation [166]. CD71 is thought to participate in the binding of pathogenic IgA1-containing immune complexes by mesangial cells in IgAN [166]. The other two receptors, integrin β1 and cell surface β1,4-galactosyltransferase, can bind IgA1 molecules, although it is not clear whether either receptor is involved in the pathogenic cellular activation in IgAN.

IgA in a soluble or aggregated form can bind to FcαRI (CD89). Although mesangial cells do not express CD89, a complex formed from IgA1 and soluble CD89 can deposit in the kidneys, as shown in an experimental animal model [179]. It is not clear whether the same mechanism may operate in some IgAN patients. In general, IgA complexes can induce immunosuppressive or pro-inflammatory responses. Soluble forms of IgA, monomers and dimers, in the circulation have low affinity for FcαRI and bind only transiently, thus mediating inhibitory signaling under homeostatic conditions [180]. Similar inhibitory effects can be induced by peptidomimetics to reduce undesirable inflammatory responses, such as those triggered by abnormal IgA-containing immune complexes in IgA-mediated blistering skin diseases [181,182].

As noted above, glomerular immune deposits in patients with IgAN are enriched for Gd-IgA1 glycoforms. A recent study provided experimental in vivo evidence to underscore the pathogenic role of IgG autoantibodies specific for Gd-IgA1 [47]. Specifically, Gd-IgA1-IgG immune complexes injected into immunodeficient mice deposited in the glomerular mesangium, together with murine complement C3, and produced glomerular injury with histological features mimicking IgAN, such as mesangioproliferative changes. Injection of the individual components (IgA1 or IgG) did not have such effects.

Transcriptome profiling of kidney tissues from mice injected with Gd-IgA1-rIgG immune complexes revealed changes concordant with findings in kidney biopsy tissue from IgAN patients. Pathway-enrichment analysis showed that immune complexes formed by Gd-IgA1 and recombinant IgG (rIgG) dysregulated expression of genes in the MAPK signaling, phagosome, complement, and coagulation pathways, as well as in cell adhesion molecules, transcriptional misregulation, PPAR and Rap1 signaling, leukocyte migration, and osteocyte differentiation [47].

These experimental approaches demonstrate the key roles of aberrantly O-glycosylated IgA1 and the corresponding IgG autoantibodies in the formation of nephritogenic immune complexes. Future studies are needed to provide additional information about processes induced by glomerular deposition of Gd-IgA1-IgG immune complexes. It is hoped that this approach can serve as a basis for development of new tools for elucidating some aspects of pathogenesis of IgAN as well as for pre-clinical testing of future therapeutic approaches.

7. IgA Nephropathy—Disease-Specific Treatment Approaches

The multi-hit hypothesis for the pathogenesis of IgAN, as described above, provides an overview of the immune players, IgG autoantibodies and Gd-IgA1, and the pathogenic immune complexes that are at the core of the disease process. Despite having discovered these players, clarified the importance of the galactose-deficient HR O-glycans for formation of immune complexes, and developed the capacity to clone and characterize IgG autoantibodies, we still lack full understanding of how such disease-causing immune complexes are formed. Coincident with this, there is a lack of disease-specific treatment for IgAN and many patients progress to ESKD. Even the new ongoing clinical trials for IgAN target specific areas of the broader disease state [for review, see [183]]. Below, we describe conceptual premises for disease-specific treatment and methods that may allow investigators to get closer to that goal.

While effective in many cases, the current treatments for IgAN fail to address the key causation of the disease, formation of pathogenic immune complexes. In principle, methods to prevent or interfere with the process can be developed. From the perspective of the IgG autoantibodies, smaller versions of IgG that retain the capacity to bind Gd-IgA1, but are reduced to monovalent interactions, could be generated (Figure 4). Examples of such reagents include Fab antigen-binding fragments, single-chain variable fragments (scFv), or single-domain nanobody fragments [31]. These small monovalent reagents could potentially reduce formation of large pathogenic immune complexes by blocking binding of IgG autoantibodies to Gd-IgA1, thereby forming smaller complexes less prone to deposit in the kidneys. An alternative to this approach is to develop glycopeptides or smaller glycosylated proteins that are analogous to the HR of Gd-IgA1 or epitopes recognized by Gd-IgA1-specific IgG (Figure 4). These Gd-IgA1 glycomimetics could bind to IgG autoantibodies and prevent formation of complexes; however, design of minimalized versions of these Gd-IgA1 analogs is hampered by gaps in our knowledgebase regarding the definitive epitope(s) on Gd-IgA1 that are recognized by IgG autoantibodies.

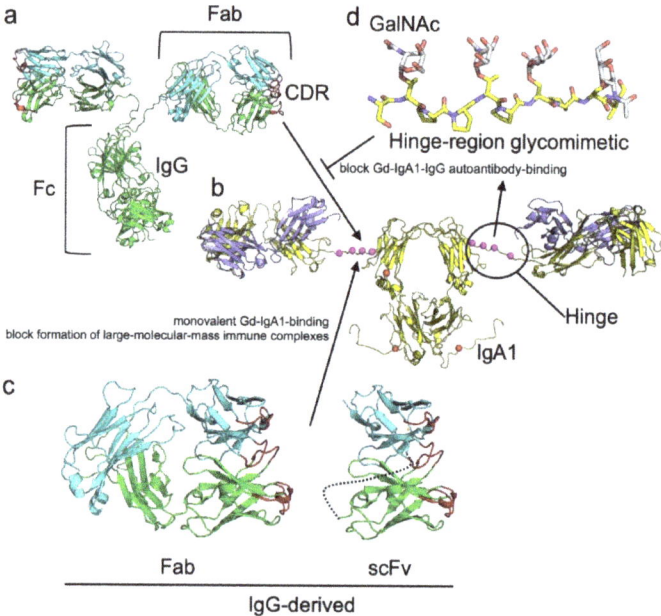

Figure 4. Structures of IgG and IgA1 with featured subdomain elements having theoretical utility to block formation of IgG-Gd-IgA1 complexes. In (**a**), an intact IgG (PDB ID: 1IGT, [184–186]) is shown in cartoon model. Heavy and light chains are green and cyan, respectively, with complementarity determining regions (CDRs) red. In (**b**), an intact IgA1 (based on PDB ID: 1IGA, [187–190]) is shown with heavy and light chains yellow and slate, respectively. Sites of O-linked (magenta) and N-linked glycans (red) are denoted by spheres. For simplicity, IgA1 is shown in monomeric rather than one of the possible polymeric forms. (**c**) Illustrates subdomain entities that could potentially be used to block IgG binding to Gd-IgA1. The Fab and scFv are both derived from the IgG and follow the same color patterns as in (**a**). The linker between VH and VL domains in the scFv is shown in dotted line. Due to the monovalent nature (single antibody-binding site) of these antibody fragments, each could bind to the Gd-IgA1, preventing IgG-binding and blocking formation of large-molecular-weight immune complexes. (**d**) A theoretical glycopeptide is shown in stick representation. The peptide, analogous to residues 224–233 of the IgA1 heavy chain, is shown with yellow carbon backbone. O-linked GalNAc (white carbon backbone) is shown linked at amino acids Thr-225, Thr-228, Ser-230, and Ser-232. This model could serve as a starting point for glycomimetic design for binding to IgG autoantibodies that target Gd-IgA1. Glycans were modeled with GLYCAM [191] and energy minimized with YASARA [192]. Images were made with PyMOL [193].

One pathway to a better understanding how these disease-causing immune complexes are formed may be the use of structural biology, an area of science that aims to define the molecular structure of proteins, protein complexes, and other biological elements to better understand the correlation between structure and function. Techniques for this pursuit include x-ray crystallography (XRC), electron microscopy (EM), small-angle x-ray scattering (SAXS), nuclear magnetic resonance spectroscopy (NMR), and mass spectrometry (MS). These tools have been critical for defining the structures of antibodies [for a recent review of structural immunology, see [194]] and the glycan composition of IgA1 (see descriptions above). The first volume structure of an immunoglobulin, an IgG, was published in 1971 [195]. This low-resolution structure (6Å resolution) showed the three-dimensional (3D) organization of the IgG domains. In subsequent years, atomic structures of individual antibody domains and segments were published: the Fab (initially at 6Å resolution [196] and later as a high-resolution structure [197]), and the fragment-crystallizable region (Fc) [198].

Individual domains were then used to resolve the 3D coordinates of the first intact antibody in 1977 [199]. Further studies led to a small-molecule Fab structure; as a result, a basis for how antibodies bind to antigens was understood [197]. Since these early structures were published, three additional intact IgG structures have been published [184–186], which have collectively confirmed a common molecular structure. Although high-resolution structures of intact IgA1 are lacking, four low-resolution bead models derived from SAXS studies have been produced [187–190]. Moreover, 3D renderings of antibodies are illustrated in Figure 4. There are nearly 5200 antibody structures in the Research Collaboratory for Structural Bioinformatics Protein Data Bank [200], 85% of which were determined with XRC. These structural data provide valuable information about antibodies in general, but more specifically provide clues as to how they interact with antigens because most antibodies are in complexes with an antigen [201].

Despite this wealth of information, there is no structure of the glycosylated HR of IgA1 or structures of IgG or Fabs derived from patients associated with IgAN. In recent years, the field of cryo-EM has undergone what has been termed the "resolution revolution", meaning that this technique has come of age, maturing to a high-resolution structural technique on par with XRC [202,203]. The advantage of cryo-EM is that the technique is amenable to proteins and protein complexes that are large and have some inherent flexibility, which can present issues with NMR and XRC techniques, respectively. Since 2020, structures of larger IgA1 segments and their complexes have been produced: Fc of secretory IgA1 in complex with J chain and the secretory component of pIgR (dimeric [204–206], tetrameric [204,206], and pentameric forms of IgA1 [204]), the dimeric form of IgA1 Fc in complex with pneumococcal adhesion protein, SpsA [206], and IgA1 in complex with the *Streptococcus pneumoniae* IgA1 protease [207]. These structures demonstrate feasibility to determine the structures of large IgA1-associated complexes using cryo-EM. The complex of IgA1 protease with IgA1 represents the first experimentally determined high-resolution partial structures of the IgA1 hinge-region, although the structure does not resolve O-glycans on the hinge-region.

As noted, a paramount goal in determining these structures is to provide a better understanding of function and, in part, to generate hypotheses on possible approaches to inhibit protein-protein associations. Still, the missing key elements in this pathway toward disease-specific therapy for IgAN include knowledge of structures of the complexes of IgG autoantibodies with Gd-IgA1autoantigen. Cryo-EM appears to be the likely avenue to acquire this information. To go a step further and better define the epitopes on Gd-IgA1, a panel of autoantibodies representing a comprehensive repertoire from patients with IgAN is needed. Each structure will presumably reveal a snapshot of a unique binding-interface. These data will provide a comprehensive topographical representation of the VH/VL surfaces involved in Gd-IgA1 recognition and differences in binding associated with IgG variability. Defining the same, overlapping, and/or distinct epitopes on the Gd-IgA1 will provide an opportunity to design strategies for disrupting the interaction of IgG and Gd-IgA1. It remains to be determined if small molecules can be designed that disrupt formation of pathogenic immune complexes, but discovery of the structures of each IgG autoantibody and Gd-IgA1 affords the opportunity to perform in silico screening of ligand libraries [208,209] in hopes of identifying, at least virtually, compounds that target critical areas of antibody-antibody binding. Compounds fitting this criterion could be validated by ELISA-based tests and further assessed in vitro (e.g., with cultured human mesangial cells) and in vivo in a small-animal model of IgAN [47]. It remains to be seen if these concepts for generating disease-specific treatments can be successfully implemented.

8. Conclusions

IgAN is characterized by glomerular immunodeposits enriched for Gd-IgA1 glycoforms and for IgG autoantibodies with specificity for the IgA1 with galactose-deficient O-glycans. These immunodeposits are thought to originate from Gd-IgA1-IgG complexes formed in the circulation. It was recently shown experimentally that human IgG autoantibodies bind to human Gd-IgA1 to form immune complexes that in a murine model induce pathogenic changes consistent with IgAN. It is hoped that a better understanding of the key players in IgAN, autoantibodies, and autoantigens, will enable development of disease-specific treatments.

Author Contributions: All authors participated in the development of the overall concept and outline. Each author was then assigned a specific section to write. B.K. combined all sections and added and formatted references. All authors reviewed and edited the final manuscript. All authors have read and agreed to the published version of the manuscript.

Funding: Supported by NIH grants AI149431, DK078244, DK082753, and DK106341, and a gift from the IGA Nephropathy Foundation of America.

Conflicts of Interest: B.A.J. and J.N. are co-inventors on US patent application 14/318,082 (assigned to UAB Research Foundation). B.A.J. and J.N. are co-founders and co-owners of and consultants for Reliant Glycosciences, LLC. Other authors declare no conflict of interest.

References

1. D'Amico, G. The commonest glomerulonephritis in the world: IgA nephropathy. *Q. J. Med.* **1987**, *64*, 709–727.
2. Berger, J.; Hinglais, N. Intercapillary deposits of IgA-IgG. *J. Urol. Nephrol.* **1968**, *74*, 694–695.
3. Conley, M.E.; Cooper, M.D.; Michael, A.F. Selective deposition of immunoglobulin A1 in immunoglobulin A nephropathy, anaphylactoid purpura nephritis, and systemic lupus erythematosus. *J. Clin. Investig.* **1980**, *66*, 1432–1436. [CrossRef] [PubMed]
4. Allen, A.C.; Bailey, E.M.; Brenchley, P.E.; Buck, K.S.; Barratt, J.; Feehally, J. Mesangial IgA1 in IgA nephropathy exhibits aberrant O-glycosylation: Observations in three patients. *Kidney Int.* **2001**, *60*, 969–973. [CrossRef] [PubMed]
5. Hiki, Y.; Odani, H.; Takahashi, M.; Yasuda, Y.; Nishimoto, A.; Iwase, H.; Shinzato, T.; Kobayashi, Y.; Maeda, K. Mass spectrometry proves under-O-glycosylation of glomerular IgA1 in IgA nephropathy. *Kidney Int.* **2001**, *59*, 1077–1085. [CrossRef]
6. Jennette, J.C. The immunohistology of IgA nephropathy. *Am. J. Kidney Dis.* **1988**, *12*, 348–352. [CrossRef]
7. Wyatt, R.J.; Julian, B.A. IgA nephropathy. *N. Engl. J. Med.* **2013**, *368*, 2402–2414. [CrossRef] [PubMed]
8. Roberts, I.S. Pathology of IgA nephropathy. *Nat. Rev. Nephrol.* **2014**, *10*, 445–454. [CrossRef]
9. D'Amico, G.; Colasanti, G.; Barbiano di Belgioioso, G.; Fellin, G.; Ragni, A.; Egidi, F.; Radaelli, L.; Fogazzi, G.; Ponticelli, C.; Minetti, L. Long-term follow-up of IgA mesangial nephropathy: Clinico-histological study in 374 patients. *Semin. Nephrol.* **1987**, *7*, 355–358.
10. D'Amico, G. Natural history of idiopathic IgA nephropathy and factors predictive of disease outcome. *Semin. Nephrol.* **2004**, *24*, 179–196. [CrossRef]
11. Barratt, J.; Feehally, J. IgA nephropathy. *J. Am. Soc. Nephrol.* **2005**, *16*, 2088–2097. [CrossRef] [PubMed]
12. Reich, H.N.; Troyanov, S.; Scholey, J.W.; Cattran, D.C.; Registry, T.G. Remission of proteinuria improves prognosis in IgA nephropathy. *J. Am. Soc. Nephrol.* **2007**, *18*, 3177–3183. [CrossRef] [PubMed]
13. Hastings, M.C.; Bursac, Z.; Julian, B.A.; Villa Baca, E.; Featherston, J.; Woodford, S.Y.; Bailey, L.; Wyatt, R.J. Life expectancy for patients from the southeastern United States with IgA nephropathy. *Kidney Int. Rep.* **2018**, *3*, 99–104. [CrossRef]
14. Woo, K.T.; Lau, Y.K.; Chan, C.M.; Wong, K.S. Angiotensin-converting enzyme inhibitor versus angiotensin 2 receptor antagonist therapy and the influence of angiotensin-converting enzyme gene polymorphism in IgA nephritis. *Ann. Acad. Med. Singap.* **2008**, *37*, 372–376.
15. Yamagata, K.; Iseki, K.; Nitta, K.; Imai, H.; Iino, Y.; Matsuo, S.; Makino, H.; Hishida, A. Chronic kidney disease perspectives in Japan and the importance of urinalysis screening. *Clin. Exp. Nephrol.* **2008**, *12*, 1–8. [CrossRef]
16. Wyatt, R.J.; Julian, B.A.; Baehler, R.W.; Stafford, C.C.; McMorrow, R.G.; Ferguson, T.; Jackson, E.; Woodford, S.Y.; Miller, P.M.; Kritchevsky, S. Epidemiology of IgA nephropathy in central and eastern Kentucky for the period 1975 through 1994. Central Kentucky Region of the Southeastern United States IgA Nephropathy DATABANK Project. *J. Am. Soc. Nephrol.* **1998**, *9*, 853–858. [CrossRef]
17. Schena, F.P. A retrospective analysis of the natural history of primary IgA nephropathy worldwide. *Am. J. Med.* **1990**, *89*, 209–215. [CrossRef]
18. Wyatt, R.J.; Kritchevsky, S.B.; Woodford, S.Y.; Miller, P.M.; Roy, S.; Holland, N.H.; Jackson, E.; Bishof, N.A. IgA nephropathy: Long-term prognosis for pediatric patients. *J. Pediatr.* **1995**, *127*, 913–919. [CrossRef]
19. Geddes, C.C.; Rauta, V.; Gronhagen-Riska, C.; Bartosik, L.P.; Jardine, A.G.; Ibels, L.S.; Pei, Y.; Cattran, D.C. A tricontinental view of IgA nephropathy. *Nephrol. Dial. Transplant.* **2003**, *18*, 1541–1548. [CrossRef]
20. Shen, A.Y.; Brar, S.S.; Khan, S.S.; Kujubu, D.A. Association of race, heart failure and chronic kidney disease. *Future Cardiol.* **2006**, *2*, 441–454. [CrossRef] [PubMed]
21. Varis, J.; Rantala, I.; Pasternack, A.; Oksa, H.; Jäntti, M.; Paunu, E.S.; Pirhonen, R. Immunoglobulin and complement deposition in glomeruli of 756 subjects who had committed suicide or met with a violent death. *J. Clin. Pathol.* **1993**, *46*, 607–610. [CrossRef]
22. Sinniah, R. Occurrence of mesangial IgA and IgM deposits in a control necropsy population. *J. Clin. Pathol.* **1983**, *36*, 276–279. [CrossRef]

23. Suzuki, K.; Honda, K.; Tanabe, K.; Toma, H.; Nihei, H.; Yamaguchi, Y. Incidence of latent mesangial IgA deposition in renal allograft donors in Japan. *Kidney Int.* **2003**, *63*, 2286–2294. [CrossRef]
24. Nakazawa, S.; Imamura, R.; Kawamura, M.; Kato, T.; Abe, T.; Namba, T.; Iwatani, H.; Yamanaka, K.; Uemura, M.; Kishikawa, H.; et al. Difference in IgA1 O-glycosylation between IgA deposition donors and IgA nephropathy recipients. *Biochem. Biophys. Res. Commun.* **2019**, *508*, 1106–1112. [CrossRef]
25. Berger, J. Recurrence of IgA nephropathy in renal allografts. *Am. J. Kidney Dis.* **1988**, *12*, 371–372. [CrossRef]
26. Floege, J. Recurrent IgA nephropathy after renal transplantation. *Semin. Nephrol.* **2004**, *24*, 287–291. [CrossRef]
27. Chandrakantan, A.; Ratanapanichkich, P.; Said, M.; Barker, C.V.; Julian, B.A. Recurrent IgA nephropathy after renal transplantation despite immunosuppressive regimens with mycophenolate mofetil. *Nephrol. Dial. Transplant.* **2005**, *20*, 1214–1221. [CrossRef]
28. Silva, F.G.; Chander, P.; Pirani, C.L.; Hardy, M.A. Disappearance of glomerular mesangial IgA deposits after renal allograft transplantation. *Transplantation* **1982**, *33*, 241–246. [PubMed]
29. Gharavi, A.G.; Moldoveanu, Z.; Wyatt, R.J.; Barker, C.V.; Woodford, S.Y.; Lifton, R.P.; Mestecky, J.; Novak, J.; Julian, B.A. Aberrant IgA1 glycosylation is inherited in familial and sporadic IgA nephropathy. *J. Am. Soc. Nephrol.* **2008**, *19*, 1008–1014. [CrossRef] [PubMed]
30. Suzuki, H.; Fan, R.; Zhang, Z.; Brown, R.; Hall, S.; Julian, B.A.; Chatham, W.W.; Suzuki, Y.; Wyatt, R.J.; Moldoveanu, Z.; et al. Aberrantly glycosylated IgA1 in IgA nephropathy patients is recognized by IgG antibodies with restricted heterogeneity. *J. Clin. Investig.* **2009**, *119*, 1668–1677. [CrossRef] [PubMed]
31. Suzuki, H.; Kiryluk, K.; Novak, J.; Moldoveanu, Z.; Herr, A.B.; Renfrow, M.B.; Wyatt, R.J.; Scolari, F.; Mestecky, J.; Gharavi, A.G.; et al. The pathophysiology of IgA nephropathy. *J. Am. Soc. Nephrol.* **2011**, *22*, 1795–1803. [CrossRef]
32. Berthoux, F.; Suzuki, H.; Thibaudin, L.; Yanagawa, H.; Maillard, N.; Mariat, C.; Tomino, Y.; Julian, B.A.; Novak, J. Autoantibodies targeting galactose-deficient IgA1 associate with progression of IgA nephropathy. *J. Am. Soc. Nephrol.* **2012**, *23*, 1579–1587. [CrossRef]
33. Zhao, N.; Hou, P.; Lv, J.; Moldoveanu, Z.; Li, Y.; Kiryluk, K.; Gharavi, A.G.; Novak, J.; Zhang, H. The level of galactose-deficient IgA1 in the sera of patients with IgA nephropathy is associated with disease progression. *Kidney Int.* **2012**, *82*, 790–796. [CrossRef]
34. Maixnerova, D.; Ling, C.; Hall, S.; Reily, C.; Brown, R.; Neprasova, M.; Suchanek, M.; Honsova, E.; Zima, T.; Novak, J.; et al. Galactose-deficient IgA1 and the corresponding IgG autoantibodies predict IgA nephropathy progression. *PLoS ONE* **2019**, *14*, e0212254. [CrossRef] [PubMed]
35. Aucouturier, P.; Monteiro, R.C.; Noël, L.H.; Preud'homme, J.L.; Lesavre, P. Glomerular and serum immunoglobulin G subclasses in IgA nephropathy. *Clin. Immunol. Immunopathol.* **1989**, *51*, 338–347. [CrossRef]
36. Placzek, W.J.; Yanagawa, H.; Makita, Y.; Renfrow, M.B.; Julian, B.A.; Rizk, D.V.; Suzuki, Y.; Novak, J.; Suzuki, H. Serum galactose-deficient-IgA1 and IgG autoantibodies correlate in patients with IgA nephropathy. *PLoS ONE* **2018**, *13*, e0190967. [CrossRef] [PubMed]
37. Berthelot, L.; Robert, T.; Vuiblet, V.; Tabary, T.; Braconnier, A.; Dramé, M.; Toupance, O.; Rieu, P.; Monteiro, R.C.; Touré, F. Recurrent IgA nephropathy is predicted by altered glycosylated IgA, autoantibodies and soluble CD89 complexes. *Kidney Int.* **2015**, *88*, 815–822. [CrossRef]
38. Maixnerova, D.; Reily, C.; Bian, Q.; Neprasova, M.; Novak, J.; Tesar, V. Markers for the progression of IgA nephropathy. *J. Nephrol.* **2016**, *29*, 535–541. [CrossRef]
39. Berthoux, F.; Suzuki, H.; Mohey, H.; Maillard, N.; Mariat, C.; Novak, J.; Julian, B.A. Prognostic value of serum biomarkers of autoimmunity for recurrence of IgA nephropathy after kidney transplantation. *J. Am. Soc. Nephrol.* **2017**, *28*, 1943–1950. [CrossRef] [PubMed]
40. Nieuwhof, C.; Kruytzer, M.; Frederiks, P.; van Breda Vriesman, P.J. Chronicity index and mesangial IgG deposition are risk factors for hypertension and renal failure in early IgA nephropathy. *Am. J. Kidney Dis.* **1998**, *31*, 962–970. [CrossRef]
41. Wada, Y.; Ogata, H.; Takeshige, Y.; Takeshima, A.; Yoshida, N.; Yamamoto, M.; Ito, H.; Kinugasa, E. Clinical significance of IgG deposition in the glomerular mesangial area in patients with IgA nephropathy. *Clin. Exp. Nephrol.* **2013**, *17*, 73–82. [CrossRef] [PubMed]
42. Shin, D.H.; Lim, B.J.; Han, I.M.; Han, S.G.; Kwon, Y.E.; Park, K.S.; Lee, M.J.; Oh, H.J.; Park, J.T.; Han, S.H.; et al. Glomerular IgG deposition predicts renal outcome in patients with IgA nephropathy. *Mod. Pathol.* **2016**, *29*, 743–752. [CrossRef]
43. Reily, C.; Stewart, T.J.; Renfrow, M.B.; Novak, J. Glycosylation in health and disease. *Nat. Rev. Nephrol.* **2019**, *15*, 346–366. [CrossRef] [PubMed]
44. Novak, J.; Julian, B.A.; Mestecky, J.; Renfrow, M.B. Glycosylation of IgA1 and pathogenesis of IgA nephropathy. *Semin. Immunopathol.* **2012**, *34*, 365–382. [CrossRef] [PubMed]
45. Bellur, S.S.; Troyanov, S.; Cook, H.T.; Roberts, I.S.; Working Group of the International IgA Nephropathy Network and the Renal Pathology Society. Immunostaining findings in IgA nephropathy: Correlation with histology and clinical outcome in the Oxford classification patient cohort. *Nephrol. Dial. Transplant.* **2011**, *26*, 2533–2536. [CrossRef]
46. Rizk, D.V.; Saha, M.K.; Hall, S.; Novak, L.; Brown, R.; Huang, Z.Q.; Fatima, H.; Julian, B.A.; Novak, J. Glomerular immunodeposits of patients with IgA nephropathy are enriched for IgG autoantibodies specific for galactose-deficient IgA1. *J. Am. Soc. Nephrol.* **2019**, *30*, 2017–2026. [CrossRef] [PubMed]
47. Moldoveanu, Z.; Suzuki, H.; Reily, C.; Satake, K.; Novak, L.; Xu, N.; Huang, Z.Q.; Knoppova, B.; Khan, A.; Hall, S.; et al. Experimental evidence of pathogenic role of IgG autoantibodies in IgA nephropathy. *J. Autoimmun.* **2021**, *118*, 102593. [CrossRef]

48. Julian, B.A.; Quiggins, P.A.; Thompson, J.S.; Woodford, S.Y.; Gleason, K.; Wyatt, R.J. Familial IgA nephropathy. Evidence of an inherited mechanism of disease. *N. Engl. J. Med.* **1985**, *312*, 202–208. [CrossRef]
49. Yeo, S.C.; Goh, S.M.; Barratt, J. Is immunoglobulin A nephropathy different in different ethnic populations? *Nephrology (Carlton)* **2019**, *24*, 885–895. [CrossRef]
50. Gharavi, A.G.; Kiryluk, K.; Choi, M.; Li, Y.; Hou, P.; Xie, J.; Sanna-Cherchi, S.; Men, C.J.; Julian, B.A.; Wyatt, R.J.; et al. Genome-wide association study identifies susceptibility loci for IgA nephropathy. *Nat. Genet.* **2011**, *43*, 321–327. [CrossRef]
51. Kiryluk, K.; Li, Y.; Sanna-Cherchi, S.; Rohanizadegan, M.; Suzuki, H.; Eitner, F.; Snyder, H.J.; Choi, M.; Hou, P.; Scolari, F.; et al. Geographic differences in genetic susceptibility to IgA nephropathy: GWAS replication study and geospatial risk analysis. *PLoS Genet.* **2012**, *8*, e1002765. [CrossRef]
52. Kiryluk, K.; Novak, J.; Gharavi, A.G. Pathogenesis of immunoglobulin A nephropathy: Recent insight from genetic studies. *Annu. Rev. Med.* **2013**, *64*, 339–356. [CrossRef]
53. Kiryluk, K.; Novak, J. The genetics and immunobiology of IgA nephropathy. *J. Clin. Investig.* **2014**, *124*, 2325–2332. [CrossRef]
54. Kiryluk, K.; Li, Y.; Scolari, F.; Sanna-Cherchi, S.; Choi, M.; Verbitsky, M.; Fasel, D.; Lata, S.; Prakash, S.; Shapiro, S.; et al. Discovery of new risk loci for IgA nephropathy implicates genes involved in immunity against intestinal pathogens. *Nat. Genet.* **2014**, *46*, 1187–1196. [CrossRef]
55. Li, M.; Wang, L.; Shi, D.C.; Foo, J.N.; Zhong, Z.; Khor, C.C.; Lanzani, C.; Citterio, L.; Salvi, E.; Yin, P.R.; et al. Genome-wide meta-analysis identifies three novel susceptibility loci and reveals ethnic heterogeneity of genetic susceptibility for IgA nephropathy. *J. Am. Soc. Nephrol.* **2020**, *31*, 2949–2963. [CrossRef]
56. Gale, D.P.; Molyneux, K.; Wimbury, D.; Higgins, P.; Levine, A.P.; Caplin, B.; Ferlin, A.; Yin, P.; Nelson, C.P.; Stanescu, H.; et al. Galactosylation of IgA1 is associated with common variation in *C1GALT1*. *J. Am. Soc. Nephrol.* **2017**, *28*, 2158–2166. [CrossRef]
57. Kiryluk, K.; Li, Y.; Moldoveanu, Z.; Suzuki, H.; Reily, C.; Hou, P.; Xie, J.; Mladkova, N.; Prakash, S.; Fischman, C.; et al. GWAS for serum galactose-deficient IgA1 implicates critical genes of the *O*-glycosylation pathway. *PLoS Genet.* **2017**, *13*, e1006609. [CrossRef]
58. Wang, Y.N.; Zhou, X.J.; Chen, P.; Yu, G.Z.; Zhang, X.; Hou, P.; Liu, L.J.; Shi, S.F.; Lv, J.C.; Zhang, H. Interaction between *GALNT12* and *C1GALT1* associates with galactose-deficient IgA1 and IgA nephropathy. *J. Am. Soc. Nephrol.* **2021**, *32*, 545–552. [CrossRef] [PubMed]
59. Maillard, N.; Wyatt, R.J.; Julian, B.A.; Kiryluk, K.; Gharavi, A.; Fremeaux-Bacchi, V.; Novak, J. Current understanding of the role of complement in IgA nephropathy. *J. Am. Soc. Nephrol.* **2015**, *26*, 1503–1512. [CrossRef] [PubMed]
60. Woof, J.M.; Russell, M.W. Structure and function relationships in IgA. *Mucosal Immunol.* **2011**, *4*, 590–597. [CrossRef] [PubMed]
61. Brandtzaeg, P.; Johansen, F.E. Mucosal B cells: Phenotypic characteristics, transcriptional regulation, and homing properties. *Immunol. Rev.* **2005**, *206*, 32–63. [CrossRef]
62. Kaetzel, C.S. The polymeric immunoglobulin receptor: Bridging innate and adaptive immune responses at mucosal surfaces. *Immunol. Rev.* **2005**, *206*, 83–99. [CrossRef]
63. Rojas, R.; Apodaca, G. Immunoglobulin transport across polarized epithelial cells. *Nat. Rev. Mol. Cell Biol.* **2002**, *3*, 944–955. [CrossRef]
64. Woof, J.M.; Mestecky, J. Mucosal immunoglobulins. *Immunol. Rev.* **2005**, *206*, 64–82. [CrossRef]
65. Franc, V.; Řehulka, P.; Raus, M.; Stulík, J.; Novak, J.; Renfrow, M.B.; Šebela, M. Elucidating heterogeneity of IgA1 hinge-region *O*-glycosylation by use of MALDI-TOF/TOF mass spectrometry: Role of cysteine alkylation during sample processing. *J. Proteom.* **2013**, *92*, 299–312. [CrossRef] [PubMed]
66. Frangione, B.; Wolfenstein-Todel, C. Partial duplication in the "hinge" region of IgA 1 myeloma proteins. *Proc. Natl. Acad. Sci. USA* **1972**, *69*, 3673–3676. [CrossRef] [PubMed]
67. Ohyama, Y.; Renfrow, M.B.; Novak, J.; Takahashi, K. Aberrantly glycosylated IgA1 in IgA nephropathy: What we know and what we don't know. *J. Clin. Med.* **2021**, *10*, 3467. [CrossRef] [PubMed]
68. Renfrow, M.B.; Cooper, H.J.; Tomana, M.; Kulhavy, R.; Hiki, Y.; Toma, K.; Emmett, M.R.; Mestecky, J.; Marshall, A.G.; Novak, J. Determination of aberrant *O*-glycosylation in the IgA1 hinge region by electron capture dissociation fourier transform-ion cyclotron resonance mass spectrometry. *J. Biol. Chem.* **2005**, *280*, 19136–19145. [CrossRef]
69. Tarelli, E.; Smith, A.C.; Hendry, B.M.; Challacombe, S.J.; Pouria, S. Human serum IgA1 is substituted with up to six *O*-glycans as shown by matrix assisted laser desorption ionisation time-of-flight mass spectrometry. *Carbohydr. Res.* **2004**, *339*, 2329–2335. [CrossRef]
70. Ju, T.; Cummings, R.D. Protein glycosylation: Chaperone mutation in Tn syndrome. *Nature* **2005**, *437*, 1252. [CrossRef] [PubMed]
71. Qin, W.; Zhou, Q.; Yang, L.C.; Li, Z.; Su, B.H.; Luo, H.; Fan, J.M. Peripheral B lymphocyte beta1,3-galactosyltransferase and chaperone expression in immunoglobulin A nephropathy. *J. Intern. Med.* **2005**, *258*, 467–477. [CrossRef]
72. Field, M.C.; Dwek, R.A.; Edge, C.J.; Rademacher, T.W. O-linked oligosaccharides from human serum immunoglobulin A1. *Biochem. Soc. Trans.* **1989**, *17*, 1034–1035. [CrossRef] [PubMed]
73. Tomana, M.; Niedermeier, W.; Mestecky, J.; Skvaril, F. The differences in carbohydrate composition between the subclasses of IgA immunoglobulins. *Immunochemistry* **1976**, *13*, 325–328. [CrossRef]
74. Reily, C.; Ueda, H.; Huang, Z.Q.; Mestecky, J.; Julian, B.A.; Willey, C.D.; Novak, J. Cellular signaling and production of galactose-deficient IgA1 in IgA nephropathy, an autoimmune disease. *J. Immunol. Res.* **2014**, *2014*, 197548. [CrossRef] [PubMed]

75. Suzuki, H.; Raska, M.; Yamada, K.; Moldoveanu, Z.; Julian, B.A.; Wyatt, R.J.; Tomino, Y.; Gharavi, A.G.; Novak, J. Cytokines alter IgA1 O-glycosylation by dysregulating C1GalT1 and ST6GalNAc-II enzymes. *J. Biol. Chem.* **2014**, *289*, 5330–5339. [CrossRef]
76. Mestecky, J.; Tomana, M.; Crowley-Nowick, P.A.; Moldoveanu, Z.; Julian, B.A.; Jackson, S. Defective galactosylation and clearance of IgA1 molecules as a possible etiopathogenic factor in IgA nephropathy. *Contrib. Nephrol.* **1993**, *104*, 172–182. [CrossRef]
77. Mestecky, J.; Tomana, M.; Moldoveanu, Z.; Julian, B.A.; Suzuki, H.; Matousovic, K.; Renfrow, M.B.; Novak, L.; Wyatt, R.J.; Novak, J. Role of aberrant glycosylation of IgA1 molecules in the pathogenesis of IgA nephropathy. *Kidney Blood Press. Res.* **2008**, *31*, 29–37. [CrossRef]
78. Hastings, M.C.; Moldoveanu, Z.; Julian, B.A.; Novak, J.; Sanders, J.T.; McGlothan, K.R.; Gharavi, A.G.; Wyatt, R.J. Galactose-deficient IgA1 in African Americans with IgA nephropathy: Serum levels and heritability. *Clin. J. Am. Soc. Nephrol.* **2010**, *5*, 2069–2074. [CrossRef]
79. Suzuki, H.; Moldoveanu, Z.; Hall, S.; Brown, R.; Vu, H.L.; Novak, L.; Julian, B.A.; Tomana, M.; Wyatt, R.J.; Edberg, J.C.; et al. IgA1-secreting cell lines from patients with IgA nephropathy produce aberrantly glycosylated IgA1. *J. Clin. Investig.* **2008**, *118*, 629–639. [CrossRef]
80. Barratt, J.; Smith, A.C.; Molyneux, K.; Feehally, J. Immunopathogenesis of IgAN. *Semin. Immunopathol.* **2007**, *29*, 427–443. [CrossRef]
81. Novak, J.; Julian, B.A.; Tomana, M.; Mestecky, J. Progress in molecular and genetic studies of IgA nephropathy. *J. Clin. Immunol.* **2001**, *21*, 310–327. [CrossRef]
82. Xing, Y.; Li, Y.; Zhang, Y.; Wang, F.; He, D.; Liu, Y.; Jia, J.; Yan, T.; Lin, S. C1GALT1 expression is associated with galactosylation of IgA1 in peripheral B lymphocyte in immunoglobulin a nephropathy. *BMC Nephrol.* **2020**, *21*, 18. [CrossRef] [PubMed]
83. Yamada, K.; Huang, Z.Q.; Raska, M.; Reily, C.; Anderson, J.C.; Suzuki, H.; Ueda, H.; Moldoveanu, Z.; Kiryluk, K.; Suzuki, Y.; et al. Inhibition of STAT3 signaling reduces IgA1 autoantigen production in IgA nephropathy. *Kidney Int. Rep.* **2017**, *2*, 1194–1207. [CrossRef] [PubMed]
84. Yamada, K.; Huang, Z.Q.; Raska, M.; Reily, C.; Anderson, J.C.; Suzuki, H.; Kiryluk, K.; Gharavi, A.G.; Julian, B.A.; Willey, C.D.; et al. Leukemia inhibitory factor signaling enhances production of galactose-deficient IgA1 in IgA nephropathy. *Kidney Dis.* **2020**, *6*, 168–180. [CrossRef] [PubMed]
85. Kiryluk, K.; Moldoveanu, Z.; Sanders, J.T.; Eison, T.M.; Suzuki, H.; Julian, B.A.; Novak, J.; Gharavi, A.G.; Wyatt, R.J. Aberrant glycosylation of IgA1 is inherited in both pediatric IgA nephropathy and Henoch-Schönlein purpura nephritis. *Kidney Int.* **2011**, *80*, 79–87. [CrossRef] [PubMed]
86. Xie, Y.X.; He, L.Y.; Chen, X.; Peng, X.F.; Ye, M.Y.; Zhao, Y.J.; Yan, W.Z.; Liu, C.; Shao, J.; Peng, Y.M. Potential diagnostic biomarkers for IgA nephropathy: A comparative study pre- and post-tonsillectomy. *Int. Urol. Nephrol.* **2016**, *48*, 1855–1861. [CrossRef]
87. Hirano, K.; Matsuzaki, K.; Yasuda, T.; Nishikawa, M.; Yasuda, Y.; Koike, K.; Maruyama, S.; Yokoo, T.; Matsuo, S.; Kawamura, T.; et al. Association between tonsillectomy and outcomes in patients with immunoglobulin A nephropathy. *JAMA Netw. Open* **2019**, *2*, e194772. [CrossRef] [PubMed]
88. Enya, T.; Miyazaki, K.; Miyazawa, T.; Oshima, R.; Morimoto, Y.; Okada, M.; Takemura, T.; Sugimoto, K. Early tonsillectomy for severe immunoglobulin A nephropathy significantly reduces proteinuria. *Pediatr. Int.* **2020**, *62*, 1054–1057. [CrossRef]
89. Kawabe, M.; Yamamoto, I.; Yamakawa, T.; Katsumata, H.; Isaka, N.; Katsuma, A.; Nakada, Y.; Kobayashi, A.; Koike, K.; Ueda, H.; et al. Association between galactose-deficient IgA1 derived from the tonsils and recurrence of IgA nephropathy in patients who underwent kidney transplantation. *Front. Immunol.* **2020**, *11*, 2068. [CrossRef]
90. Aratani, S.; Matsunobu, T.; Shimizu, A.; Okubo, K.; Kashiwagi, T.; Sakai, Y. Tonsillectomy combined with steroid pulse therapy prevents the progression of chronic kidney disease in patients with immunoglobulin A (IgA) nephropathy in a single Japanese institution. *Cureus* **2021**, *13*, e15736. [CrossRef]
91. Nakata, J.; Suzuki, Y.; Suzuki, H.; Sato, D.; Kano, T.; Yanagawa, H.; Matsuzaki, K.; Horikoshi, S.; Novak, J.; Tomino, Y. Changes in nephritogenic serum galactose-deficient IgA1 in IgA nephropathy following tonsillectomy and steroid therapy. *PLoS ONE* **2014**, *9*, e89707. [CrossRef]
92. Kawamura, T.; Yoshimura, M.; Miyazaki, Y.; Okamoto, H.; Kimura, K.; Hirano, K.; Matsushima, M.; Utsunomiya, Y.; Ogura, M.; Yokoo, T.; et al. A multicenter randomized controlled trial of tonsillectomy combined with steroid pulse therapy in patients with immunoglobulin A nephropathy. *Nephrol. Dial. Transplant.* **2014**, *29*, 1546–1553. [CrossRef] [PubMed]
93. Feehally, J.; Coppo, R.; Troyanov, S.; Bellur, S.S.; Cattran, D.; Cook, T.; Roberts, I.S.; Verhave, J.C.; Camilla, R.; Vergano, L.; et al. Tonsillectomy in a European cohort of 1,147 patients with IgA nephropathy. *Nephron* **2016**, *132*, 15–24. [CrossRef]
94. Kim, M.J.; Schaub, S.; Molyneux, K.; Koller, M.T.; Stampf, S.; Barratt, J. Effect of immunosuppressive drugs on the changes of serum galactose-deficient IgA1 in patients with IgA nephropathy. *PLoS ONE* **2016**, *11*, e0166830. [CrossRef] [PubMed]
95. Kosztyu, P.; Hill, M.; Jemelkova, J.; Czernekova, L.; Kafkova, L.R.; Hruby, M.; Matousovic, K.; Vondrak, K.; Zadrazil, J.; Sterzl, I.; et al. Glucocorticoids reduce aberrant O-glycosylation of IgA1 in IgA nephropathy patients. *Kidney Blood Press. Res.* **2018**, *43*, 350–359. [CrossRef]
96. Rauen, T.; Fitzner, C.; Eitner, F.; Sommerer, C.; Zeier, M.; Otte, B.; Panzer, U.; Peters, H.; Benck, U.; Mertens, P.R.; et al. Effects of two immunosuppressive treatment protocols for IgA nephropathy. *J. Am. Soc. Nephrol.* **2018**, *29*, 317–325. [CrossRef] [PubMed]
97. Fellström, B.C.; Barratt, J.; Cook, H.; Coppo, R.; Feehally, J.; de Fijter, J.W.; Floege, J.; Hetzel, G.; Jardine, A.G.; Locatelli, F.; et al. Targeted-release budesonide versus placebo in patients with IgA nephropathy (NEFIGAN): A double-blind, randomised, placebo-controlled phase 2b trial. *Lancet* **2017**, *389*, 2117–2127. [CrossRef]

98. Coppo, R. Biomarkers and targeted new therapies for IgA nephropathy. *Pediatr. Nephrol.* **2017**, *32*, 725–731. [CrossRef]
99. Coppo, R.; Mariat, C. Systemic corticosteroids and mucosal-associated lymphoid tissue-targeted therapy in immunoglobulin A nephropathy: Insight from the NEFIGAN study. *Nephrol. Dial. Transplant.* **2020**, *35*, 1291–1294. [CrossRef] [PubMed]
100. Tomana, M.; Kulhavy, R.; Mestecky, J. Receptor-mediated binding and uptake of immunoglobulin A by human liver. *Gastroenterology* **1988**, *94*, 762–770. [CrossRef]
101. Mestecky, J.; Moldoveanu, Z.; Tomana, M.; Epps, J.M.; Thorpe, S.R.; Phillips, J.O.; Kulhavy, R. The role of the liver in catabolism of mouse and human IgA. *Immunol. Investig.* **1989**, *18*, 313–324. [CrossRef] [PubMed]
102. Baenziger, J.U.; Maynard, Y. Human hepatic lectin. Physiochemical properties and specificity. *J. Biol. Chem.* **1980**, *255*, 4607–4613. [CrossRef]
103. Tomana, M.; Phillips, J.O.; Kulhavy, R.; Mestecky, J. Carbohydrate-mediated clearance of secretory IgA from the circulation. *Mol. Immunol.* **1985**, *22*, 887–892. [CrossRef]
104. Basset, C.; Devauchelle, V.; Durand, V.; Jamin, C.; Pennec, Y.L.; Youinou, P.; Dueymes, M. Glycosylation of immunoglobulin A influences its receptor binding. *Scand. J. Immunol.* **1999**, *50*, 572–579. [CrossRef] [PubMed]
105. Park, E.I.; Mi, Y.; Unverzagt, C.; Gabius, H.J.; Baenziger, J.U. The asialoglycoprotein receptor clears glycoconjugates terminating with sialic acid alpha 2,6GalNAc. *Proc. Natl. Acad. Sci. USA* **2005**, *102*, 17125–17129. [CrossRef]
106. Steirer, L.M.; Park, E.I.; Townsend, R.R.; Baenziger, J.U. The asialoglycoprotein receptor regulates levels of plasma glycoproteins terminating with sialic acid alpha2,6-galactose. *J. Biol. Chem.* **2009**, *284*, 3777–3783. [CrossRef]
107. Roccatello, D.; Picciotto, G.; Torchio, M.; Ropolo, R.; Ferro, M.; Franceschini, R.; Quattrocchio, G.; Cacace, G.; Coppo, R.; Sena, L.M. Removal systems of immunoglobulin A and immunoglobulin A containing complexes in IgA nephropathy and cirrhosis patients. The role of asialoglycoprotein receptors. *Lab. Investig.* **1993**, *69*, 714–723. [PubMed]
108. Tomana, M.; Matousovic, K.; Julian, B.A.; Radl, J.; Konecny, K.; Mestecky, J. Galactose-deficient IgA1 in sera of IgA nephropathy patients is present in complexes with IgG. *Kidney Int.* **1997**, *52*, 509–516. [CrossRef] [PubMed]
109. Suzuki, H.; Moldoveanu, Z.; Hall, S.; Brown, R.; Julian, B.A.; Wyatt, R.J.; Tomana, M.; Tomino, Y.; Novak, J.; Mestecky, J. IgA nephropathy: Characterization of IgG antibodies specific for galactose-deficient IgA1. *Contrib. Nephrol.* **2007**, *157*, 129–133. [CrossRef]
110. Cisar, J.O.; Sandberg, A.L.; Reddy, G.P.; Abeygunawardana, C.; Bush, C.A. Structural and antigenic types of cell wall polysaccharides from viridans group streptococci with receptors for oral actinomyces and streptococcal lectins. *Infect. Immun.* **1997**, *65*, 5035–5041. [CrossRef] [PubMed]
111. Johnson, D.C.; Spear, P.G. O-linked oligosaccharides are acquired by herpes simplex virus glycoproteins in the Golgi apparatus. *Cell* **1983**, *32*, 987–997. [CrossRef]
112. Kieff, E.; Dambaugh, T.; Heller, M.; King, W.; Cheung, A.; van Santen, V.; Hummel, M.; Beisel, C.; Fennewald, S.; Hennessy, K.; et al. The biology and chemistry of Epstein-Barr virus. *J. Infect. Dis.* **1982**, *146*, 506–517. [CrossRef] [PubMed]
113. Wertz, G.W.; Krieger, M.; Ball, L.A. Structure and cell surface maturation of the attachment glycoprotein of human respiratory syncytial virus in a cell line deficient in O glycosylation. *J. Virol.* **1989**, *63*, 4767–4776. [CrossRef] [PubMed]
114. Yanagawa, H.; Suzuki, H.; Suzuki, Y.; Kiryluk, K.; Gharavi, A.G.; Matsuoka, K.; Makita, Y.; Julian, B.A.; Novak, J.; Tomino, Y. A panel of serum biomarkers differentiates IgA nephropathy from other renal diseases. *PLoS ONE* **2014**, *9*, e98081. [CrossRef]
115. Hamel, K.M.; Liarski, V.M.; Clark, M.R. Germinal center B-cells. *Autoimmunity* **2012**, *45*, 333–347. [CrossRef]
116. Huang, Z.Q.; Raska, M.; Stewart, T.J.; Reily, C.; King, R.G.; Crossman, D.K.; Crowley, M.R.; Hargett, A.; Zhang, Z.; Suzuki, H.; et al. Somatic mutations modulate autoantibodies against galactose-deficient IgA1 in IgA nephropathy. *J. Am. Soc. Nephrol.* **2016**, *27*, 3278–3284. [CrossRef]
117. Tomana, M.; Novak, J.; Julian, B.A.; Matousovic, K.; Konecny, K.; Mestecky, J. Circulating immune complexes in IgA nephropathy consist of IgA1 with galactose-deficient hinge region and antiglycan antibodies. *J. Clin. Investig.* **1999**, *104*, 73–81. [CrossRef]
118. Springer, G.F.; Tegtmeyer, H. Origin of anti-Thomsen-Friedenreich (T) and Tn agglutinins in man and in White Leghorn chicks. *Br. J. Haematol.* **1981**, *47*, 453–460. [CrossRef]
119. Mestecky, J.; Novak, J.; Moldoveanu, Z.; Raska, M. IgA nephropathy enigma. *Clin. Immunol.* **2016**, *172*, 72–77. [CrossRef]
120. Raška, M.; Zadražil, J.; Horynová, M.S.; Kafková, L.R.; Vráblíková, A.; Matoušovic, K.; Novak, J.; Městecký, J. IgA nephropathy-research-generated questions. *Vnitrni Lekarstvi* **2016**, *62* (Suppl. 6), 67–77.
121. Ito, S.; Misaki, T.; Naka, S.; Wato, K.; Nagasawa, Y.; Nomura, R.; Otsugu, M.; Matsumoto-Nakano, M.; Nakano, K.; Kumagai, H.; et al. Specific strains of Streptococcus mutans, a pathogen of dental caries, in the tonsils, are associated with IgA nephropathy. *Sci. Rep.* **2019**, *9*, 20130. [CrossRef]
122. Yamaguchi, H.; Goto, S.; Takahashi, N.; Tsuchida, M.; Watanabe, H.; Yamamoto, S.; Kaneko, Y.; Higashi, K.; Mori, H.; Nakamura, Y.; et al. Aberrant mucosal immunoreaction to tonsillar microbiota in immunoglobulin A nephropathy. *Nephrol. Dial. Transplant.* **2021**, *36*, 75–86. [CrossRef]
123. Muthana, S.M.; Gildersleeve, J.C. Factors affecting anti-glycan IgG and IgM repertoires in human serum. *Sci. Rep.* **2016**, *6*, 19509. [CrossRef] [PubMed]
124. Huflejt, M.E.; Vuskovic, M.; Vasiliu, D.; Xu, H.; Obukhova, P.; Shilova, N.; Tuzikov, A.; Galanina, O.; Arun, B.; Lu, K.; et al. Anti-carbohydrate antibodies of normal sera: Findings, surprises and challenges. *Mol. Immunol.* **2009**, *46*, 3037–3049. [CrossRef] [PubMed]

125. New, J.S.; Dizon, B.L.P.; Fucile, C.F.; Rosenberg, A.F.; Kearney, J.F.; King, R.G. Neonatal exposure to commensal-bacteria-derived antigens directs polysaccharide-specific B-1 B cell repertoire development. *Immunity* **2020**, *53*, 172–186 e176. [CrossRef] [PubMed]
126. Stuchlová Horynová, M.; Raška, M.; Clausen, H.; Novak, J. Aberrant O-glycosylation and anti-glycan antibodies in an autoimmune disease IgA nephropathy and breast adenocarcinoma. *Cell Mol. Life Sci.* **2013**, *70*, 829–839. [CrossRef]
127. Springer, G.F.; Taylor, C.R.; Howard, D.R.; Tegtmeyer, H.; Desai, P.R.; Murthy, S.M.; Felder, B.; Scanlon, E.F. Tn, a carcinoma-associated antigen, reacts with anti-Tn of normal human sera. *Cancer* **1985**, *55*, 561–569. [CrossRef]
128. Dobrochaeva, K.; Khasbiullina, N.; Shilova, N.; Antipova, N.; Obukhova, P.; Ovchinnikova, T.; Galanina, O.; Blixt, O.; Kunz, H.; Filatov, A.; et al. Specificity of human natural antibodies referred to as anti-Tn. *Mol. Immunol.* **2020**, *120*, 74–82. [CrossRef]
129. Zlocowski, N.; Grupe, V.; Garay, Y.C.; Nores, G.A.; Lardone, R.D.; Irazoqui, F.J. Purified human anti-Tn and anti-T antibodies specifically recognize carcinoma tissues. *Sci. Rep.* **2019**, *9*, 8097. [CrossRef]
130. Gendler, S.J.; Lancaster, C.A.; Taylor-Papadimitriou, J.; Duhig, T.; Peat, N.; Burchell, J.; Pemberton, L.; Lalani, E.N.; Wilson, D. Molecular cloning and expression of human tumor-associated polymorphic epithelial mucin. *J. Biol. Chem.* **1990**, *265*, 15286–15293. [CrossRef]
131. Blixt, O.; Clo, E.; Nudelman, A.S.; Sorensen, K.K.; Clausen, T.; Wandall, H.H.; Livingston, P.O.; Clausen, H.; Jensen, K.J. A high-throughput O-glycopeptide discovery platform for seromic profiling. *J. Proteome Res.* **2010**, *9*, 5250–5261. [CrossRef]
132. Karsten, U.; Serttas, N.; Paulsen, H.; Danielczyk, A.; Goletz, S. Binding patterns of DTR-specific antibodies reveal a glycosylation-conditioned tumor-specific epitope of the epithelial mucin (MUC1). *Glycobiology* **2004**, *14*, 681–692. [CrossRef] [PubMed]
133. Fiedler, W.; DeDosso, S.; Cresta, S.; Weidmann, J.; Tessari, A.; Salzberg, M.; Dietrich, B.; Baumeister, H.; Goletz, S.; Gianni, L.; et al. A phase I study of PankoMab-GEX, a humanised glyco-optimised monoclonal antibody to a novel tumour-specific MUC1 glycopeptide epitope in patients with advanced carcinomas. *Eur. J. Cancer* **2016**, *63*, 55–63. [CrossRef]
134. Wu, G.; Maharjan, S.; Kim, D.; Kim, J.N.; Park, B.K.; Koh, H.; Moon, K.; Lee, Y.; Kwon, H.J. A novel monoclonal antibody targets mucin1 and attenuates growth in pancreatic cancer model. *Int. J. Mol. Sci.* **2018**, *19*, 2004. [CrossRef]
135. Danielczyk, A.; Stahn, R.; Faulstich, D.; Loffler, A.; Marten, A.; Karsten, U.; Goletz, S. PankoMab: A potent new generation anti-tumour MUC1 antibody. *Cancer Immunol. Immunother.* **2006**, *55*, 1337–1347. [CrossRef] [PubMed]
136. Doi, M.; Yokoyama, A.; Kondo, K.; Ohnishi, H.; Ishikawa, N.; Hattori, N.; Kohno, N. Anti-tumor effect of the anti-KL-6/MUC1 monoclonal antibody through exposure of surface molecules by MUC1 capping. *Cancer Sci.* **2006**, *97*, 420–429. [CrossRef] [PubMed]
137. de Bono, J.S.; Rha, S.Y.; Stephenson, J.; Schultes, B.C.; Monroe, P.; Eckhardt, G.S.; Hammond, L.A.; Whiteside, T.L.; Nicodemus, C.F.; Cermak, J.M.; et al. Phase I trial of a murine antibody to MUC1 in patients with metastatic cancer: Evidence for the activation of humoral and cellular antitumor immunity. *Ann. Oncol.* **2004**, *15*, 1825–1833. [CrossRef]
138. Berlyn, K.A.; Schultes, B.; Leveugle, B.; Noujaim, A.A.; Alexander, R.B.; Mann, D.L. Generation of CD4(+) and CD8(+) T lymphocyte responses by dendritic cells armed with PSA/anti-PSA (antigen/antibody) complexes. *Clin. Immunol.* **2001**, *101*, 276–283. [CrossRef] [PubMed]
139. Gordon, A.N.; Schultes, B.C.; Gallion, H.; Edwards, R.; Whiteside, T.L.; Cermak, J.M.; Nicodemus, C.F. CA125- and tumor-specific T-cell responses correlate with prolonged survival in oregovomab-treated recurrent ovarian cancer patients. *Gynecol. Oncol.* **2004**, *94*, 340–351. [CrossRef]
140. Iwase, H.; Yokozeki, Y.; Hiki, Y.; Tanaka, A.; Kokubo, T.; Sano, T.; Ishii-Karakasa, I.; Hisatani, K.; Kobayashi, Y.; Hotta, K. Human serum immunoglobulin G3 subclass bound preferentially to asialo-, agalactoimmunoglobulin A1/Sepharose. *Biochem. Biophys. Res. Commun.* **1999**, *264*, 424–429. [CrossRef]
141. Kokubo, T.; Hiki, Y.; Iwase, H.; Tanaka, A.; Nishikido, J.; Hotta, K.; Kobayashi, Y. Exposed peptide core of IgA1 hinge region in IgA nephropathy. *Nephrol. Dial. Transplant.* **1999**, *14*, 81–85. [CrossRef] [PubMed]
142. Cederholm, B.; Wieslander, J.; Bygren, P.; Heinegård, D. Circulating complexes containing IgA and fibronectin in patients with primary IgA nephropathy. *Proc. Natl. Acad. Sci. USA* **1988**, *85*, 4865–4868. [CrossRef]
143. Jennette, J.C.; Wieslander, J.; Tuttle, R.; Falk, R.J. Serum IgA-fibronectin aggregates in patients with IgA nephropathy and Henoch-Schönlein purpura: Diagnostic value and pathogenic implications. The Glomerular Disease Collaborative Network. *Am. J. Kidney Dis.* **1991**, *18*, 466–471. [CrossRef]
144. Nakamura, I.; Iwase, H.; Ohba, Y.; Hiki, Y.; Katsumata, T.; Kobayashi, Y. Quantitative analysis of IgA1 binding protein prepared from human serum by hypoglycosylated IgA1/Sepharose affinity chromatography. *J. Chromatogr. B Analyt. Technol. Biomed. Life Sci.* **2002**, *776*, 101–106. [CrossRef]
145. Novak, J.; Tomana, M.; Matousovic, K.; Brown, R.; Hall, S.; Novak, L.; Julian, B.A.; Wyatt, R.J.; Mestecky, J. IgA1-containing immune complexes in IgA nephropathy differentially affect proliferation of mesangial cells. *Kidney Int.* **2005**, *67*, 504–513. [CrossRef]
146. Novak, J.; Raskova Kafkova, L.; Suzuki, H.; Tomana, M.; Matousovic, K.; Brown, R.; Hall, S.; Sanders, J.T.; Eison, T.M.; Moldoveanu, Z.; et al. IgA1 immune complexes from pediatric patients with IgA nephropathy activate cultured human mesangial cells. *Nephrol. Dial. Transplant.* **2011**, *26*, 3451–3457. [CrossRef]
147. Yanagihara, T.; Brown, R.; Hall, S.; Moldoveanu, Z.; Goepfert, A.; Tomana, M.; Julian, B.A.; Mestecky, J.; Novak, J. In vitro-generated immune complexes containing galactose-deficient IgA1 stimulate proliferation of mesangial cells. *Results Immunol.* **2012**, *2*, 166–172. [CrossRef]

148. Czerkinsky, C.; Koopman, W.J.; Jackson, S.; Collins, J.E.; Crago, S.S.; Schrohenloher, R.E.; Julian, B.A.; Galla, J.H.; Mestecky, J. Circulating immune complexes and immunoglobulin A rheumatoid factor in patients with mesangial immunoglobulin A nephropathies. *J. Clin. Investig.* **1986**, *77*, 1931–1938. [CrossRef] [PubMed]
149. Maillard, N.; Boerma, L.; Hall, S.; Huang, Z.Q.; Mrug, M.; Moldoveanu, Z.; Julian, B.A.; Renfrow, M.B.; Novak, J. Proteomic analysis of engineered IgA1-IgG immune complexes reveals association with activated complement C3. *J. Am. Soc. Nephrol.* **2013**, *24*, 490A.
150. Wyatt, R.J.; Kanayama, Y.; Julian, B.A.; Negoro, N.; Sugimoto, S.; Hudson, E.C.; Curd, J.G. Complement activation in IgA nephropathy. *Kidney Int.* **1987**, *31*, 1019–1023. [CrossRef]
151. Rizk, D.V.; Maillard, N.; Julian, B.A.; Knoppova, B.; Green, T.J.; Novak, J.; Wyatt, R.J. The emerging role of complement proteins as a target for therapy of IgA nephropathy. *Front. Immunol.* **2019**, *10*, 504. [CrossRef] [PubMed]
152. Medjeral-Thomas, N.R.; Cook, H.T.; Pickering, M.C. Complement activation in IgA nephropathy. *Semin. Immunopathol.* **2021**, *31*, 1019–1023. [CrossRef]
153. Xu, B.; Zhu, L.; Wang, Q.; Zhao, Y.; Jia, M.; Shi, S.; Liu, L.; Lv, J.; Lai, W.; Ji, J.; et al. Mass spectrometry-based screening identifies circulating immunoglobulin A-α1-microglobulin complex as potential biomarker in immunoglobulin A nephropathy. *Nephrol. Dial. Transplant.* **2021**, *36*, 782–792. [CrossRef] [PubMed]
154. Coppo, R.; Basolo, B.; Martina, G.; Rollino, C.; De Marchi, M.; Giacchino, F.; Mazzucco, G.; Messina, M.; Piccoli, G. Circulating immune complexes containing IgA, IgG and IgM in patients with primary IgA nephropathy and with Henoch-Schoenlein nephritis. Correlation with clinical and histologic signs of activity. *Clin. Nephrol.* **1982**, *18*, 230–239.
155. Schena, F.P.; Pastore, A.; Ludovico, N.; Sinico, R.A.; Benuzzi, S.; Montinaro, V. Increased serum levels of IgA1-IgG immune complexes and anti-F(ab')2 antibodies in patients with primary IgA nephropathy. *Clin. Exp. Immunol.* **1989**, *77*, 15–20.
156. Kemper, C.; Pangburn, M.K.; Fishelson, Z. Complement nomenclature 2014. *Mol. Immunol.* **2014**, *61*, 56–58. [CrossRef]
157. Floege, J.; Daha, M.R. IgA nephropathy: New insights into the role of complement. *Kidney Int.* **2018**, *94*, 16–18. [CrossRef]
158. Novak, J.; Rizk, D.; Takahashi, K.; Zhang, X.; Bian, Q.; Ueda, H.; Ueda, Y.; Reily, C.; Lai, L.Y.; Hao, C.; et al. New Insights into the Pathogenesis of IgA Nephropathy. *Kidney Dis.* **2015**, *1*, 8–18. [CrossRef]
159. Knoppova, B.; Reily, C.; Maillard, N.; Rizk, D.V.; Moldoveanu, Z.; Mestecky, J.; Raska, M.; Renfrow, M.B.; Julian, B.A.; Novak, J. The origin and activities of IgA1-containing immune complexes in IgA nephropathy. *Front. Immunol.* **2016**, *7*, 117. [CrossRef]
160. Chen, A.; Chen, W.P.; Sheu, L.F.; Lin, C.Y. Pathogenesis of IgA nephropathy: In vitro activation of human mesangial cells by IgA immune complex leads to cytokine secretion. *J. Pathol.* **1994**, *173*, 119–126. [CrossRef]
161. Coppo, R.; Amore, A.; Cirina, P.; Messina, M.; Basolo, B.; Segoloni, G.; Berthoux, F.; Boulahrouz, R.; Egido, J.; Alcazar, R. Characteristics of IgA and macromolecular IgA in sera from IgA nephropathy transplanted patients with and without IgAN recurrence. *Contrib. Nephrol.* **1995**, *111*, 85–92. [CrossRef] [PubMed]
162. Amore, A.; Cirina, P.; Conti, G.; Brusa, P.; Peruzzi, L.; Coppo, R. Glycosylation of circulating IgA in patients with IgA nephropathy modulates proliferation and apoptosis of mesangial cells. *J. Am. Soc. Nephrol.* **2001**, *12*, 1862–1871. [CrossRef]
163. Leung, J.C.; Tsang, A.W.; Chan, L.Y.; Tang, S.C.; Lam, M.F.; Lai, K.N. Size-dependent binding of IgA to HepG2, U937, and human mesangial cells. *J. Lab. Clin. Med.* **2002**, *140*, 398–406. [CrossRef] [PubMed]
164. Novak, J.; Vu, H.L.; Novak, L.; Julian, B.A.; Mestecky, J.; Tomana, M. Interactions of human mesangial cells with IgA and IgA-containing immune complexes. *Kidney Int.* **2002**, *62*, 465–475. [CrossRef] [PubMed]
165. Leung, J.C.; Tang, S.C.; Chan, L.Y.; Tsang, A.W.; Lan, H.Y.; Lai, K.N. Polymeric IgA increases the synthesis of macrophage migration inhibitory factor by human mesangial cells in IgA nephropathy. *Nephrol. Dial. Transplant.* **2003**, *18*, 36–45. [CrossRef]
166. Moura, I.C.; Arcos-Fajardo, M.; Sadaka, C.; Leroy, V.; Benhamou, M.; Novak, J.; Vrtovsnik, F.; Haddad, E.; Chintalacharuvu, K.R.; Monteiro, R.C. Glycosylation and size of IgA1 are essential for interaction with mesangial transferrin receptor in IgA nephropathy. *J. Am. Soc. Nephrol.* **2004**, *15*, 622–634. [CrossRef]
167. Leung, J.C.; Tang, S.C.; Chan, L.Y.; Chan, W.L.; Lai, K.N. Synthesis of TNF-alpha by mesangial cells cultured with polymeric anionic IgA–role of MAPK and NF-kappaB. *Nephrol. Dial. Transplant.* **2008**, *23*, 72–81. [CrossRef]
168. Lai, K.N.; Leung, J.C.; Chan, L.Y.; Saleem, M.A.; Mathieson, P.W.; Tam, K.Y.; Xiao, J.; Lai, F.M.; Tang, S.C. Podocyte injury induced by mesangial-derived cytokines in IgA nephropathy. *Nephrol. Dial. Transplant.* **2009**, *24*, 62–72. [CrossRef]
169. Tam, K.Y.; Leung, J.C.K.; Chan, L.Y.Y.; Lam, M.F.; Tang, S.C.W.; Lai, K.N. Macromolecular IgA1 taken from patients with familial IgA nephropathy or their asymptomatic relatives have higher reactivity to mesangial cells in vitro. *Kidney Int.* **2009**, *75*, 1330–1339. [CrossRef]
170. Coppo, R.; Fonsato, V.; Balegno, S.; Ricotti, E.; Loiacono, E.; Camilla, R.; Peruzzi, L.; Amore, A.; Bussolati, B.; Camussi, G. Aberrantly glycosylated IgA1 induces mesangial cells to produce platelet-activating factor that mediates nephrin loss in cultured podocytes. *Kidney Int.* **2010**, *77*, 417–427. [CrossRef]
171. Tamouza, H.; Chemouny, J.M.; Raskova Kafkova, L.; Berthelot, L.; Flamant, M.; Demion, M.; Mesnard, L.; Paubelle, E.; Walker, F.; Julian, B.A.; et al. The IgA1 immune complex-mediated activation of the MAPK/ERK kinase pathway in mesangial cells is associated with glomerular damage in IgA nephropathy. *Kidney Int.* **2012**, *82*, 1284–1296. [CrossRef]
172. Novak, J.; Moldoveanu, Z.; Julian, B.A.; Raska, M.; Wyatt, R.J.; Suzuki, Y.; Tomino, Y.; Gharavi, A.G.; Mestecky, J.; Suzuki, H. Aberrant glycosylation of IgA1 and anti-glycan antibodies in IgA nephropathy: Role of mucosal immune system. *Adv. Otorhinolaryngol.* **2011**, *72*, 60–63. [CrossRef]

173. Novak, J.; Barratt, J.; Julian, B.A.; Renfrow, M.B. Aberrant glycosylation of the IgA1 molecule in IgA nephropathy. *Semin. Nephrol.* **2018**, *38*, 461–476. [CrossRef]
174. Moura, I.C.; Arcos-Fajardo, M.; Gdoura, A.; Leroy, V.; Sadaka, C.; Mahlaoui, N.; Lepelletier, Y.; Vrtovsnik, F.; Haddad, E.; Benhamou, M.; et al. Engagement of transferrin receptor by polymeric IgA1: Evidence for a positive feedback loop involving increased receptor expression and mesangial cell proliferation in IgA nephropathy. *J. Am. Soc. Nephrol.* **2005**, *16*, 2667–2676. [CrossRef]
175. Moura, I.C.; Centelles, M.N.; Arcos-Fajardo, M.; Malheiros, D.M.; Collawn, J.F.; Cooper, M.D.; Monteiro, R.C. Identification of the transferrin receptor as a novel immunoglobulin (Ig)A1 receptor and its enhanced expression on mesangial cells in IgA nephropathy. *J. Exp. Med.* **2001**, *194*, 417–425. [CrossRef]
176. Tamouza, H.; Vende, F.; Tiwari, M.; Arcos-Fajardo, M.; Vrtovsnik, F.; Benhamou, M.; Monteiro, R.C.; Moura, I.C. Transferrin receptor engagement by polymeric IgA1 induces receptor expression and mesangial cell proliferation: Role in IgA nephropathy. *Contrib. Nephrol.* **2007**, *157*, 144–147. [CrossRef] [PubMed]
177. Kaneko, Y.; Otsuka, T.; Tsuchida, Y.; Gejyo, F.; Narita, I. Integrin α1/β1 and α2/β1 as a receptor for IgA1 in human glomerular mesangial cells in IgA nephropathy. *Int. Immunol.* **2012**, *24*, 219–232. [CrossRef]
178. Molyneux, K.; Wimbury, D.; Pawluczyk, I.; Muto, M.; Bhachu, J.; Mertens, P.R.; Feehally, J.; Barratt, J. β1,4-galactosyltransferase 1 is a novel receptor for IgA in human mesangial cells. *Kidney Int.* **2017**, *92*, 1458–1468. [CrossRef] [PubMed]
179. Launay, P.; Grossetête, B.; Arcos-Fajardo, M.; Gaudin, E.; Torres, S.P.; Beaudoin, L.; Patey-Mariaud de Serre, N.; Lehuen, A.; Monteiro, R.C. Fcalpha receptor (CD89) mediates the development of immunoglobulin A (IgA) nephropathy (Berger's disease). Evidence for pathogenic soluble receptor-IgA complexes in patients and CD89 transgenic mice. *J. Exp. Med.* **2000**, *191*, 1999–2009. [CrossRef] [PubMed]
180. Hansen, I.S.; Baeten, D.L.P.; den Dunnen, J. The inflammatory function of human IgA. *Cell Mol. Life Sci.* **2019**, *76*, 1041–1055. [CrossRef] [PubMed]
181. Heineke, M.H.; van Egmond, M. Immunoglobulin A: Magic bullet or Trojan horse? *Eur. J. Clin. Investig.* **2017**, *47*, 184–192. [CrossRef]
182. Breedveld, A.; van Egmond, M. IgA and FcαRI: Pathological roles and therapeutic opportunities. *Front. Immunol.* **2019**, *10*, 553. [CrossRef]
183. Cheung, C.K.; Rajasekaran, A.; Barratt, J.; Rizk, D.V. An update on the current state of management and clinical trials for IgA nephropathy. *J. Clin. Med.* **2021**, *10*, 2493. [CrossRef]
184. Harris, L.J.; Larson, S.B.; Hasel, K.W.; McPherson, A. Refined structure of an intact IgG2a monoclonal antibody. *Biochemistry* **1997**, *36*, 1581–1597. [CrossRef]
185. Harris, L.J.; Skaletsky, E.; McPherson, A. Crystallographic structure of an intact IgG1 monoclonal antibody. *J. Mol. Biol.* **1998**, *275*, 861–872. [CrossRef] [PubMed]
186. Saphire, E.O.; Parren, P.W.; Pantophlet, R.; Zwick, M.B.; Morris, G.M.; Rudd, P.M.; Dwek, R.A.; Stanfield, R.L.; Burton, D.R.; Wilson, I.A. Crystal structure of a neutralizing human IgG against HIV-1: A template for vaccine design. *Science* **2001**, *293*, 1155–1159. [CrossRef] [PubMed]
187. Boehm, M.K.; Woof, J.M.; Kerr, M.A.; Perkins, S.J. The Fab and Fc fragments of IgA1 exhibit a different arrangement from that in IgG: A study by X-ray and neutron solution scattering and homology modelling. *J. Mol. Biol.* **1999**, *286*, 1421–1447. [CrossRef] [PubMed]
188. Almogren, A.; Furtado, P.B.; Sun, Z.; Perkins, S.J.; Kerr, M.A. Purification, properties and extended solution structure of the complex formed between human immunoglobulin A1 and human serum albumin by scattering and ultracentrifugation. *J. Mol. Biol.* **2006**, *356*, 413–431. [CrossRef] [PubMed]
189. Bonner, A.; Furtado, P.B.; Almogren, A.; Kerr, M.A.; Perkins, S.J. Implications of the near-planar solution structure of human myeloma dimeric IgA1 for mucosal immunity and IgA nephropathy. *J. Immunol.* **2008**, *180*, 1008–1018. [CrossRef] [PubMed]
190. Bonner, A.; Almogren, A.; Furtado, P.B.; Kerr, M.A.; Perkins, S.J. Location of secretory component on the Fc edge of dimeric IgA1 reveals insight into the role of secretory IgA1 in mucosal immunity. *Mucosal Immunol.* **2009**, *2*, 74–84. [CrossRef]
191. Woods Group. GLYCAM Web. Complex. Carbohydrate Research Center, University of Georgia, Athens, Georgia, 2005–2021. Available online: http://glycam.org (accessed on 8 August 2021).
192. Krieger, E.; Joo, K.; Lee, J.; Lee, J.; Raman, S.; Thompson, J.; Tyka, M.; Baker, D.; Karplus, K. Improving physical realism, stereochemistry, and side-chain accuracy in homology modeling: Four approaches that performed well in CASP8. *Proteins* **2009**, *77* (Suppl. 9), 114–122. Available online: http://www.yasara.org (accessed on 20 August 2021). [CrossRef]
193. DeLano, W.L. *The PyMOL Molecular Graphics System*; Version 1.7.1.1; Schrödinger, LLC.: New York, NY, USA, 2002; Available online: http://www.pymol.org (accessed on 17 November 2019).
194. Wilson, I.A.; Stanfield, R.L. 50 Years of structural immunology. *J. Biol. Chem.* **2021**, *296*, 100745. [CrossRef]
195. Sarma, V.R.; Silverton, E.W.; Davies, D.R.; Terry, W.D. The three-dimensional structure at 6 A resolution of a human gamma Gl immunoglobulin molecule. *J. Biol. Chem.* **1971**, *246*, 3753–3759. [CrossRef]
196. Poljak, R.J.; Amzel, L.M.; Avey, H.P.; Becka, L.N. Structure of Fab′ New at 6 A resolution. *Nat. New Biol.* **1972**, *235*, 137–140. [CrossRef] [PubMed]
197. Amzel, L.M.; Poljak, R.J.; Saul, F.; Varga, J.M.; Richards, F.F. The three dimensional structure of a combining region-ligand complex of immunoglobulin NEW at 3.5-A resolution. *Proc. Natl. Acad. Sci. USA* **1974**, *71*, 1427–1430. [CrossRef] [PubMed]

198. Deisenhofer, J. Crystallographic refinement and atomic models of a human Fc fragment and its complex with fragment B of protein A from Staphylococcus aureus at 2.9- and 2.8-A resolution. *Biochemistry* **1981**, *20*, 2361–2370. [CrossRef] [PubMed]
199. Silverton, E.W.; Navia, M.A.; Davies, D.R. Three-dimensional structure of an intact human immunoglobulin. *Proc. Natl. Acad. Sci. USA* **1977**, *74*, 5140–5144. [CrossRef] [PubMed]
200. Berman, H.M.; Westbrook, J.; Feng, Z.; Gilliland, G.; Bhat, T.N.; Weissig, H.; Shindyalov, I.N.; Bourne, P.E. The Protein Data Bank. *Nucleic Acids Res.* **2000**, *28*, 235–242. [CrossRef]
201. Dunbar, J.; Krawczyk, K.; Leem, J.; Baker, T.; Fuchs, A.; Georges, G.; Shi, J.; Deane, C.M. SAbDab: The structural antibody database. *Nucleic Acids Res.* **2014**, *42*, D1140–D1146. [CrossRef]
202. Kuhlbrandt, W. Biochemistry. The resolution revolution. *Science* **2014**, *343*, 1443–1444. [CrossRef]
203. Callaway, E. The revolution will not be crystallized: A new method sweeps through structural biology. *Nature* **2015**, *525*, 172–174. [CrossRef] [PubMed]
204. Kumar, N.; Arthur, C.P.; Ciferri, C.; Matsumoto, M.L. Structure of the secretory immunoglobulin A core. *Science* **2020**, *367*, 1008–1014. [CrossRef] [PubMed]
205. Kumar Bharathkar, S.; Parker, B.W.; Malyutin, A.G.; Haloi, N.; Huey-Tubman, K.E.; Tajkhorshid, E.; Stadtmueller, B.M. The structures of secretory and dimeric immunoglobulin A. *eLife* **2020**, *9*, e56098. [CrossRef] [PubMed]
206. Wang, Y.; Wang, G.; Li, Y.; Zhu, Q.; Shen, H.; Gao, N.; Xiao, J. Structural insights into secretory immunoglobulin A and its interaction with a pneumococcal adhesin. *Cell Res.* **2020**, *30*, 602–609. [CrossRef]
207. Wang, Z.; Rahkola, J.; Redzic, J.S.; Chi, Y.C.; Tran, N.; Holyoak, T.; Zheng, H.; Janoff, E.; Eisenmesser, E. Mechanism and inhibition of Streptococcus pneumoniae IgA1 protease. *Nat. Commun.* **2020**, *11*, 6063. [CrossRef] [PubMed]
208. Trott, O.; Olson, A.J. AutoDock Vina: Improving the speed and accuracy of docking with a new scoring function, efficient optimization, and multithreading. *J. Comput. Chem.* **2010**, *31*, 455–461. [CrossRef]
209. Shin, W.H.; Christoffer, C.W.; Wang, J.; Kihara, D. PL-PatchSurfer2: Improved local surface matching-based virtual screening method that is tolerant to target and ligand structure variation. *J. Chem. Inf. Model.* **2016**, *56*, 1676–1691. [CrossRef]

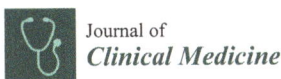

Review

The Contribution of Complement to the Pathogenesis of IgA Nephropathy: Are Complement-Targeted Therapies Moving from Rare Disorders to More Common Diseases?

Felix Poppelaars [1,*], Bernardo Faria [1,2], Wilhelm Schwaeble [3] and Mohamed R. Daha [1,4]

[1] Department of Internal Medicine, Division of Nephrology, University Medical Center Groningen, University of Groningen, 9700 AD Groningen, The Netherlands; faria_bernardo@yahoo.com (B.F.); M.R.Daha@lumc.nl (M.R.D.)
[2] Nephrology and Infectious Disease R&D Group, INEB, Institute of Investigation and Innovation in Health (i3S), University of Porto, 4200-135 Porto, Portugal
[3] Department of Veterinary Medicine, University of Cambridge, Cambridge CB3 0ES, UK; hws24@cam.ac.uk
[4] Department of Nephrology, Leiden University Medical Center, University of Leiden, 2300 RC Leiden, The Netherlands
* Correspondence: f.poppelaars@umcg.nl

Abstract: Primary IgA nephropathy (IgAN) is a leading cause of chronic kidney disease and kidney failure for which there is no disease-specific treatment. However, this could change, since novel therapeutic approaches are currently being assessed in clinical trials, including complement-targeting therapies. An improved understanding of the role of the lectin and the alternative pathway of complement in the pathophysiology of IgAN has led to the development of these treatment strategies. Recently, in a phase 2 trial, treatment with a blocking antibody against mannose-binding protein-associated serine protease 2 (MASP-2, a crucial enzyme of the lectin pathway) was suggested to have a potential benefit for IgAN. Now in a phase 3 study, this MASP-2 inhibitor for the treatment of IgAN could mark the start of a new era of complement therapeutics where common diseases can be treated with these drugs. The clinical development of complement inhibitors requires a better understanding by physicians of the biology of complement, the pathogenic role of complement in IgAN, and complement-targeted therapies. The purpose of this review is to provide an overview of the role of complement in IgAN, including the recent discovery of new mechanisms of complement activation and opportunities for complement inhibitors as the treatment of IgAN.

Keywords: complement; kidney; nephrology

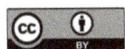

1. Introduction to the Complement System

The complement system forms a major arm of innate immunity and is comprised of a large number of circulating and membrane-bound proteins [1]. The majority of these proteins circulate in an inactive form, but in response to pathogen-associated molecular patterns (PAMPs) and/or danger-associated molecular patterns (DAMPs), become activated through sequential enzymatic reactions [2,3]. Detection of these molecular patterns by the complement system is achieved via various pattern recognition molecules, and subsequent complement activation is realized by their associated serine proteases [4]. Complement activation can arise through three major pathways, including the classical pathway, the lectin pathway, and the alternative pathway, which all lead to the cleavage of C3, thereby forming C3a and C3b [5]. In the nomenclature of the complement system, when proteins are activated and cleaved into smaller fragments, the minor fragment is assigned the letter "a", while the major fragment is assigned the letter "b". The classical pathway recognizes immune complexes of IgM or hexameric IgG via C1q (the pattern recognition molecule of this pathway) together with the associated serine proteases C1r and C1s [6,7]. The lectin pathway contains six pattern recognition molecules: mannose-binding lectin (MBL), ficolin-1 (previously M-ficolin), ficolin-2 (previously L-ficolin), ficolin-3 (previously H-ficolin), collectin-10 (previously collectin liver 1), and collectin-11 (previously collectin kidney 1). These form a complex with MBL-associated serine proteases (MASPs) and recognize carbohydrate and acetylated structures on pathogens [8,9]. The alternative pathway continuously maintains low-level activity by the spontaneous hydrolysis of C3, called the 'tick-over', and thereby generates C3b, which can then covalently bind to various proteins, lipids, and carbohydrate structures on microbial surfaces [10]. Properdin has also been postulated to act as a pattern recognition molecule, thereby initiating alternative pathway activation [11,12], although these findings have not been consistent among studies and experimental conditions [13]. Besides PAMPs, complement activation is also brought about by DAMPs, e.g., activation of the classical pathway by C-reactive protein (CRP) or pentraxin-3 [14,15]. Other examples are the activation of the lectin pathway by L-fucose on stressed cells and cleavage of C3 by the neutrophil enzymes elastase or myeloperoxidase (MPO), resulting in alternative pathway activation [12,16,17].

Regardless of the pathway, progressive C3 activation results in the formation of the C5-convertases. Correspondingly, the C5-convertases cleave C5 into C5a, an extremely potent inflammatory mediator, and C5b. C5b is the initiator of the terminal step, and, together with the components C6 through C9, assembles the membrane attack complex (MAC), also called C5b-9 [18]. Traditionally, the MAC was found to be formed on Gram-negative bacteria such as Neisseria meningitidis, leading to cell lysis. However, the MAC can also assemble on the surface of other pathogens, erythrocytes, or damaged host cells. Moreover, on host cells, the amount of C9 in the MAC determines the pore size and thereby the function, which ranges from pro-inflammatory effects to cell death [19]. Complement activation also leads to the generation of other effector molecules, such as opsonins (C4b, C4d, C3b, iC3b, and C3dg) and anaphylatoxins (C3a, C5a), which can interact with their respective complement receptors (complement receptors (CR), C3a receptors (C3aR) as well as C5a receptors (C5aR)). To better understand the complement system, it is important to realize that activation can take place in the blood, called the fluid phase, as well as on surfaces, called the solid phase. However, under normal conditions, this system is tightly controlled by regulators present in the blood (fluid-phase regulators) and on cell surfaces (solid-phase regulators) [20]. Examples of solid-phase regulators include membrane cofactor protein (CD46), decay acceleration factor (CD55), the C3b receptor CR1 (CD35), and membrane attack complex-inhibitory protein (CD59), which are widely expressed on human cells. On the other hand, C1-inhibitor, C4b-binding protein (C4bp), Factor H, and Factor I are major fluid-phase regulators present in the blood.

2. Novel Insights into an Old Defense System

Today, our appreciation of the complement system has advanced immensely. As a result, it is easy to assume that its role has been completely unraveled. However, recent reports have identified novel players and unexpected functions of the complement system and have demonstrated that there is more to it than we now know. Important recent discoveries include: (i) the cross-talk between the lectin and alternative pathways, in particular by MASP-3; and (ii) the capacity of Factor H-related proteins (FHRs) to antagonize the ability of Factor H to regulate complement activation (Figure 1). These discoveries are important for a better understanding of the involvement of the complement system in IgAN.

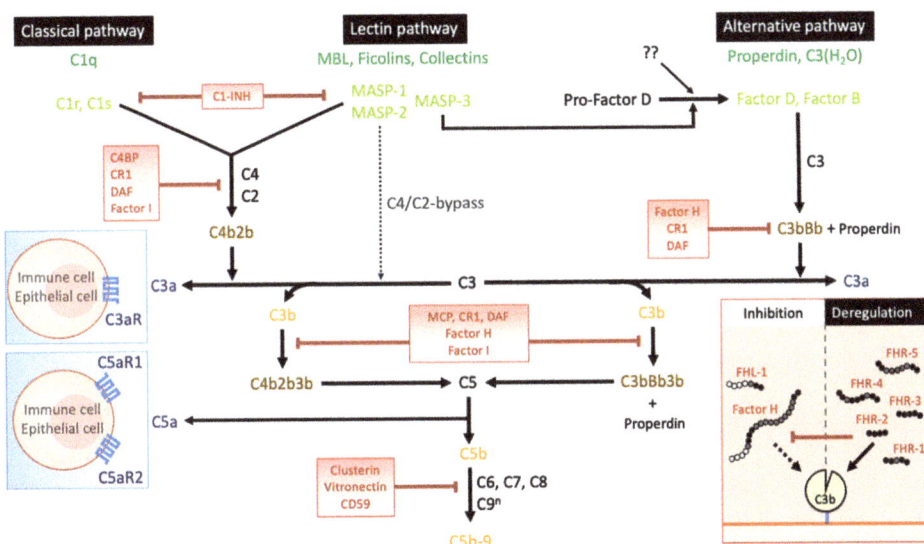

Figure 1. Overview of the complement system. Complement activation can be initiated via three different pathways: the classical pathway, the lectin pathway, and the alternative pathway. The classical pathway begins with the activation of C1, a complex composed of one C1q molecule (the pattern recognition molecule—dark green) as well as two C1r molecules and two C1s molecules (the serine proteases—light green). The lectin pathway begins via any of its pattern recognition molecules (dark green); that is, mannose-binding lectin (MBL), ficolins, or certain collectins, which work together with MBL-associated serine protease 1 (MASP-1) and 2 (MASP-2). Activation of either the classical or the lectin pathway leads to the cleavage of C4 and C2 and the formation of the C4bC2a complex, also known as the C3-convertase (gold). In the alternative pathway, activation occurs via the spontaneously thioester-hydrolyzed form of C3 ($C3(H_2O)$) or via surface interactions of properdin (the pattern recognition molecules—dark green), which acts with Factor B and Factor D (the serine proteases—light green) to form the C3-convertase C3bBb (gold). Overall, all three pathways lead to the formation of their respective C3-convertases (gold), which in turn cleave C3 into C3a (an anaphylatoxin—blue) and the opsonin C3b (yellow). MASP-2 has also been shown to directly cleave native C3, thereby bypassing C2 and C4 in the activation of the lectin pathway; this is also known as the C4/C2 bypass mechanism (grey). Recently, MASP-3 was revealed to cleave pro-Factor D into Factor D, establishing a novel link between the lectin and alternative pathway. Although MASP-3 is responsible for the main activation of pro-Factor D, there is also an unknown alternative pro-Factor D activator. Increasing densities of C3b through activation of C3 by the C3-convertases favors the formation of the C5-convertases (gold). In the classical and lectin pathways, C5-convertase is formed by a complex of C3b with C4b and C2a known as C4b2b3b. In the alternative pathway, an additional C3b binds to the C3 convertase (C3bBb) to form the C5-convertase C3bBb3b. Properdin is a key positive regulator of complement activity which acts by stabilizing alternative pathway C3- and C5-convertases. The C5-convertases (C4b2b3b and/or C3bBb3b, respectively) cleave C5 to generate the potent chemoattractant C5a (an anaphylatoxin—blue) and C5b (yellow), the initial component of the membrane attack complex. Next, C6, C7, C8, and C9 bind serially to surface-bound C5b to form the final complex, C5b-9 (yellow). Further interactions with additional C9 molecules, up to 17 molecules, widens the inner pore of the membrane attack complex. In addition, the anaphylatoxins C3a and C5a bind to their respective receptor (blue), C3a-receptor (C3aR), C5a receptor 1 (C5aR1), and C5a receptor 2 (C5aR2) on target cells to mediate a variety of inflammatory responses. In parallel to these activation pathways, complement regulation is established through membrane-bound and soluble complement inhibitors. In the classical and lectin pathway, C1-inhibitor (C1-INH) regulates the activity of the pattern recognition molecules and associated serine proteases, whereas C4b-binding protein (C4BP) inhibits activation at the C4 level. Factor I and Factor H act on C3- and C5-convertases. In addition, the membrane-bound inhibitors complement receptor 1 (CR1/CD35) and membrane cofactor protein (MCP/CD46) act as co-factors for Factor I, whereas decay-accelerating factor (DAF/CD55) accelerates the decay of C3-convertases. The membrane-bound regulator CD59, as well as soluble regulators clusterin and vitronectin, impair the formation of C5b-9. The Factor H protein family consists of Factor H, Factor H-like protein 1 (FHL-1), and five Factor H-related proteins (FHR). Factor H consists of 20 domains. The first four domains (white) provide the inhibitory function of the protein, while the

internal region (black) and the last two units (black) are needed for binding to cells and tissue sites. FHL-1 is composed of the first 7 domains of Factor H, whereas the FHRs have structural homology to binding domains (black) of Factor H. The current belief is therefore that FHRs compete with Factor H (and FHL-1) for binding to certain surfaces. The binding of Factor H (and FHL-1) will lead to complement inhibition, whereas binding of the FHRs will further enhance complement activation.

Although the complement system is presented as three separate and clearly outlined pathways, multiple reports have demonstrated that the pathways are closely connected and intertwined. Earlier studies demonstrated that initial complement activation by the classical pathway, as well as the lectin pathway, is amplified by the alternative pathway, and this amplification loop is estimated to contribute up to ~80% of the achieved complement activation [21,22]. Recently, the contrary has also been demonstrated, as the lectin pathway was shown to be indispensable for efficient alternative pathway activation [23]. In the lectin pathway, binding of MBL, ficolins, or collectins to their ligands leads to autoactivation of MASP-1, which thereafter activates MASP-2 [8]. Subsequently, MASP-2 cleaves C4, whereas C2 is cleaved by both MASPs, resulting in the formation of C3-convertases (i.e., C4bC2a) [24]. These convertases can then cleave C3 into C3a and C3b. Recently, another serine protease was discovered, namely MASP-3. This third serine protease is an alternative splicing product of the MASP-1 gene, and its functional significance remained an enigma until recently. In an elegant series of experiments, Dobo et al. revealed that activated MASP-3 cleaves pro-Factor D into Factor D, thereby establishing a crucial link between the lectin and the alternative pathway [25]. Using a specific MASP-3 inhibitor, they were able to block the conversion of pro-Factor D into Factor D. Additionally, Factor D isoforms were analyzed in MASP-1/3-deficient Malpuech–Michels–Mingarelli–Carnevale patients and MASP-1/3$^{-/-}$ mice [26]. These experiments demonstrated that MASP-3 is responsible for the main activation of pro-Factor D, while also stressing that an alternative pro-Factor D activator exists [23]. In a follow-up study by the same authors, MASP-3 was shown to be mostly present as an active enzyme in blood under normal circumstances [27]. Proprotein convertase subtilisin/kexin 6 (PCSK6) was later identified as the main activator of MASP-3, thus completing the elucidation of this novel axis which is involved in the activation of the alternative pathway [28].

Dysregulation of the complement system is a causal factor in the development of various inflammatory and autoimmune diseases [29]. The complement regulatory protein Factor H is a key player in maintaining balance [30]. The discovery that Factor H consists of 20 units, known as "short consensus repeats" (SCR), has helped to attribute the different functions of Factor H to specific domains within the protein [31]. The first 4 units (SCRs 1–4) provide the inhibitory function of the protein, while the internal region (SCRs 6–8) and the last 2 units (SCRs 19, 20) are needed for binding to cells and tissue sites [32–34]. Genetic and acquired factors can cause distinct molecular defects in Factor H and can thereby give rise to different diseases [35]. For example, mutations that cause a complete Factor H deficiency lead to uncontrolled complement activation in the fluid phase and are linked to C3 glomerulopathy (C3G), a heterogeneous histopathological entity characterized by glomerular C3 deposition [36]. Heterozygous mutations in Factor H only lead to partial deficiencies, and these are associated with C3G but also with other diseases such as age-related macular degeneration (AMD), atypical hemolytic uremic syndrome (aHUS), and IgAN [37]. Alternatively, mutations or autoantibodies that affect the binding sites of Factor H give rise to aHUS because they impair the ability of Factor H to control complement activation on surfaces without modifying complement regulation in the fluid phase [38–41]. In addition to Factor H, humans also have five FHRs: FHR-1, FHR-2, FHR-3, FHR-4 and FHR-5 [42]. The genes for the FHRs are believed to have arisen during evolution through duplication events of the Factor H gene [43]. Subsequently, the FHRs have structural homology to Factor H, but they all lack the first four units of Factor H (i.e., the inhibitory region). Thus, based on their structure, FHRs were originally predicted to be irrelevant for maintaining immune homeostasis. However, recent work has opposed this notion. Genetic studies have revealed that variants of FHRs are strongly associated with human pathology, mostly those involving the kidney and retina [44]. These findings indicate that the FHRs could be involved in their pathophysiology. Nevertheless, the distinct molecular mechanisms by which FHRs contribute to disease are poorly understood. All FHRs are predicted to bind similar ligands as Factor H but lack its regulatory activity. The current belief, therefore, is that the FHRs antagonize the ability of Factor H to regulate complement activation [30,42]. Thus, FHRs act as de-regulators of the complement system by competing with Factor H for binding to surfaces that require protection. Notably, clear differences exist among the different FHRs [37]. For instance, FHR-1, FHR-2, and FHR-5 can dimerize to form homodimers. Conversely, FHR-3 and FHR-4 lack this dimerization motif in their N-terminal domains. Initial work proposed that, in addition to homodimers, heterodimers could also be formed between FHR-1 and FHR-2 as well as FHR-1 and FHR-5, whereas FHR-2/FHR-5 heterodimers would only occur if FHR-1 was absent [45]. However, recently, another study proposed that only four dimers are present in the blood: FHR-1, FHR-2, and FHR-5 homodimers, as well as heterodimers of FHR-1/FHR-2 [46]. Additional studies are thus needed to verify the compositions of these dimers in the circulation, together with the exact function of these dimers. Currently, these dimers are believed to have increased avidity for tissue-bound complement fragments, enabling them to more efficiently compete with Factor H [45].

3. The Unique Susceptibility of the Kidney to Complement-Mediated Injury

The complement system is more than a defense system against pathogens, as it also acts as a surveillance system to preserve tissue homeostasis and stimulate repair [4]. As a consequence, complement can be the initiator or aggravating factor in renal diseases. The complement system contributes to kidney disease via different mechanisms: excessive or inappropriate activation, insufficient regulation, or ineffective clearance [29]. Overwhelming activation can be triggered when the complement system is exposed to vast amounts of PAMPs or DAMPs, as seen in sepsis and brain death [47,48]. Separately, immune recognition of apparently innocent materials or biological surfaces can create inappropriate complement activation, as seen in hemodialysis and transplantation [49–53]. Independently, loss of complement regulation due to genetic alterations can lead to an imbalance that can cause tissue damage, as seen in C3G and aHUS [31,54]. Finally, ineffective removal of immune complexes and cellular debris due to deficiencies in complement components can induce autoimmune diseases such as lupus nephritis [31,55]. A combination of these mechanisms is also possible (e.g., initial insufficient regulation that leads to excessive activation), reflecting the complexity of complement-mediated renal diseases.

The kidney is particularly susceptible to complement-mediated injury, possibly due to the high blood flow, ultrafiltration, relatively low expression of complement receptors, and local variations in electrolyte concentrations and pH [56]. In addition, the local synthesis of complement proteins in the kidney seems to be of major significance [57,58]. The main source for complement factors is the liver, with the exception of C1q, properdin, and C7, predominantly produced by leukocytes, and Factor D synthesized by adipocytes [59–64]. However, accumulating evidence indicates that a wide range of cell types in the kidney are also able to produce complement components [58]. Renal tubular epithelial cells can produce virtually all complement proteins and are the main renal source of complement [65,66]. Under basal conditions, the kidney produces up to 5% of the circulating C3, but this can increase up to 16% during inflammation [67]. In renal diseases, complement activation can therefore occur in different compartments, namely systemically (i.e., in blood) or locally (i.e., in the kidney). Local production of complement proteins seems to be predominantly important at serum-restricted sites, such as the renal interstitium [68]. Local complement activation will lead to increased local vascular permeability, subsequently resulting in the leakage of systemic complement proteins and the initiation of the immune response [8]. Recently, a possible new compartment has been suggested, namely intracellular complement activation [69,70]. However, the occurrence of intracellular complement activation in renal disease and its relevance remains to be investigated.

4. The Complement System in IgA Nephropathy

IgAN is the most common form of glomerulonephritis and an important cause of kidney failure [71]. The diagnosis is confirmed by a kidney biopsy, revealing predominant deposition of IgA1 in the renal mesangium. IgAN is believed to have a multi-hit pathogenesis, namely: genetically determined high circulating levels of galactose-deficient IgA1, subsequent synthesis of antibodies directed against these galactose-deficient IgA, binding of these autoantibodies to IgA1 to form immune complexes, and finally, deposition of the immune complexes in the renal mesangium, leading to immune activation and renal damage [72]. The presence of complement activation in patients with IgAN was reported almost five decades ago [73]. However, the relevance of the complement system to the pathophysiology was not immediately recognized. Recent advances have increased our knowledge of the role of the complement system in the pathophysiology of IgAN (Figure 2). Additionally, these developments have enabled the development of novel therapeutic strategies for IgAN that are currently being tested in clinical trials.

4.1. Local Complement Activation

Very early on, in the initial reports about the disease, complement deposition was already described in renal biopsies of IgAN patients [73]. These first descriptions of the disease reported mesangial deposition of IgA and C3 in renal biopsies in more than 90% of cases. However, the importance of local complement deposition in IgAN was not recognized until later reports revealed that the extent of C3 deposits in the mesangium correlated with the severity and progression of IgAN [49,74–77]. In these recent studies, glomerular C3 deposition was observed in 71 to 100% of IgAN patients [78–81]. Next to glomerular IgA and C3 deposits, properdin and C5b-9 are almost always present, while C1q is typically absent [49,73,82–84]. Local complement activation in IgAN was therefore thought to result from the alternative pathway. In accordance, early studies demonstrated the ability of IgA to activate the alternative pathway in vitro [85,86]. The mechanism behind IgA-induced alternative pathway activation is poorly understood, but the polymerization of IgA is critical. Other proteins of the alternative pathway have also been identified in kidney biopsies of patients with IgAN, including Factor B, Factor H, and the FHRs [87–93]. Multiple studies have also investigated the utility of urinary Factor H levels for the assessment of disease activity and prognosis in patients with IgAN [89,93–95]. Surprisingly, urinary levels of Factor H were positively associated with markers of IgAN severity and disease progression. It is noteworthy to mention that because of the structural homology between Factor H and FHRs, it is very well possible that these Factor H assays also detected the FHRs and thereby confound the results [37]. Proteomic analysis of microdissected glomeruli in IgAN biopsies have verified the presence of Factor H, FHR-1, FHR-2, FHR-3, and FHR-5 [96]. Moreover, FHR-2 and FHR-5 were significantly more abundant in the glomeruli of patients with progressive IgAN compared to non-progressive IgAN. The presence of FHRs in IgAN was first mentioned 20 years ago by Murphy et al., who described glomerular FHR-5 deposits in a range of renal biopsy specimens including IgAN [97]. Mesangial deposition of FHR-5 was detected in all 20 IgAN cases, and the pattern of FHR-5 deposition was comparable, but not always identical, to that of IgA, C3, and sC5b-9. Recently, increased glomerular staining for FHR-5 was shown to be associated with progressive disease, while a trend was seen for greater FHR1 staining [88]. In contrast, glomerular Factor H staining was significantly reduced in patients with progressive IgAN in comparison to stable disease. Glomerular FHR5 deposition positively correlated with glomerular staining of C3 activation fragments, C5b-9, and absent Factor H staining.

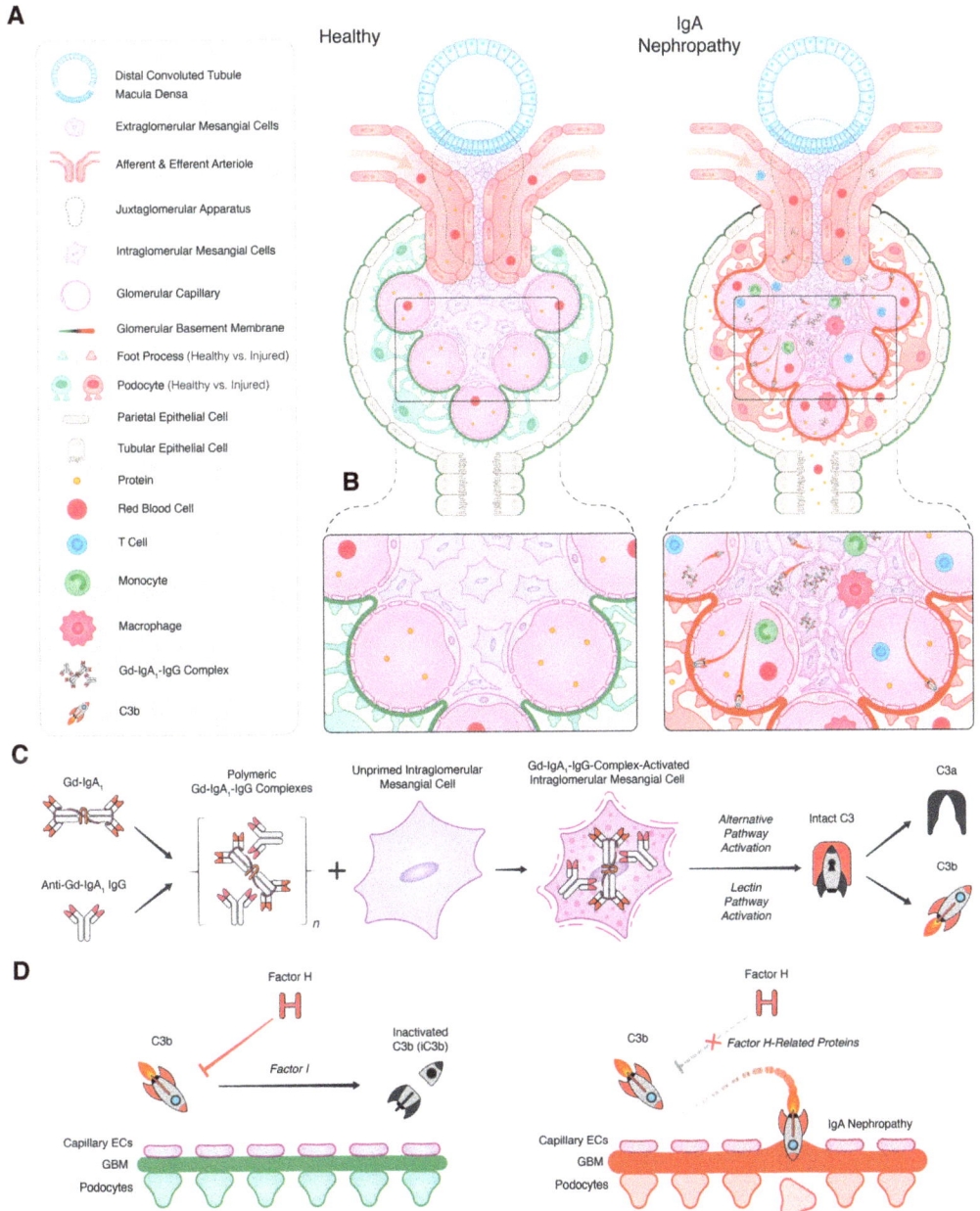

Figure 2. The role of complement activation in IgA nephropathy. (**A**) In a healthy glomerulus, filtration of blood occurs, and intact podocytes prevent the loss of proteins. In IgA nephropathy (IgAN), deposition occurs of immune complexes containing polymeric galactose-deficient IgA1 in the glomerular mesangium. (**B**) This leads to immune activation and induces proliferation of mesangial cells, increases the synthesis of extracellular matrix, and causes glomerular basement membrane (GBM) thickening, podocyte injury and protein loss. (**C**) Polymeric IgA1 and IgA1-containing immune complexes can activate both the alternative and lectin pathway, leading to the cleavage of intact C3, thereby forming C3a and C3b. (**D**) Factor H is a key regulator of the complement system, and together with Factor I, Factor H cleaves C3b to iC3b. Lastly, the Factor H-related proteins can compete with the regulatory functions of Factor H, thereby promoting complement activation.

These results are in line with the hypothesis that FHRs compete with Factor H, thereby amplifying complement activation. No association was seen between glomerular staining for FHR-1 and IgAN severity. Similarly, a Chinese cohort found mesangial staining of FHR-5 in 57.1% of IgAN cases, and FHR-5 deposition was associated with histologic injury [98]. FHR-5 co-localized and correlated with IgA as well as C3 deposits. IgAN patients with endocapillary hypercellularity and segmental glomerulosclerosis had greater glomerular FHR-5 staining. Interestingly, the authors reported sex differences in glomerular FHR-5 depositions, with greater staining in male IgAN patients. These data indicate that FHR-5 might be a key contributor to complement dysregulation in IgAN (Table 1). It is important to mention that FHR-5 detection by immunohistochemistry in the study by Medjeral-Thomas et al. and by Guo et al. was achieved by using rabbit polyclonal antibodies against FHR-5 [88,98], creating the possibility of cross-reactivity with other FHRs [37].

Table 1. The role of the Factor H protein family in IgA nephropathy.

	Evidence for the Involvement of the Factor H Protein Family in the Pathogenesis of IgA Nephropathy		
	Genetic	Histologic	Serologic
Factor H	Genetic variants of Factor H associated with lower plasma levels may contribute to genetic susceptibility to IgAN [99].	Glomerular deposition of Factor H staining is reduced in patients with progressive IgAN compared to stable disease. Absence of glomerular Factor H deposition is associated with progressive disease [88].	Plasma Factor H levels are not altered in IgAN patients, and these levels are not associated with disease severity, but the plasma FHR-1/Factor H ratio is associated with disease progression [99,100].
Factor H-related protein 1 (FHR-1)	The deletion of complement factor H-related proteins 3 and 1 genes (CFHR3,1Δ) is associated with protection against IgAN [101–104].	Proteomics showed that FHR-1 is more abundant in the glomeruli of IgAN patients compared to controls. Glomerular FHR-1 deposits have also been identified in IgAN, but no association is seen with IgAN severity [88,96].	Plasma FHR-1 levels are elevated in IgAN patients compared to healthy controls, and the plasma FHR-1/Factor H ratio is associated with disease progression of the disease [99,100].
Factor H-related protein 2 (FHR-2)	N.D.	Proteomic analysis revealed that FHR-2 is more abundant in the glomeruli of patients with progressive IgAN compared to non-progressive IgAN [96].	N.D.
Factor H-related protein 3 (FHR-3)	The deletion of complement factor H-related proteins 3 and 1 genes (CFHR3,1Δ) is associated with protection against IgAN [101–104].	Proteomic analysis demonstrated that FHR-3 is more abundant in the glomeruli of IgAN patients compared to controls [96].	N.D.
Factor H-related protein 4 (FHR-4)	N.D.	N.D.	N.D.
Factor H-related protein 5 (FHR-5)	Rare genetic variants in FHR-5 may contribute to the genetic susceptibility to IgAN [105].	Glomerular FHR-5 deposits have been identified in IgAN and correlate with C3 and C5b-9 deposits. Increased glomerular staining for FHR-5 is associated with more severe histology and progressive disease [88,96–98].	Serum FHR-5 levels are higher in IgAN patients compared to healthy controls and are associated with more severe histology, unresponsiveness to immunosuppression, and disease progression [100,106].

An overview of all the available evidence of the involvement of the Factor H protein family in IgA nephropathy. Abbreviations: N.D, not determined; IgAN, IgA Nephropathy; FHR-1, Factor H-related protein 1; FHR-2, Factor H-related protein 2; FHR-3, Factor H-related protein 3; FHR-4, Factor H-related protein 4; FHR-5, Factor H-related protein 5.

Although previous studies had shown that the role of the classical pathway is limited in IgAN, little attention had initially been paid to the lectin pathway until the group of Fujita et al. demonstrated glomerular deposition of MBL and MASP-1 in IgAN which co-localized with C3b and C5b-9 deposits [107]. A follow-up study showed mesangial deposits of MBL, MASP-1, and C4 in over half of the IgAN cases, and also showed that IgA2 co-localized with MBL and MASP-1 in the mesangium of these patients [108]. Later, additional components of the lectin pathway, such as ficolin-2 deposition, were also demonstrated in IgAN [78,109]. In agreement with these results, IgA was shown to induce activation of the lectin pathway in vitro [16]. Interestingly, lectin pathway presence in renal biopsies is only seen in a subset of IgAN patients [78,107,108]. In the landmark paper by Roos et al., glomerular deposition of Ficolin-2 and MBL was shown to be associated with a higher level of histological damage, demonstrated by increased mesangial and extracapillary proliferation, interstitial infiltration, and glomerular sclerosis, as well as with heavier proteinuria [78]. Urine levels of MBL and C4d have also been shown to be associated with markers of disease activity and severity in IgAN, and urinary levels of these complement proteins correlate with their respective mesangial deposits [110,111]. These findings were further supported by the association of mesangial C4d deposition with disease progression and lower renal survival in IgAN patients [80,81,109,112]. Espinosa et al. was the first to demonstrate that mesangial C4d staining and absent C1q (indicative of lectin pathway activation) in IgAN patients was associated with progression to kidney failure [112]. In a follow-up study, they assessed the prognostic value of glomerular C4d staining in IgAN in a larger cohort [80]. Mesangial C4d deposits were identified in 39% of the 283 patients and C4d-positive staining was an independent risk factor for the development of kidney failure in IgAN. These results had important practical implications, because C4d staining is already routinely used in clinical practice for the diagnosis of antibody-mediated humoral rejection in biopsies from kidney transplant patients [113]. Various studies have subsequently investigated the use of C4d staining in IgAN as an indicator of disease severity and as a risk factor for kidney outcomes in different geographical populations, stages of chronic kidney disease, and degree of proteinuria [77,81,109,114]. Recently, a meta-analysis was performed on IgAN studies evaluating the relationship between glomerular C4d deposits and kidney outcomes, and the authors found that glomerular C4d deposition in IgAN was associated with higher histological disease activity, faster decline in eGFR, and kidney failure [115]. However, C4d deposition in IgAN is not limited to the glomeruli and has also been documented in the vasculature of the kidney. Arteriolar C4d deposits in IgAN are also associated with faster disease progression, and the association with progressive kidney disease was found to be stronger than glomerular C4d deposits [79]. In accordance, in IgAN, C3 deposition is also routinely found in extraglomerular areas such as in Bowman's capsule and in the arterioles, and these C3 deposits also seem to be associated with worse outcome [116].

Glomerular C5b-9 deposition in IgAN was first reported over 3 decades ago by Rauterberg and colleagues [84]. Terminal pathway activation, as shown by C5b-9, was present in all IgAN cases, but not in controls. Furthermore, mesangial deposits of C5b-9 co-localized with both IgA and C3d deposition. Correspondingly, Medjeral-Thomas et al. reported that mesangial C5b-9 staining significantly correlated with both mesangial C3b/iC3b/C3c and C3d staining [117]. C5b-9 deposition in the glomeruli has been suggested to contribute to podocyte injury and subsequent proteinuria in IgAN [118]. Furthermore, decreased expression of CR1 (also known as CD35) on podocytes correlated with glomerular C5b-9 deposition in IgAN. These findings insinuate that reduced CR1 expression perhaps increases the sensitivity of podocytes to complement attack in IgAN [118]. However, decreased CR1 expression on podocytes is a shared histopathological feature among glomerular diseases and is not specific to IgAN [119]. In addition to the mesangium, C5b-9 can also be found along the capillary wall in the glomerulus, Bowman's capsule, the tubular basement membrane, and the vascular wall [120]. In recent studies, the presence of C5b-9 in IgAN biopsies has been confirmed by proteomics analysis of microdissected glomeruli [96]. Terminal pathway components were significantly more abundant in IgAN biopsies than in healthy controls, as well as in IgAN cases with progressive disease compared to IgAN with non-progressive disease. Furthermore, terminal pathway components were associated with a higher histological score and lower kidney function. In accordance, multiple studies have found a relationship between C5b-9 staining in IgAN and histological lesions as well as clinical outcomes [120]. Overall, glomerular C5b-9 deposition in IgAN correlates with the extent of glomerulosclerosis, mesangial expansion, hypercellularity, interstitial inflammation, and fibrosis as well as tubular atrophy, whereas tubular C5b-9 staining is associated with the extent of tubular atrophy, interstitial inflammation, and interstitial fibrosis [121–129]. Regarding clinical outcome, glomerular and tubular staining of C5b-9 has been associated with kidney function, proteinuria, and progressive IgAN [84,117,124,125,127,130,131]. Correspondingly, increased C5aR1 expression has also been reported in renal biopsies of IgAN cases, and C5aR1 staining also correlates with histological injury, proteinuria, and kidney function [132]. C5aR1 staining in IgAN was mainly found on glomerular mesangial cells, tubular epithelial cells, and interstitial infiltrating cells. Similarly, urine levels of C5a and soluble C5b-9 (sC5b-9) have been found to be associated with markers of disease activity in IgAN, thereby further supporting the significance of the terminal pathway [93,132].

4.2. Systemic Complement Activation

In addition to local complement activation in IgAN, systemic complement activation has also been evaluated. Although plasma C3 levels are usually normal, activation fragments of C3 are elevated in some patients and correlate with the levels of IgA-containing immune complexes, histology, and disease progression [133–136]. However, most of these studies were performed in the 1980s and 1990s. Proteomics analysis of circulating deglycosylated IgA-immune complexes confirmed the presence of C3 activation fragments, such as iC3b, C3c, and C3dg [137]. More recently, systemic C3 levels were investigated in 343 IgAN patients [76]. Only 19% had serum C3 levels below the normal range. However, IgAN patients with decreased C3 levels had higher extents of mesangial C3 deposits in their renal biopsy than those with normal C3 levels. Furthermore, serum C3 levels were significantly associated with progression to kidney failure, but the predictive value of serum C3 was lower than clinical markers such as proteinuria and eGFR. In contrast, a separate study of 496 patients with IgAN, of whom 22% had low levels of C3, reported that serum C3 levels did not associate with disease progression [138]. Others have suggested that for IgAN, serum IgA1/C3 ratio may be a better marker for disease activity and progression than serum C3 levels alone [139,140]. Subsequently, Chen et al. investigated the relationship between the serum galactose-deficient IgA1/C3 ratio and disease progression in 1210 IgAN patients [141]. The galactose-deficient IgA1/C3 ratio had a much stronger association with disease progression than either marker alone, and the risk of kidney failure increased continuously with the ratio. These findings do not only show the potential of galactose-deficient IgA1/C3 ratios for risk assessment in IgAN, but also suggest that the complement-activating ability of the galactose-deficient IgA1 immune complexes determines disease severity. Terminal pathway activation leading to the generation of C5a and sC5b-9 has also been evaluated in IgAN, although much less extensively. A single study performed by Zwirner et al. found no differences in plasma sC5b-9 levels between patients with IgAN, Henoch–Schonlein purpura, and non-immune kidney disease [135]. In addition, none of the sC5b-9 values in IgAN patients exceeded the normal range, as defined by levels in the non-immune renal disease group. In a larger Taiwanese cohort, plasma levels of C5a were found to be higher in IgAN patients [87]. However, these patients were compared to healthy controls and patients with primary focal segmental sclerosis. Interestingly, IgAN patients who received immunosuppression had lower levels of C5a as early as 1 month after treatment.

Serologic evidence of alternative pathway activation (and/or the amplification loop) has also been documented in IgAN. Overall, IgAN patients seem to have higher systemic levels of alternative pathway components, as well as complement regulators [117,142]. Plasma levels of Ba, the smaller activation fragment of Factor B, were shown to be increased in IgAN patients compared to healthy controls and patients with primary focal segmental sclerosis [87]. Additionally, plasma Ba levels positively correlated with plasma levels of

C5a levels, as well as weakly (yet statistically significantly) with the degree of proteinuria and impaired renal function. Recent work has investigated circulating levels of the FHRs in IgAN. Plasma levels of FHR-1 were shown to be elevated in Spanish IgAN patients compared to controls, whereas Factor H levels were normal [99]. In accordance, FHR-1/Factor H ratios were also elevated in IgAN, and the highest FHR-1 levels and FHR-1/Factor H ratios were found in patients with IgAN with disease progression. A separate study confirmed these results and demonstrated that plasma FHR-1 and the plasma FHR-1/Factor H ratio were increased in IgAN and associated with progression of the disease [100]. In addition, two independent studies showed that serum levels of FHR-5 were significantly higher in IgAN patients than in control patients [100,106]. In a British cohort, serum levels of FHR-5 were associated with more severe histology and unresponsiveness to immunosuppression, but not with progressive disease [100]. In a Chinese cohort, serum levels of FHR-5 were also associated with increased histological injury [106]. However, in contrast to the British cohort, Zhu et al. did report an association between serum FHR-5 levels and the risk of progressive disease. Whether these differences are due to dissimilar definitions of progressive disease or the consequence of ethnic/geographical differences remains to be determined. Nevertheless, these data, therefore, support the hypothesis that FHR-1 and FHR-5 compete with the regulatory function of Factor H. Factor H tips the balance towards alternative pathway inhibition and reduces the severity of the inflammatory injury, whereas these FHRs amplify alternative pathway activation and thereby stimulate IgAN development and progression of the disease (Table 1) [143].

Circulating levels of lectin pathway components have also been linked to IgAN severity. However, this association was complex and U-shaped, indicating that both low and high MBL levels associate with a higher risk, whereas IgAN patients with midrange levels are protected [144]. MBL deficiency in IgAN patients was associated with 50% loss of kidney function or kidney failure, whereas high levels of MBL (>3540 ng/mL) was associated with various markers of disease severity, including cellular crescents in the kidney biopsy and the degree of proteinuria, although the significance was lost after adjustment for other clinical variables. Furthermore, circulating levels of MBL do not seem to correlate with glomerular MBL deposits in the kidney biopsy [78]. Plasma levels of other lectin pathway components have also been investigated in IgAN. Circulating levels of ficolin-1, ficolin-2, MASP-1, and MBL-associated protein 2 (MAP-2) were increased in IgAN patients compared to healthy controls, but did not differ between IgAN patients with stable and progressive disease [117]. MAP-2 (previously MAp19) is an alternative splice product of the MASP-2 gene, and since this truncated form of 19 kDa lacks the serine protease domain, little is known about its function [145]. Earlier studies also reported systemic C4 activation in IgAN patients. Plasma C4d/C4 ratios, as a marker of C4 activation, were increased on at least one occasion in 28% of the adult IgAN patients [136]. Unfortunately, these studies have not been repeated since then. It would be especially interesting to see if plasma C4d levels in IgAN patients correlate with the extent of glomerular C4d deposits, since this has been demonstrated for other types of glomerulonephritis [146]. Initially, serum levels of C4bp were reported to be higher in IgAN patients than controls [90]. Others were not able to confirm these results, but did find that C4bp levels were higher in IgAN patients with worse prognoses [142]. Recently, Medjeral-Thomas et al. demonstrated that IgAN patients have reduced levels of MASP-3 compared to healthy controls [117]. Moreover, reduced MASP-3 levels were associated with the progression of IgAN [90]. These findings warrant further investigation, since MASP-3 is a vital player in the interaction between LP and AP and could clarify the connection between these two pathways in IgAN [25].

4.3. Genetic Variants in Complement Genes

Numerous studies support a strong genetic contribution to IgAN, and it was through these genetic studies that the concept of an autoimmune etiology originated [147]. Genome-wide association studies (GWAS) have revealed that disease susceptibility is greatly impacted by genetic variants in the antigen processing and presentation pathway, as well as the mucosal defense system [101,102,148]. Furthermore, GWAS highlighted the involvement of the complement system in IgAN [101–103]. These studies identified a common deletion within the Factor H gene locus as protective against IgAN (Table 1). This protective deletion results in the loss of the genes for FHR-3 and FHR-1 (CFHR3,1Δ) while leaving the gene for Factor H intact, and each copy of the deletion reduces the risk of IgAN by nearly 40% [101,103]. Interestingly, CFHR3,1Δ has been found with a relatively high prevalence, and the population frequency ranges from 0% in East Asians to 20% in Europeans, and up to 50% in certain African populations [149]. Moreover, CFHR3,1Δ has been associated with a lower risk for the development of AMD and IgAN, whereas it increases the risk for systemic lupus erythematosus (SLE) and aHUS (because of anti-Factor H autoantibodies) [101,150–152]. Fine mapping of the Factor H gene cluster in Chinese cohorts confirmed that CFHR3,1Δ is strongly protective against IgAN [104]. Furthermore, in IgAN patients, the deletion was associated with a lower prevalence of glomerular segmental sclerosis, tubular atrophy and interstitial fibrosis [104]. Further mechanistic studies revealed that CFHR3,1Δ in IgAN is associated with reduced mesangial C3 deposition and higher circulating levels of Factor H and C3, together with lower circulating C3a levels [153,154]. Recently, CFHR3,1Δ was also shown to be associated with better graft survival in patients who received a kidney transplant for IgAN [155]. In conclusion, the mechanism behind the protective effect of CFHR3,1Δ in IgAN is thought to arise from the reduced competition of FHRs with Factor H, thereby promoting inhibition rather than activation and accordingly reducing inflammation. In conformity, genetic variants of Factor H associated with lower plasma levels have also been identified in IgAN patients, suggesting that impaired regulation due to Factor H deficiencies could equally increase disease susceptibility [99]. Rare genetic variants of FHR-5 have also been described in IgAN, and allele frequencies differed significantly from that in controls [105]. The exact mechanism behind the association of these variants with IgAN remains unclear, but the FHR-5 variants are suggested to have increased binding capacity for C3b [105].

Genetics have also been utilized to advance the understanding of the lectin pathway in IgAN susceptibility and severity, especially for MBL. In the general population, there is a wide variation in circulating levels of MBL due to common genetic variants in the MBL gene (MBL2) [156]. The incidence of a MBL deficiency differs among populations, with the highest reported prevalence of more than 60% found in certain South American Indian groups [157]. The influence of MBL polymorphisms in IgAN was first investigated in a cohort of 77 IgAN patients and 140 controls [158]. Although no major conclusions could be drawn from this initial study, it is interesting to note that certain allele frequencies were lower in IgAN patients compared to controls. Conversely, Shi et al. found that IgAN patients with an MBL polymorphism in codon 54, which is associated with lower plasma levels, had a worse prognosis [159]. A separate study of Chinese patients investigated the impact of MBL2 gene polymorphisms on IgAN in a cohort of 749 IgAN patients and 489 controls [144]. The study found no differences in MBL2 haplotypes between IgAN patients and healthy controls, although a tendency was seen for a lower frequency of the O allele, which leads to a reduction in MBL functionality. These findings would suggest a protective role for low-producing MBL variants. Recently, the impact of MBL2 and ficolin-2 gene (FCN2) polymorphisms on disease progression were explored in over 1000 IgAN patients [160]. After screening for candidate variants through complete genetic sequencing of MBL2 and FCN2 in a small subset of patients, 7 expression-associated variations were further assessed in the discovery cohort. After adjustment for clinical and pathologic risk factors in multivariate analysis, only one variant in MBL2 (rs1800450) was associated with progression to kidney failure in IgAN patients. Moreover, the association remained significant in their validation cohort. The minor allele of rs1800450 G > A polymorphism was found to be associated with lower plasma levels of MBL, and homozygous IgAN patients had no detectable MBL levels, no glomerular deposition of MBL, increased histological injury as well as an increased risk of disease progression to kidney failure. Overall, the impact of MBL2 variants on IgAN can therefore not be unequivocally defined, since low-producing variants have both been suggested to be detrimental and beneficial.

5. Therapeutic Complement Inhibition in IgA Nephropathy

The growing body of evidence linking complement activation to the pathogenesis of IgAN has encouraged the study of complement-targeted therapies in this disease. To date, multiple clinical trials are ongoing to evaluate the safety and efficacy of different complement inhibitors in IgAN (Table 2). The targets of these therapies include MASP-2, C3, Factor B, C5, and C5aR1. Unfortunately, limited information has thus far been made available regarding these trials. The impressive panel of compounds currently pursued in IgAN is slightly surprising, since little data exist on preclinical complement inhibition in IgAN due to the lack of appropriate animal models. Zhang et al. demonstrated in a mouse model of IgAN that C3aR and C5aR1 deficiency leads to improved histology and reduced proteinuria [161]. These data, together with the fact that renal expression of C3aR and C5aR1 in IgAN patients correlates with disease activity and severity of renal injury, suggests that targeting C3aR or C5aR1 pharmaceutically could form a successful treatment option [132]. In accordance, preliminary data from the open-label phase II trial with avacopan, a C5aR1 antagonist, demonstrated reduced proteinuria and clinical improvement in 3 of the 7 IgAN patients (NCT02384317) [162]. In a Phase III trial involving patients with ANCA-associated vasculitis, avacopan was shown to be superior compared to prednisone in regards to remission rates, and the U.S. Food and Drug Administration (FDA) has approved avacopan as an adjunctive treatment for ANCA-associated vasculitis [163]. Effects of Eeulizumab treatment, a monoclonal antibody against C5, in IgAN were evaluated in two case reports as well as in a patient with IgAN recurrence after kidney donation with inconsistent results [164–166]. Nevertheless, ravulizumab, a long-acting anti-C5 blocking antibody engineered from eculizumab, is currently being evaluated in a Phase II trial for the treatment of IgAN (NCT04564339). Furthermore, small interfering RNA-targeting C5 (ALN-CC5) is also being evaluated in a Phase II trial in IgAN (NCT03841448). In addition to targeting the terminal pathway, inhibition of C3 with APL-2 is also being tested as a treatment option for IgAN (NCT03453619). APL-2 (pegcetacoplan) is a compstatin derivative that prevents C3 activation and has recently been approved by the FDA for the treatment of paroxysmal nocturnal hemoglobinuria (PNH) [167]. Efforts to specifically block activation of the alternative pathway (as well as the amplification loop) have led to the development of inhibitors that target Factor B. To this end, both Novartis and Ionis Pharmaceuticals are testing their Factor B inhibitors in phase II/III clinical trials in IgAN (NCT03373461, NCT04014335). The antisense Factor B inhibitor IONIS-FB-LRx (Ionis Pharmaceuticals) targets the production of Factor B, thereby effectively reducing circulating levels [168]. Meanwhile, Novartis has a small molecule inhibitor of Factor B that blocks the active site of Factor B and the Bb fragment [169]. From a different standpoint, targeting the lectin pathway through MASP-2 inhibition is also being pursued as a treatment option for IgAN. Blockage of MASP-2 would hamper glomerular lectin pathway activation, while still enabling C3 activation through the classical and alternative pathway. Narsoplimab (OMS721) is a humanized monoclonal antibody that blocks MASP-2; this antibody has been clinically developed by Omeros. Data of the phase II clinical trial with narsoplimab (OMS721) in IgAN were recently published [170]. First, 4 patients with corticosteroid-dependent IgAN were treated with 12 weekly infusions in a single-arm open-label substudy. After four weeks of initial Narsoplimab treatment, patients underwent steroid taper for the next four weeks, while the tapered steroid dose was maintained for the last four weeks. Next, these patients were followed up for six weeks after the last Narsoplimab infusion. Overall, the daily corticosteroid dose was reduced from 45 mg to 5 mg, and a median reduction of 72% was seen in 24-h urine protein excretion, while kidney function remained stable in all patients. Secondly, twelve patients with IgAN who were not receiving corticosteroids were randomized 1:1 to receive weekly narsoplimab infusions or vehicle for 12 weeks in a double-blind design. Once again, patients were followed for 6 weeks after the last treatment. After this follow-up period, all patients could enter dosing extension and receive narsoplimab. Overall reduction in proteinuria between the narsoplimab and vehicle groups was similar. However, for the eight patients that continued in the narsoplimab dosing extension (3 of which had initially received the vehicle), there was an overall decrease in proteinuria of 61.4%, suggesting a potential benefit. Interim analysis of both sub-studies indicated that the drug was safe and well-tolerated. Following up on these results, combined with a breakthrough therapy designation for IgAN by the FDA, the MASP-2 inhibitor is currently being tested in a Phase III, double-blind, randomized, and placebo-controlled study of IgAN patients with more than 1 g/day proteinuria (NCT03608033). A key unresolved question regarding the design of this trial remains whether MASP-2 inhibition will be equally effective in all IgAN patients, since histological lectin pathway activation is only seen in a subset of patients.

Table 2. Clinical trials with complement inhibitors in IgA nephropathy.

Trail ID	Target	Compound	Company	Design	Status
NCT03608033	MASP-2	Monoclonal antibody, intravenous injection	Omeros	Randomized, double-blind, placebo-controlled, Phase 3 study	Ongoing
NCT03453619	C3	Pegylated peptide, subcutaneous injection	Apellis Pharmaceuticals	Single arm open-label Phase 2 study	Ongoing
NCT04578834	Factor B	Small molecule, orally administered	Novartis	Multi-center, randomized, double-blind, placebo-controlled, Phase 3 study	Ongoing
NCT04014335	Factor B	Antisense oligonucleotide, subcutaneous injection	Ionis Pharmaceuticals	Single arm open-label Phase 2 study	Ongoing
NCT04564339	C5	Monoclonal antibody, intravenous injection	Alexion Pharmaceuticals	Randomized, double-blind, placebo-controlled Phase 2 study	Ongoing
NCT03841448	C5	Small interfering RNA, subcutaneous injection	Alnylam Pharmaceuticals	Randomized, double-blind, placebo-controlled Phase 2 study	Ongoing
NCT02384317	C5aR1	Small molecule, orally administered	Chemocentryx	Single arm open-label Phase 2 study	Completed

An overview of complement inhibitors that are currently being evaluated in clinical trials of IgA nephropathy. Last updated on 1 September 2021. Abbreviations: C5aR1, C5a receptor 1; MASP-2, mannose-binding protein-associated serine protease 2.

6. Conclusions and Future Perspective

During the last few decades, a vast body of data has demonstrated the importance of the complement system, specifically the lectin and alternative pathway, as key drivers of pathology in IgAN. Complement activation has been shown to occur on circulating galactose-deficient IgA-immune complexes and in the glomerular mesangium after their deposition, thereby initiating and/or amplifying glomerular inflammation and kidney injury. Furthermore, acquired and inherited complement abnormalities that lead to complement dysregulation or a more active complement system alter disease susceptibility and the risk of progression. Despite these major advances, IgAN remains a challenging disease for physicians because of its heterogeneity and the risk to cause kidney failure. Complement measurements and histology for complement proteins could help to determine disease activity and severity. Additionally, this could enable personalized approaches by selecting patients for complement targeted therapies or other novel treatments. Multiple clinical trials with an impressive panel of complement inhibitors are currently ongoing, giving an exciting glimpse at the potential of using complement inhibitors for the treatment of IgAN. The approval of complement inhibitors for IgAN would be a major milestone for multiple reasons. It is also worth mentioning that IgAN could be the first common disease to be treated with complement inhibitors, since previous complement drugs have all been granted to rare and orphan diseases (e.g., aHUS and PNH). Moreover, any discussion of the use of complement inhibitors in patients with IgAN also needs to consider the costs. The excessive costs of current complement inhibitors, such as eculizumab, cannot be overlooked (approximately $500,000 per year per patient). Such pricing may be acceptable for rare indications, but not for a common disease such as IgAN. However, lower drug pricing could be achieved by extending the applications of complement-targeted therapies to a larger patient population, such as those with IgAN or other forms of glomerulonephritis.

Author Contributions: Conceptualization, F.P., W.S. and M.R.D.; investigation, F.P. and B.F.; writing—original draft preparation, F.P. and B.F.; writing—review and editing, W.S. and M.R.D. All authors have read and agreed to the published version of the manuscript.

Funding: The European Union's Horizon 2020 Future and Emerging Technologies (FET) Open programme under grant agreement ID 899163 (SciFiMed project) The European Renal Association–European Dialysis and Transplantation Association (ERA–EDTA), on behalf of its Research Fellowship Program, to Bernardo Faria.

Acknowledgments: The illustrations of Figure 2 were made by Siawosh K. Eskandari.

Conflicts of Interest: F.P. owns stock in Chemocentryx. W.S. has been involved as a consultant for Omeros and owns stock in Omeros. B.F. and M.R.D. have no conflict of interest to declare. The funders had no role in the interpretation of data, in the writing of the manuscript, or in the decision to publish the results.

References

1. Ricklin, D.; Hajishengallis, G.; Yang, K.; Lambris, J.D. Complement: A key system for immune surveillance and homeostasis. *Nat. Immunol.* **2010**, *11*, 785–797. [CrossRef]
2. Walport, M.J. Complement. First of two parts. *N. Engl. J. Med.* **2001**, *344*, 1058–1066. [CrossRef] [PubMed]
3. Walport, M.J. Complement. Second of two parts. *N. Engl. J. Med.* **2001**, *344*, 1140–1144. [CrossRef] [PubMed]
4. Ricklin, D.; Reis, E.S.; Lambris, J.D. Complement in disease: A defence system turning offensive. *Nat. Rev. Nephrol.* **2016**, *12*, 383–401. [CrossRef] [PubMed]
5. Noris, M.; Remuzzi, G. Overview of Complement Activation and Regulation. *Semin. Nephrol.* **2013**, *33*, 479–492. [CrossRef]
6. Garcia, B.L.; Zwarthoff, S.A.; Rooijakkers, S.H.M.; Geisbrecht, B.V. Novel Evasion Mechanisms of the Classical Complement Pathway. *J. Immunol.* **2016**, *197*, 2051–2060. [CrossRef]
7. Diebolder, C.; Beurskens, F.J.; de Jong, R.N.; Koning, R.; Strumane, K.; Lindorfer, M.A.; Voorhorst, M.; Ugurlar, D.; Rosati, S.; Heck, A.; et al. Complement Is Activated by IgG Hexamers Assembled at the Cell Surface. *Science* **2014**, *343*, 1260–1263. [CrossRef]
8. Da Costa, M.G.; Poppelaars, F.; Berger, S.P.; Daha, M.R.; Seelen, M.A. The lectin pathway in renal disease: Old concept and new insights. *Nephrol. Dial. Transplant.* **2018**, *33*, 2073–2079. [CrossRef]
9. Garred, P.; Genster, N.; Pilely, K.; Bayarri-Olmos, R.B.; Rosbjerg, A.; Ma, Y.J.; Skjoedt, M.O. A journey through the lectin pathway of complement-MBL and beyond. *Immunol. Rev.* **2016**, *274*, 74–97. [CrossRef]
10. Lachmann, P.J. The Amplification Loop of the Complement Pathways. In *Advances in Immunology*; Elsevier BV: Amsterdam, The Netherlands, 2009; Volume 104, pp. 115–149.
11. Kemper, C.; Atkinson, J.P.; Hourcade, D.E. Properdin: Emerging Roles of a Pattern-Recognition Molecule. *Annu. Rev. Immunol.* **2010**, *28*, 131–155. [CrossRef]
12. O'Flynn, J.; Kotimaa, J.; Faber-Krol, R.; Koekkoek, K.; Klar-Mohamad, N.; Koudijs, A.; Schwaeble, W.J.; Stover, C.; Daha, M.R.; van Kooten, C. Properdin binds independent of complement activation in an in vivo model of anti-glomerular basement membrane disease. *Kidney Int.* **2018**, *94*, 1141–1150. [CrossRef]
13. Harboe, M.; Johnson, C.; Nymo, S.; Ekholt, K.; Schjalm, C.; Lindstad, J.K.; Pharo, A.; Hellerud, B.C.; Ekdahl, K.N.; Mollnes, T.E.; et al. Properdin binding to complement activating surfaces depends on initial C3b deposition. *Proc. Natl. Acad. Sci. USA* **2017**, *114*, e534–e539. [CrossRef]
14. Du Clos, T.W.; Mold, C. Pentraxins (CRP, SAP) in the process of complement activation and clearance of apoptotic bodies through Fcγ receptors. *Curr. Opin. Organ Transplant.* **2011**, *16*, 15–20. [CrossRef]
15. Inforzato, A.; Doni, A.; Barajon, I.; Leone, R.; Garlanda, C.; Bottazzi, B.; Mantovani, A. PTX3 as a paradigm for the interaction of pentraxins with the Complement system. *Semin. Immunol.* **2013**, *25*, 79–85. [CrossRef]
16. Roos, A.; Bouwman, L.H.; Van Gijlswijk-Janssen, D.J.; Faber-Krol, M.C.; Stahl, G.; Daha, M.R. Human IgA Activates the Complement System Via the Mannan-Binding Lectin Pathway. *J. Immunol.* **2001**, *167*, 2861–2868. [CrossRef]
17. Farrar, C.A.; Tran, D.; Li, K.; Wuding, Z.; Peng, Q.; Schwaeble, W.; Zhou, W.; Sacks, S.H. Collectin-11 detects stress-induced L-fucose pattern to trigger renal epithelial injury. *J. Clin. Investig.* **2016**, *126*, 1911–1925. [CrossRef]
18. Bayly-Jones, C.; Bubeck, D.; Dunstone, M.A. The mystery behind membrane insertion: A review of the complement membrane attack complex. *Philos. Trans. R. Soc. B Biol. Sci.* **2017**, *372*, 20160221. [CrossRef]
19. Ramm, L.E.; Whitlow, M.B.; Mayer, M.M. The relationship between channel size and the number of C9 molecules in the C5b-9 complex. *J. Immunol.* **1985**, *134*, 2594–2599.

20. Zipfel, P.F.; Skerka, C. Complement regulators and inhibitory proteins. *Nat. Rev. Immunol.* **2009**, *9*, 729–740. [CrossRef]
21. Harboe, M.; Ulvund, G.; Vien, L.; Fung, M.; Mollnes, T.E. The quantitative role of alternative pathway amplification in classical pathway induced terminal complement activation. *Clin. Exp. Immunol.* **2004**, *138*, 439–446. [CrossRef]
22. Harboe, M.; Garred, P.; Borgen, M.S.; Stahl, G.L.; Roos, A.; Mollnes, T.E. Design of a complement mannose-binding lectin pathway-specific activation system applicable at low serum dilutions. *Clin. Exp. Immunol.* **2006**, *144*, 512–520. [CrossRef] [PubMed]
23. Dobó, J.; Kocsis, A.; Gál, P. Be on target: Strategies of targeting alternative and lectin pathway components in comple-ment-mediated diseases. *Front. Immunol.* **2018**, *9*, 1. [CrossRef] [PubMed]
24. Heja, D.; Kocsis, A.; Dobo, J.; Szilagyi, K.; Szasz, R.; Zavodszky, P.; Pál, G.; Gal, P. Revised mechanism of complement lectin-pathway activation revealing the role of serine protease MASP-1 as the exclusive activator of MASP-2. *Proc. Natl. Acad. Sci. USA* **2012**, *109*, 10498–10503. [CrossRef] [PubMed]
25. Dobó, J.; Szakács, D.; Oroszlán, G.; Kortvely, E.; Kiss, B.; Boros, E.; Szász, R.; Závodszky, P.; Gál, P.; Pál, G. MASP-3 is the exclusive pro-factor D activator in resting blood: The lectin and the alternative complement pathways are fundamentally linked. *Sci. Rep.* **2016**, *6*, 31877. [CrossRef]
26. Pihl, R.; Jensen, L.; Hansen, A.G.; Thøgersen, I.B.; Andres, S.; Dagnæs-Hansen, F.; Oexle, K.; Enghild, J.J.; Thiel, S. Analysis of Factor D Isoforms in Malpuech–Michels–Mingarelli–Carnevale Patients Highlights the Role of MASP-3 as a Maturase in the Alternative Pathway of Complement. *J. Immunol.* **2017**, *199*, 2158–2170. [CrossRef]
27. Oroszlán, G.; Dani, R.; Szilágyi, A.; Závodszky, P.; Thiel, S.; Gál, P.; Dobó, J. Extensive Basal Level Activation of Complement Mannose-Binding Lectin-Associated Serine Protease-3: Kinetic Modeling of Lectin Pathway Activation Provides Possible Mechanism. *Front. Immunol.* **2017**, *8*, 1821. [CrossRef]
28. Oroszlán, G.; Dani, R.; Végh, B.M.; Varga, D.; Ács, A.V.; Pál, G.; Závodszky, P.; Farkas, H.; Gál, P.; Dobó, J. Proprotein Convertase Is the Highest-Level Activator of the Alternative Complement Pathway in the Blood. *J. Immunol.* **2021**, *206*, 2198–2205. [CrossRef]
29. Ricklin, D.; Mastellos, D.C.; Reis, E.S.; Lambris, J.D. The renaissance of complement therapeutics. *Nat. Rev. Nephrol.* **2018**, *14*, 26–47. [CrossRef]
30. Sánchez-Corral, P.; Pouw, R.B.; López-Trascasa, M.; Józsi, M. Self-Damage Caused by Dysregulation of the Complement Alternative Pathway: Relevance of the Factor H Protein Family. *Front. Immunol.* **2018**, *9*, 1607. [CrossRef]
31. Poppelaars, F.; Thurman, J.M. Complement-mediated kidney diseases. *Mol. Immunol.* **2020**, *128*, 175–187. [CrossRef]
32. Zipfel, P.F. Complement Factor H: Physiology and Pathophysiology. *Semin. Thromb. Hemost.* **2001**, *27*, 191–200. [CrossRef]
33. Parente, R.; Clark, S.; Inforzato, A.; Day, A.J. Complement factor H in host defense and immune evasion. *Cell. Mol. Life Sci.* **2017**, *74*, 1605–1624. [CrossRef]
34. Ferreira, V.P.; Pangburn, M.K.; Cortes, C. Complement control protein factor H: The good, the bad, and the inadequate. *Mol. Immunol.* **2010**, *47*, 2187–2197. [CrossRef]
35. De Córdoba, S.R.; De Jorge, E.G. Translational Mini-Review Series on Complement Factor H: Genetics and disease associations of human complement factor H. *Clin. Exp. Immunol.* **2007**, *151*, 1–13. [CrossRef]
36. Smith, R.J.H.; Appel, G.B.; Blom, A.M.; Cook, H.T.; D'Agati, V.D.; Fakhouri, F.; Fremeaux-Bacchi, V.; Józsi, M.; Kavanagh, D.; Lambris, J.; et al. C3 glomerulopathy — understanding a rare complement-driven renal disease. *Nat. Rev. Nephrol.* **2019**, *15*, 129–143. [CrossRef]
37. Poppelaars, F.; de Jorge, E.G.; Jongerius, I.; Baeumner, A.J.; Steiner, M.-S.; Józsi, M.; Toonen, E.J.M.; Pauly, D. The SciFiMed consortium A Family Affair: Addressing the Challenges of Factor H and the Related Proteins. *Front. Immunol.* **2021**, *12*, 12. [CrossRef]
38. Sánchez-Corral, P.; González-Rubio, C.; De Cordoba, S.R.; López-Trascasa, M. Functional analysis in serum from atypical Hemolytic Uremic Syndrome patients reveals impaired protection of host cells associated with mutations in factor H. *Mol. Immunol.* **2004**, *41*, 81–84. [CrossRef]
39. Nester, C.M.; Barbour, T.; de Cordoba, S.R.; Dragon-Durey, M.-A.; Fremeaux-Bacchi, V.; Goodship, T.H.; Kavanagh, D.; Noris, M.; Pickering, M.; Sanchez-Corral, P.; et al. Atypical aHUS: State of the art. *Mol. Immunol.* **2015**, *67*, 31–42. [CrossRef]
40. Józsi, M.; Heinen, S.; Hartmann, A.; Ostrowicz, C.W.; Hälbich, S.; Richter, H.; Kunert, A.; Licht, C.; Saunders, R.E.; Perkins, S.J.; et al. Factor H and Atypical Hemolytic Uremic Syndrome: Mutations in the C-Terminus Cause Structural Changes and Defective Recognition Functions. *J. Am. Soc. Nephrol.* **2005**, *17*, 170–177. [CrossRef]
41. Manuelian, T.; Hellwage, J.; Meri, S.; Caprioli, J.; Noris, M.; Heinen, S.; Jozsi, M.; Neumann, H.P.; Remuzzi, G.; Zipfel, P.F. Mutations in factor H reduce binding affinity to C3b and heparin and surface attachment to endothelial cells in hemolytic uremic syndrome. *J. Clin. Investig.* **2003**, *111*, 1181–1190. [CrossRef]
42. Cserhalmi, M.; Papp, A.; Brandus, B.; Uzonyi, B.; Józsi, M. Regulation of regulators: Role of the complement factor H-related proteins. *Semin. Immunol.* **2019**, *45*, 101341. [CrossRef]
43. Cantsilieris, S.; Nelson, B.J.; Huddleston, J.; Baker, C.; Harshman, L.; Penewit, K.; Munson, K.; Sorensen, M.; Welch, A.E.; Dang, V.; et al. Recurrent structural variation, clustered sites of selection, and disease risk for the complement factor H (CFH) gene family. *Proc. Natl. Acad. Sci. USA* **2018**, *115*, e4433–e4442. [CrossRef]
44. Jozsi, M.; Meri, S. Factor H-Related Proteins. *Methods Mol. Biol.* **2014**, *1100*, 225–236. [CrossRef] [PubMed]

45. De Jorge, E.G.; Caesar, J.J.E.; Malik, T.H.; Patel, M.; Colledge, M.; Johnson, S.; Hakobyan, S.; Morgan, P.; Harris, C.L.; Pickering, M.; et al. Dimerization of complement factor H-related proteins modulates complement activation in vivo. *Proc. Natl. Acad. Sci. USA* **2013**, *110*, 4685–4690. [CrossRef] [PubMed]
46. Van Beek, A.E.; Pouw, R.B.; Brouwer, M.C.; Van Mierlo, G.; Geissler, J.; Heer, P.O.-D.; De Boer, M.; Van Leeuwen, K.; Rispens, T.; Wouters, D.; et al. Factor H-Related (FHR)-1 and FHR-2 Form Homo- and Heterodimers, while FHR-5 Circulates Only As Homodimer in Human Plasma. *Front. Immunol.* **2017**, *8*. [CrossRef] [PubMed]
47. Poppelaars, F.; Seelen, M.A. Complement-mediated inflammation and injury in brain dead organ donors. *Mol. Immunol.* **2017**, *84*, 77–83. [CrossRef] [PubMed]
48. Rittirsch, D.; Flierl, M.A.; Nadeau, B.A.; Day, D.E.; Huber-Lang, M.; Mackay, C.; Zetoune, F.S.; Gerard, N.P.; Cianflone, K.; Koehl, J.; et al. Functional roles for C5a receptors in sepsis. *Nat. Med.* **2008**, *14*, 551–557. [CrossRef] [PubMed]
49. Maillard, N.; Wyatt, R.J.; Julian, B.A.; Kiryluk, K.; Gharavi, A.; Fremeaux-Bacchi, V.; Novak, J. Current Understanding of the Role of Complement in IgA Nephropathy. *J. Am. Soc. Nephrol.* **2015**, *26*, 1503–1512. [CrossRef] [PubMed]
50. Poppelaars, F.; Da Costa, M.G.; Faria, B.; Berger, S.P.; Assa, S.; Daha, M.R.; Pestana, J.O.M.; Van Son, W.J.; Franssen, C.; Seelen, M.A. Intradialytic Complement Activation Precedes the Development of Cardiovascular Events in Hemodialysis Patients. *Front. Immunol.* **2018**, *9*, 2070. [CrossRef]
51. Jager, N.M.; Poppelaars, F.; Daha, M.R.; Seelen, M.A. Complement in renal transplantation: The road to translation. *Mol. Immunol.* **2017**, *89*, 22–35. [CrossRef]
52. Poppelaars, F.; Faria, B.; Da Costa, M.G.; Franssen, C.F.M.; Van Son, W.J.; Berger, S.P.; Daha, M.R.; Seelen, M.A. The Complement System in Dialysis: A Forgotten Story? *Front. Immunol.* **2018**, *9*, 71. [CrossRef]
53. Poppelaars, F.; da Costa, M.G.; Berger, S.P.; Assa, S.; Meter-Arkema, A.H.; Daha, M.R.; van Son, W.J.; Franssen, C.F.M.; Seelen, M.A.J. Strong predictive value of mannose-binding lectin levels for cardiovascular risk of hemodialysis patients. *J. Transl. Med.* **2016**, *14*, 1–12. [CrossRef]
54. Grumach, A.S.; Kirschfink, M. Are complement deficiencies really rare? Overview on prevalence, clinical importance and modern diagnostic approach. *Mol. Immunol.* **2014**, *61*, 110–117. [CrossRef]
55. Bao, L.; Cunningham, P.N.; Quigg, R.J. Complement in Lupus Nephritis: New Perspectives. *Kidney Dis.* **2015**, *1*, 91–99. [CrossRef]
56. Sacks, S.; Zhou, W. New Boundaries for Complement in Renal Disease. *J. Am. Soc. Nephrol.* **2008**, *19*, 1865–1869. [CrossRef]
57. Pratt, J.R.; Basheer, S.A.; Sacks, S.H. Local synthesis of complement component C3 regulates acute renal transplant rejection. *Nat. Med.* **2002**, *8*, 582–587. [CrossRef]
58. Zhou, W.; Marsh, J.E.; Sacks, S.H. Intrarenal synthesis of complement. *Kidney Int.* **2001**, *59*, 1227–1235. [CrossRef]
59. Lubbers, R.; van Essen, M.; Van Kooten, C.; Trouw, L.A. Production of complement components by cells of the immune system. *Clin. Exp. Immunol.* **2017**, *188*, 183–194. [CrossRef]
60. Wu, X.; Hutson, I.; Akk, A.M.; Mascharak, S.; Pham, C.T.N.; Hourcade, D.E.; Brown, R.; Atkinson, J.P.; Harris, C.A. Contribution of Adipose-Derived Factor D/Adipsin to Complement Alternative Pathway Activation: Lessons from Lipodystrophy. *J. Immunol.* **2018**, *200*, 2786–2797. [CrossRef]
61. Schwaeble, W.; Huemer, H.P.; Most, J.; Dierich, M.P.; Strobel, M.; Claus, C.; Reid5, K.B.M.; Loms Ziegler-Heitbrock, H.W. Expression of properdin in human monocytes. *Eur. J. Biochem.* **1994**, *219*, 759–764. [CrossRef]
62. Petry, F.; Botto, M.; Holtappels, R.; Walport, M.J.; Loos, M. Reconstitution of the complement function in C1q-deficient (C1qa-/-) mice with wild-type bone marrow cells. *J. Immunol.* **2001**, *167*, 4033–4037. [CrossRef]
63. Naughton, M.A.; Walport, M.J.; Würzner, R.; Carter, M.J.; Alexander, G.J.M.; Goldman, J.M.; Botto, M. Organ-specific contribution to circulating C7 levels by the bone marrow and liver in humans. *Eur. J. Immunol.* **1996**, *26*, 2108–2112. [CrossRef]
64. White, R.T.; Damm, D.; Hancock, N.; Rosen, B.S.; Lowell, B.B.; Usher, P.; Flier, J.S.; Spiegelman, B.M. Human adipsin is identical to complement factor D and is expressed at high levels in adipose tissue. *J. Biol. Chem.* **1992**, *267*, 9210–9213. [CrossRef]
65. Daha, M.R.; van Kooten, C. Is the proximal tubular cell a proinflammatory cell? *Nephrol. Dial. Transplant* **2000**, *15* (Suppl. 6), 41–43. [CrossRef]
66. Daha, M.R.; van Kooten, C. Is there a role for locally produced complement in renal disease? *Nephrol. Dial. Transplant* **2000**, *15*, 1506–1509. [CrossRef]
67. Tang, S.C.W.; Zhou, W.; Sheerin, N.S.; Vaughan, R.W.; Sacks, S. Contribution of renal secreted complement C3 to the circulating pool in humans. *J. Immunol.* **1999**, *162*, 4336–4341.
68. Marsh, J.E.; Zhou, W.; Sacks, S.H. Local tissue complement synthesis—Fine tuning a blunt instrument. *Arch. Immunol. Ther. Exp.* **2001**, *49*, 41–46.
69. Liszewski, M.K.; Kolev, M.; Le Friec, G.; Leung, M.; Bertram, P.G.; Fara, A.F.; Subias, M.; Pickering, M.C.; Drouet, C.; Meri, S.; et al. Intracellular Complement Activation Sustains T Cell Homeostasis and Mediates Effector Differentiation. *Immunity* **2013**, *39*, 1143–1157. [CrossRef] [PubMed]
70. Arbore, G.; Kemper, C.; Kolev, M. Intracellular complement—The complosome—In immune cell regulation. *Mol. Immunol.* **2017**, *89*, 2–9. [CrossRef] [PubMed]
71. Wyatt, R.J.; Julian, B.A. IgA Nephropathy. *N. Engl. J. Med.* **2013**, *368*, 2402–2414. [CrossRef] [PubMed]
72. Suzuki, H.; Kiryluk, K.; Novak, J.; Moldoveanu, Z.; Herr, A.; Renfrow, M.B.; Wyatt, R.; Scolari, F.; Mestecky, J.; Gharavi, A.G.; et al. The Pathophysiology of IgA Nephropathy. *J. Am. Soc. Nephrol.* **2011**, *22*, 1795–1803. [CrossRef]

73. Evans, D.J.; Williams, D.G.; Peters, D.K.; Sissons, J.G.P.; Boulton-Jones, J.M.; Ogg, C.S.; Cameron, J.S.; Hoffbrand, B.I. Glomerular Deposition of Properdin in Henoch-Schonlein Syndrome and Idiopathic Focal Nephritis. *BMJ* **1973**, *3*, 326–328. [CrossRef]
74. Lang, Y.; Song, S.; Zhao, L.; Yang, Y.; Liu, T.; Shen, Y.; Wang, W. Serum IgA/C3 ratio and glomerular C3 staining predict progression of IgA nephropathy in children. *Transl. Pediatr.* **2021**, *10*, 666–672. [CrossRef]
75. Wu, D.; Li, X.; Yao, X.; Zhang, N.; Lei, L.; Zhang, H.; Tang, M.; Ni, J.; Ling, C.; Chen, Z.; et al. Mesangial C3 deposition and serum C3 levels predict renal outcome in IgA nephropathy. *Clin. Exp. Nephrol.* **2021**, *25*, 641–651. [CrossRef]
76. Kim, S.J.; Koo, H.M.; Lim, B.J.; Oh, H.J.; Yoo, D.E.; Shin, D.H.; Lee, M.J.; Doh, F.M.; Park, J.T.; Yoo, T.-H.; et al. Decreased Circulating C3 Levels and Mesangial C3 Deposition Predict Renal Outcome in Patients with IgA Nephropathy. *PLoS ONE* **2012**, *7*, e40495. [CrossRef]
77. Nam, K.H.; Joo, Y.S.; Lee, C.; Lee, S.; Kim, J.; Yun, H.-R.; Park, J.T.; Chang, T.I.; Ryu, D.-R.; Yoo, T.-H.; et al. Predictive value of mesangial C3 and C4d deposition in IgA nephropathy. *Clin. Immunol.* **2020**, *211*, 108331. [CrossRef]
78. Roos, A.; Rastaldi, M.P.; Calvaresi, N.; Oortwijn, B.D.; Schlagwein, N.; Van Gijlswijk-Janssens, D.J.; Stahl, G.; Matsushita, M.; Fujita, T.; van Kooten, C.; et al. Glomerular Activation of the Lectin Pathway of Complement in IgA Nephropathy Is Associated with More Severe Renal Disease. *J. Am. Soc. Nephrol.* **2006**, *17*, 1724–1734. [CrossRef]
79. Faria, B.; Canão, P.; Cai, Q.; Henriques, C.; Matos, A.C.; Poppelaars, F.; da Costa, M.G.; Daha, M.R.; Silva, R.; Pestana, M.; et al. Arteriolar C4d in IgA Nephropathy: A Cohort Study. *Am. J. Kidney Dis.* **2020**, *76*, 669–678. [CrossRef]
80. Espinosa, M.; Ortega, R.; Sánchez, M.; Segarra, A.; Salcedo, M.T.; González, F.; Camacho, R.; Valdivia, M.A.; Cabrera, R.; López, K.; et al. Association of C4d Deposition with Clinical Outcomes in IgA Nephropathy. *Clin. J. Am. Soc. Nephrol.* **2014**, *9*, 897–904. [CrossRef]
81. Segarra, A.; Romero, K.; Agraz, I.; Ramos, N.; Madrid, A.; Carnicer, C.; Jatem, E.; Vilalta, R.; Lara, L.E.; Ostos, E.; et al. Mesangial C4d Deposits in Early IgA Nephropathy. *Clin. J. Am. Soc. Nephrol.* **2017**, *13*, 258–264. [CrossRef]
82. McCoy, R.C.; Abramowsky, C.R.; Tisher, C.C. IgA nephropathy. *Am. J. Pathol.* **1974**, *76*, 123–144. [PubMed]
83. Lee, H.-J.; Choi, S.Y.; Jeong, K.H.; Sung, J.-Y.; Moon, S.K.; Moon, J.-Y.; Lee, S.-H.; Lee, T.-W.; Ihm, C.-G. Association of C1q deposition with renal outcomes in IgA nephropathy. *Clin. Nephrol.* **2013**, *80*, 98–104. [CrossRef]
84. Rauterberg, E.W.; Lieberknecht, H.M.; Wingen, A.M.; Ritz, E. Complement membrane attack (MAC) in idiopathic IgA-glomerulonephritis. *Kidney Int.* **1987**, *31*, 820–829. [CrossRef]
85. Hiemstra, P.S.; Gorter, A.; Stuurman, M.E.; Van Es, L.A.; Daha, M.R. Activation of the alternative pathway of complement by human serum IgA. *Eur. J. Immunol.* **1987**, *17*, 321–326. [CrossRef]
86. Russell, M.W.; Mansa, B. Complement-fixing properties of human IgA antibodies. Alternative pathway complement activa-tion by plastic-bound, but not specific antigen-bound, IgA. *Scand. J. Immunol.* **1989**, *30*, 175–183. [CrossRef]
87. Chiu, Y.-L.; Lin, W.-C.; Shu, K.-H.; Fang, Y.-W.; Chang, F.-C.; Chou, Y.-H.; Wu, C.-F.; Chiang, W.-C.; Lin, S.-L.; Chen, Y.-M.; et al. Alternative Complement Pathway Is Activated and Associated with Galactose-Deficient IgA1 Antibody in IgA Nephropathy Patients. *Front. Immunol.* **2021**, *12*. [CrossRef]
88. Medjeral-Thomas, N.R.; Moffitt, H.; Lomax-Browne, H.J.; Constantinou, N.; Cairns, T.; Cook, H.T.; Pickering, M.C. Glomerular Complement Factor H–Related Protein 5 (FHR5) Is Highly Prevalent in C3 Glomerulopathy and Associated With Renal Impairment. *Kidney Int. Rep.* **2019**, *4*, 1387–1400. [CrossRef]
89. Zhang, J.-J.; Jiang, L.; Liu, G.; Wang, S.-X.; Zou, W.-Z.; Zhang, H.; Zhao, M.-H. Levels of Urinary Complement Factor H in Patients with IgA Nephropathy are Closely Associated with Disease Activity. *Scand. J. Immunol.* **2009**, *69*, 457–464. [CrossRef]
90. Miyazaki, R.; Kuroda, M.; Akiyama, T.; Otani, I.; Tofuku, Y.; Takeda, R. Glomerular deposition and serum levels of complement control proteins in patients with IgA nephropathy. *Clin. Nephrol.* **1984**, *21*, 335–340.
91. Tomino, Y.; Endoh, M.; Nomoto, Y.; Sakai, H. Double immunofluorescence studies of immunoglobulins, complement components and their control proteins in patients with IgA nephropathy. *Pathol. Int.* **1982**, *32*, 251–256. [CrossRef]
92. Tomino, Y.; Sakai, H.; Nomoto, Y.; Endoh, M.; Arimori, S.; Fujita, T. Deposition of C4-binding protein and β 1H globulin in kidneys of patients with IgA nephropathy. *Tokai J. Exp. Clin. Med.* **1981**, *6*, 217–222. [PubMed]
93. Onda, K.; Ohsawa, I.; Ohi, H.; Tamano, M.; Mano, S.; Wakabayashi, M.; Toki, A.; Horikoshi, S.; Fujita, T.; Tomino, Y. Excretion of complement proteins and its activation marker C5b-9 in IgA nephropathy in relation to renal function. *BMC Nephrol.* **2011**, *12*, 64. [CrossRef] [PubMed]
94. Wen, L.; Zhao, Z.; Wang, Z.; Xiao, J.; Birn, H.; Gregersen, J.W. High levels of urinary complement proteins are associated with chronic renal damage and proximal tubule dysfunction in immunoglobulin A nephropathy. *Nephrology* **2018**, *24*, 703–710. [CrossRef] [PubMed]
95. Liu, M.; Chen, Y.; Zhou, J.; Liu, Y.; Wang, F.; Shi, S.; Zhao, Y.; Wang, S.; Liu, L.; Lv, J.; et al. Implication of Urinary Complement Factor H in the Progression of Immunoglobulin A Nephropathy. *PLoS ONE* **2015**, *10*, e0126812. [CrossRef]
96. Paunas, T.I.F.; Finne, K.; Leh, S.; Marti, H.-P.; Mollnes, T.E.; Berven, F.; Vikse, B.E. Glomerular abundance of complement proteins characterized by proteomic analysis of laser-captured microdissected glomeruli associates with progressive disease in IgA nephropathy. *Clin. Proteom.* **2017**, *14*, 30. [CrossRef]
97. Murphy, B.; Georgiou, T.; Machet, D.; Hill, P.; McRae, J. Factor H-related protein-5: A novel component of human glomerular immune deposits. *Am. J. Kidney Dis.* **2002**, *39*, 24–27. [CrossRef]
98. Guo, W.-Y.; Sun, L.-J.; Dong, H.-R.; Wang, G.-Q.; Xu, X.-Y.; Zhao, Z.-R.; Cheng, H. Glomerular Complement Factor H–Related Protein 5 is Associated with Histologic Injury in Immunoglobulin A Nephropathy. *Kidney Int. Rep.* **2021**, *6*, 404–413. [CrossRef]

99. Tortajada, A.; Gutiérrez, E.; De Jorge, E.G.; Anter, J.; Segarra, A.; Espinosa, M.; Blasco, M.; Roman, E.; Marco, H.; Quintana, L.F.; et al. Elevated factor H–related protein 1 and factor H pathogenic variants decrease complement regulation in IgA nephropathy. *Kidney Int.* **2017**, *92*, 953–963. [CrossRef]
100. Medjeral-Thomas, N.R.; Lomax-Browne, H.J.; Beckwith, H.; Willicombe, M.; McLean, A.G.; Brookes, P.; Pusey, C.D.; Falchi, M.; Cook, H.T.; Pickering, M.C. Circulating complement factor H–related proteins 1 and 5 correlate with disease activity in IgA nephropathy. *Kidney Int.* **2017**, *92*, 942–952. [CrossRef]
101. Gharavi, A.G.; Kiryluk, K.; Choi, M.; Li, Y.; Hou, P.; Xie, J.; Sanna-Cherchi, S.; Men, C.J.; Julian, B.A.; Wyatt, R.; et al. Genome-wide association study identifies susceptibility loci for IgA nephropathy. *Nat. Genet.* **2011**, *43*, 321–327. [CrossRef]
102. Kiryluk, K.; Li, Y.; Scolari, F.; Sanna-Cherchi, S.; Choi, M.; Verbitsky, M.; Fasel, D.; Lata, S.; Prakash, S.; Shapiro, S.; et al. Discovery of new risk loci for IgA nephropathy implicates genes involved in immunity against intestinal pathogens. *Nat. Genet.* **2014**, *46*, 1187–1196. [CrossRef]
103. Kiryluk, K.; Li, Y.; Sanna-Cherchi, S.; Rohanizadegan, M.; Suzuki, H.; Eitner, F.; Snyder, H.J.; Choi, M.; Hou, P.; Scolari, F.; et al. Geographic Differences in Genetic Susceptibility to IgA Nephropathy: GWAS Replication Study and Geospatial Risk Analysis. *PLoS Genet.* **2012**, *8*, e1002765. [CrossRef]
104. Xie, J.; Kiryluk, K.; Li, Y.; Mladkova, N.; Zhu, L.; Hou, P.; Ren, H.; Wang, W.; Zhang, H.; Chen, N.; et al. Fine Mapping Implicates a Deletion of CFHR1 and CFHR3 in Protection from IgA Nephropathy in Han Chinese. *J. Am. Soc. Nephrol.* **2016**, *27*, 3187–3194. [CrossRef]
105. Zhai, Y.-L.; Meng, S.-J.; Zhu, L.; Shi, S.-F.; Wang, S.-X.; Liu, L.-J.; Lv, J.-C.; Yu, F.; Zhao, M.-H.; Zhang, H. Rare Variants in the Complement Factor H–Related Protein 5 Gene Contribute to Genetic Susceptibility to IgA Nephropathy. *J. Am. Soc. Nephrol.* **2016**, *27*, 2894–2905. [CrossRef]
106. Zhu, L.; Guo, W.-Y.; Shi, S.-F.; Liu, L.-J.; Lv, J.-C.; Medjeral-Thomas, N.R.; Lomax-Browne, H.J.; Pickering, M.C.; Zhang, H. Circulating complement factor H–related protein 5 levels contribute to development and progression of IgA nephropathy. *Kidney Int.* **2018**, *94*, 150–158. [CrossRef]
107. Endo, M.; Ohi, H.; Ohsawa, I.; Fujita, T.; Matsushita, M. Glomerular deposition of mannose-binding lectin (MBL) indicates a novel mechanism of complement activation in IgA nephropathy. *Nephrol. Dial. Transplant.* **1998**, *13*, 1984–1990. [CrossRef]
108. Hisano, S.; Matsushita, M.; Fujita, T.; Endo, Y.; Takebayashi, S. Mesangial IgA2 deposits and lectin pathway-mediated complement activation in IgA glomerulonephritis. *Am. J. Kidney Dis.* **2001**, *38*, 1082–1088. [CrossRef]
109. Faria, B.; Henriques, C.; Matos, A.; Daha, M.R.; Pestana, M.; Seelen, M. Combined C4d and CD3 immunostaining predicts immunoglobulin (Ig)A nephropathy progression. *Clin. Exp. Immunol.* **2015**, *179*, 354–361. [CrossRef]
110. Liu, L.-L.; Jiang, Y.; Wang, L.-N.; Liu, N. Urinary mannose-binding lectin is a biomarker for predicting the progression of immunoglobulin (Ig)A nephropathy. *Clin. Exp. Immunol.* **2012**, *169*, 148–155. [CrossRef]
111. Segarra-Medrano, A.; Carnicer-Caceres, C.; Valtierra-Carmeno, N.; Agraz-Pamplona, I.; Terrades, N.R.; Escalante, E.J.; Ostos-Roldan, E. Estudio de las variables asociadas a la activación local del complemento en la nefropatía IgA idiopática. *Nefrologia* **2017**, *37*, 320–329. [CrossRef]
112. Espinosa, M.; Ortega, R.; Gómez-Carrasco, J.M.; López-Rubio, F.; López-Andreu, M.; López-Oliva, M.O.; Aljama, P. Mesangial C4d deposition: A new prognostic factor in IgA nephropathy. *Nephrol. Dial. Transplant.* **2008**, *24*, 886–891. [CrossRef]
113. Haas, M.; Loupy, A.; Lefaucheur, C.; Roufosse, C.; Glotz, D.; Seron, D.; Nankivell, B.J.; Halloran, P.F.; Colvin, R.B.; Akalin, E.; et al. The Banff 2017 Kidney Meeting Report: Revised diagnostic criteria for chronic active T cell–mediated rejection, anti-body-mediated rejection, and prospects for integrative endpoints for next-generation clinical trials. *Am. J. Transplant.* **2018**, *18*, 293–307. [CrossRef]
114. Baek, H.S.; Han, M.H.; Kim, Y.J.; Cho, M.H. Clinical Relevance of C4d Deposition in Pediatric Immunoglobulin A Nephropathy. *Fetal Pediatr. Pathol.* **2018**, *37*, 326–336. [CrossRef]
115. Jiang, Y.; Zan, J.; Shi, S.; Hou, W.; Zhao, W.; Zhong, X.; Zhou, X.; Lv, J.; Zhang, H. Glomerular C4d Deposition and Kidney Disease Progression in IgA Nephropathy: A Systematic Review and Meta-analysis. *Kidney Med.* **2021**. [CrossRef]
116. Ohsawa, I.; Kusaba, G.; Ishii, M.; Sato, N.; Inoshita, H.; Onda, K.; Hashimoto, A.; Nagamachi, S.; Suzuki, H.; Shimamoto, M.; et al. Extraglomerular C3 deposition and metabolic impacts in patients with IgA nephropathy. *Nephrol. Dial. Transplant.* **2012**, *28*, 1856–1864. [CrossRef]
117. Medjeral-Thomas, N.R.; Troldborg, A.; Constantinou, N.; Lomax-Browne, H.J.; Hansen, A.G.; Willicombe, M.; Pusey, C.D.; Cook, H.T.; Thiel, S.; Pickering, M.C. Progressive IgA Nephropathy Is Associated With Low Circulating Mannan-Binding Lectin–Associated Serine Protease-3 (MASP-3) and Increased Glomerular Factor H–Related Protein-5 (FHR5) Deposition. *Kidney Int. Rep.* **2018**, *3*, 426–438. [CrossRef]
118. Xu, L.; Yang, H.-C.; Hao, C.-M.; Lin, S.-T.; Gu, Y.; Ma, J. Podocyte number predicts progression of proteinuria in IgA nephropathy. *Mod. Pathol.* **2010**, *23*, 1241–1250. [CrossRef]
119. Moll, S.; Miot, S.; Sadallah, S.; Gudat, F.; Mihatsch, M.J.; Schifferli, J.A. No complement receptor 1 stumps on podocytes in human glomerulopathies. *Kidney Int.* **2001**, *59*, 160–168. [CrossRef]
120. Koopman, J.J.E.; van Essen, M.F.; Rennke, H.G.; de Vries, A.P.J.; van Kooten, C. Deposition of the Membrane Attack Complex in Healthy and Diseased Human Kidneys. *Front. Immunol.* **2021**, *11*, 3802. [CrossRef]
121. Ootaka, T.; Suzuki, M.; Sudo, K.; Sato, H.; Seino, J.; Saito, T.; Yoshinaga, K. Histologic Localization of Terminal Complement Complexes in Renal Diseases: An Immunohistochemical Study. *Am. J. Clin. Pathol.* **1989**, *91*, 144–151. [CrossRef]

122. Bariety, J.; Hinglais, N.; Bhakdi, S.; Mandet, C.; Rouchon, M.; Kazatchkine, M.D. Immunohistochemical study of complement S protein (Vitronectin) in normal and diseased human kidneys: Relationship to neoantigens of the C5b-9 terminal complex. *Clin. Exp. Immunol.* **1989**, *75*, 76–81. [PubMed]
123. Hinglais, N.; Kazatchkine, M.D.; Bhakdi, S.; Appay, M.; Mandet, C.; Grossetete, J.; Bariéty, J. Immunohistochemical study of the C5b-9 complex of complement in human kidneys. *Kidney Int.* **1986**, *30*, 399–410. [CrossRef] [PubMed]
124. Alexopoulos, E.; Papaghianni, A.; Papadimitriou, M. The pathogenetic significance of C5b-9 in IgA nephropathy. *Nephrol. Dial. Transplant.* **1995**, *10*, 1166–1172. [CrossRef] [PubMed]
125. Stangou, M.; Alexopoulos, E.; Pantzaki, A.; Leonstini, M.; Memmos, D. C5b-9 glomerular deposition and tubular α3β1-integrin expression are implicated in the development of chronic lesions and predict renal function outcome in immunoglobulin A nephropathy. *Scand. J. Urol. Nephrol.* **2008**, *42*, 373–380. [CrossRef]
126. Pratt, J.R.; Abe, K.; Miyazaki, M.; Zhou, W.; Sacks, S.H. In Situ Localization of C3 Synthesis in Experimental Acute Renal Allograft Rejection. *Am. J. Pathol.* **2000**, *157*, 825–831. [CrossRef]
127. Abe, K.; Miyazaki, M.; Koji, T.; Furusu, A.; Shioshita, K.; Tsukasaki, S.; Ozono, Y.; Harada, T.; Sakai, H.; Kohno, S. Intraglomerular synthesis of complement C3 and its activation products in IgA nephropathy. *Nephron* **2001**, *87*, 231–239. [CrossRef]
128. Eguchi, K.; Tomino, Y.; Yagame, M.; Miyazaki, M.; Takiura, F.; Miura, M.; Suga, T.; Endoh, M.; Nomoto, Y.; Sakai, H. Double immunofluorescence studies of IgA and poly C9 (MAC) in glomeruli from patients with IgA nephropathy. *Tokai J. Exp. Clin. Med.* **1987**, *12*, 331–335.
129. Mosolits, S.; Magyarlaki, T.; Nagy, J. Membrane Attack Complex and Membrane Cofactor Protein Are Related to Tubulointerstitial Inflammation in Various Human Glomerulopathies. *Nephron* **1997**, *75*, 179–187. [CrossRef]
130. Dumont, C.; Mérouani, A.; Ducruet, T.; Benoit, G.; Clermont, M.-J.; Lapeyraque, A.L.; Phan, V.; Patey, N. Clinical relevance of membrane attack complex deposition in children with IgA nephropathy and Henoch-Schönlein purpura. *Pediatr. Nephrol.* **2020**, *35*, 843–850. [CrossRef]
131. Takahashi, T.; Inaba, S.; Okada, T. Vitronectin in children with renal disease—1. Immunofluorescence study of vitronectin and C5b-9 in childhood IgA nephropathy. *Nihon Jinzo Gakkai Shi* **1995**, *37*, 213–223.
132. Liu, L.; Zhang, Y.; Duan, X.; Peng, Q.; Liu, Q.; Zhou, Y.; Quan, S.; Xing, G. C3a, C5a Renal Expression and Their Receptors are Correlated to Severity of IgA Nephropathy. *J. Clin. Immunol.* **2014**, *34*, 224–232. [CrossRef]
133. Tanaka, C.; Suhara, Y.; Kikkawa, Y. Circulating immune complexes and complement breakdown products in childhood IgA nephropathy. *Nihon Jinzo Gakkai Shi* **1991**, *33*, 709–717.
134. Wyatt, R.J.; Julian, B.A. Activation of Complement in IgA Nephropathy. *Am. J. Kidney Dis.* **1988**, *12*, 437–442. [CrossRef]
135. Zwirner, J.; Burg, M.; Schulze, M.; Brunkhorst, R.; Götze, O.; Koch, K.-M.; Floege, J. Activated complement C3: A potentially novel predictor of progressive IgA nephropathy. *Kidney Int.* **1997**, *51*, 1257–1264. [CrossRef]
136. Wyatt, R.; Kanayama, Y.; Julian, B.A.; Negoro, N.; Sugimoto, S.; Hudson, E.C.; Curd, J.G. Complement activation in IgA nephropathy. *Kidney Int.* **1987**, *31*, 1019–1023. [CrossRef]
137. Knoppova, B.; Reily, C.; Maillard, N.; Rizk, D.V.; Moldoveanu, Z.; Mestecky, J.; Raska, M.; Renfrow, M.B.; Julian, B.A.; Novak, J. The Origin and Activities of IgA1-Containing Immune Complexes in IgA Nephropathy. *Front. Immunol.* **2016**, *7*, 117. [CrossRef]
138. Yang, X.; Wei, R.-B.; Wang, Y.; Su, T.-Y.; Li, Q.-P.; Yang, T.; Huang, M.-J.; Li, K.-Y.; Chen, X.-M. Decreased Serum C3 Levels in Immunoglobulin A (IgA) Nephropathy with Chronic Kidney Disease: A Propensity Score Matching Study. *Med. Sci. Monit.* **2017**, *23*, 673–681. [CrossRef]
139. Kawasaki, Y.; Maeda, R.; Ohara, S.; Suyama, K.; Hosoya, M. Serum IgA/C3 and glomerular C3 staining predict severity of IgA nephropathy. *Pediatr. Int.* **2017**, *60*, 162–167. [CrossRef]
140. Mizerska-Wasiak, M.; Małdyk, J.; Rybi-Szuminska, A.; Wasilewska, A.; Miklaszewska, M.; Pietrzyk, J.; Firszt-Adamczyk, A.; Stankiewicz, R.; Bieniaś, B.; Zajączkowska, M.; et al. Relationship between serum IgA/C3 ratio and severity of histological lesions using the Oxford classification in children with IgA nephropathy. *Pediatr. Nephrol.* **2015**, *30*, 1113–1120. [CrossRef]
141. Chen, P.; Yu, G.; Zhang, X.; Xie, X.; Wang, J.; Shi, S.; Liu, L.; Lv, J.; Zhang, H. Plasma Galactose-Deficient IgA1 and C3 and CKD Progression in IgA Nephropathy. *Clin. J. Am. Soc. Nephrol.* **2019**, *14*, 1458–1465. [CrossRef]
142. Onda, K.; Ohi, H.; Tamano, M.; Ohsawa, I.; Wakabayashi, M.; Horikoshi, S.; Fujita, T.; Tomino, Y. Hypercomplementemia in adult patients with IgA nephropathy. *J. Clin. Lab. Anal.* **2007**, *21*, 77–84. [CrossRef]
143. Thurman, J.M.; Laskowski, J. Complement factor H–related proteins in IgA nephropathy—sometimes a gentle nudge does the trick. *Kidney Int.* **2017**, *92*, 790–793. [CrossRef]
144. Guo, W.-Y.; Zhu, L.; Meng, S.-J.; Shi, S.-F.; Liu, L.-J.; Lv, J.-C.; Zhang, H. Mannose-Binding Lectin Levels Could Predict Prognosis in IgA Nephropathy. *J. Am. Soc. Nephrol.* **2017**, *28*, 3175–3181. [CrossRef]
145. Degn, S.E.; Thiel, S.; Nielsen, O.; Hansen, A.G.; Steffensen, R.; Jensenius, J.C. MAp19, the alternative splice product of the MASP2 gene. *J. Immunol. Methods* **2011**, *373*, 89–101. [CrossRef]
146. Martin, M.; Trattner, R.; Nilsson, S.C.; Björk, A.; Zickert, A.; Blom, A.M.; Gunnarsson, I. Plasma C4d Correlates with C4d Deposition in Kidneys and With Treatment Response in Lupus Nephritis Patients. *Front. Immunol.* **2020**, *11*, 582737. [CrossRef] [PubMed]
147. Kiryluk, K.; Novak, J. The genetics and immunobiology of IgA nephropathy. *J. Clin. Investig.* **2014**, *124*, 2325–2332. [CrossRef] [PubMed]

148. Yu, X.-Q.; Li, M.; Zhang, H.; Low, H.-Q.; Wei, X.; Wang, J.-Q.; Sun, L.-D.; Sim, K.S.; Li, Y.; Foo, J.N.; et al. A genome-wide association study in Han Chinese identifies multiple susceptibility loci for IgA nephropathy. *Nat. Genet.* **2012**, *44*, 178–182. [CrossRef] [PubMed]
149. Holmes, L.V.; Strain, L.; Staniforth, S.J.; Moore, I.; Marchbank, K.; Kavanagh, D.; Goodship, J.A.; Cordell, H.J.; Goodship, T.H.J. Determining the Population Frequency of the CFHR3/CFHR1 Deletion at 1q32. *PLoS ONE* **2013**, *8*, e60352. [CrossRef]
150. Zhao, J.; Wu, H.; Khosravi, M.; Cui, H.; Qian, X.; Kelly, J.; Kaufman, K.M.; Langefeld, C.D.; Williams, A.H.; Comeau, M.E.; et al. Association of Genetic Variants in Complement Factor H and Factor H-Related Genes with Systemic Lupus Erythematosus Susceptibility. *PLoS Genet.* **2011**, *7*, e1002079. [CrossRef]
151. Zipfel, P.F.; Edey, M.; Heinen, S.; Józsi, M.; Richter, H.; Misselwitz, J.; Hoppe, B.; Routledge, D.; Strain, L.; Hughes, A.E.; et al. Deletion of Complement Factor H–Related Genes CFHR1 and CFHR3 Is Associated with Atypical Hemolytic Uremic Syndrome. *PLoS Genet.* **2007**, *3*, e41. [CrossRef]
152. Hughes, A.E.; Orr, N.; Esfandiary, H.; Diaz-Torres, M.; Goodship, T.; Chakravarthy, U. A common CFH haplotype, with deletion of CFHR1 and CFHR3, is associated with lower risk of age-related macular degeneration. *Nat. Genet.* **2006**, *38*, 1173–1177. [CrossRef]
153. Zhu, L.; Zhai, Y.-L.; Wang, F.-M.; Hou, P.; Lv, J.-C.; Xu, D.-M.; Shi, S.-F.; Liu, L.-J.; Yu, F.; Zhao, M.-H.; et al. Variants in Complement Factor H and Complement Factor H-Related Protein Genes, CFHR3 and CFHR1, Affect Complement Activation in IgA Nephropathy. *J. Am. Soc. Nephrol.* **2014**, *26*, 1195–1204. [CrossRef]
154. Jullien, P.; Laurent, B.; Claisse, G.; Masson, I.; Dinic, M.; Thibaudin, D.; Berthoux, F.; Alamartine, E.; Mariat, C.; Maillard, N. Deletion Variants of CFHR1 and CFHR3 Associate with Mesangial Immune Deposits but Not with Progression of IgA Nephropathy. *J. Am. Soc. Nephrol.* **2018**, *29*, 661–669. [CrossRef]
155. Pesce, F.; Stea, E.D.; Divella, C.; Accetturo, M.; Laghetti, P.; Gallo, P.; Rossini, M.; Cianciotta, F.; Crispino, L.; Granata, A.; et al. DelCFHR3-1 influences graft survival in transplant patients with IgA nephropathy via complement-mediated cellular senescence. *Arab. Archaeol. Epigr.* **2021**, *21*, 838–845. [CrossRef]
156. Garred, P. Mannose-binding lectin deficiency—Revisited. *Mol. Immunol.* **2003**, *40*, 73–84. [CrossRef]
157. Garred, P.; Larsen, F.; Seyfarth, J.; Fujita, R.; Madsen, H.O. Mannose-binding lectin and its genetic variants. *Genes Immun.* **2006**, *7*, 85–94. [CrossRef]
158. Gong, Z.L.R. Mannose-binding Lectin Gene Polymorphism Associated with the Patterns of Glomerular Immune Deposition in IgA Nephropathy. *Scand. J. Urol. Nephrol.* **2001**, *35*, 228–232. [CrossRef]
159. Shi, B.; Wang, L.; Mou, S.; Zhang, M.; Wang, Q.; Qi, C.; Cao, L.; Che, X.; Fang, W.; Gu, L.; et al. Identification of mannose-binding lectin as a mechanism in progressive immunoglobulin A nephropathy. *Int. J. Clin. Exp. Pathol.* **2015**, *8*, 1889–1899.
160. Ouyang, Y.; Zhu, L.; Shi, M.; Yu, S.; Jin, Y.; Wang, Z.; Ma, J.; Yang, M.; Zhang, X.; Pan, X.; et al. A Rare Genetic Defect of MBL2 Increased the Risk for Progression of IgA Nephropathy. *Front. Immunol.* **2019**, *10*. [CrossRef]
161. Zhang, Y.; Yan, X.; Zhao, T.; Xu, Q.; Peng, Q.; Hu, R.; Quan, S.; Zhou, Y.; Xing, G. Targeting C3a/C5a receptors inhibits human mesangial cell proliferation and alleviates immunoglobulin A nephropathy in mice. *Clin. Exp. Immunol.* **2017**, *189*, 60–70. [CrossRef]
162. Bruchfeld, A.; Nachman, P.; Parikh, S.; Lafayette, R.; Potarca, A.; Diehl, J.; Lohr, L.; Miao, S.; Schall, T.; Bekker, P. TO012C5A Receptor Inhibitor avacopan in Iga Nephropathy study. *Nephrol. Dial. Transplant.* **2017**, *32*, iii82. [CrossRef]
163. Jayne, D.R.; Merkel, P.A.; Schall, T.J.; Bekker, P. Avacopan for the Treatment of ANCA—Associated Vasculitis. *N. Engl. J. Med.* **2021**, *384*, 599–609. [CrossRef] [PubMed]
164. Rosenblad, T.; Rebetz, J.; Johansson, M.; Békássy, Z.; Sartz, L.; Karpman, D. Eculizumab treatment for rescue of renal function in IgA nephropathy. *Pediatr. Nephrol.* **2014**, *29*, 2225–2228. [CrossRef] [PubMed]
165. Ring, T.; Pedersen, B.B.; Salkus, G.; Goodship, T.H. Use of eculizumab in crescentic IgA nephropathy: Proof of principle and conundrum? *Clin. Kidney J.* **2015**, *8*, 489–491. [CrossRef]
166. Herzog, A.; Wanner, C.; Amann, K.; Lopau, K. First Treatment of Relapsing Rapidly Progressive IgA Nephropathy With Eculizumab After Living Kidney Donation: A Case Report. *Transplant. Proc.* **2017**, *49*, 1574–1577. [CrossRef]
167. Hillmen, P.; Szer, J.; Weitz, I.; Röth, A.; Höchsmann, B.; Panse, J.; Usuki, K.; Griffin, M.; Kiladjian, J.-J.; de Castro, C.; et al. Pegcetacoplan versus Eculizumab in Paroxysmal Nocturnal Hemoglobinuria. *N. Engl. J. Med.* **2021**, *384*, 1028–1037. [CrossRef]
168. Systemic Pharmacodynamic Efficacy of a Complement Factor B Antisense Oligonucleotide in Preclinical and Phase 1 Clinical Studies. IOVS. ARVO Journals. Available online: https://iovs.arvojournals.org/article.aspx?articleid=2639711 (accessed on 2 September 2021).
169. Schubart, A.; Anderson, K.; Mainolfi, N.; Sellner, H.; Ehara, T.; Adams, C.M.; Mac Sweeney, A.; Liao, S.-M.; Crowley, M.; Littlewood-Evans, A.; et al. Small-molecule factor B inhibitor for the treatment of complement-mediated diseases. *Proc. Natl. Acad. Sci. USA* **2019**, *116*, 7926–7931. [CrossRef]
170. Lafayette, R.A.; Rovin, B.H.; Reich, H.N.; Tumlin, J.A.; Floege, J.; Barratt, J. Safety, Tolerability and Efficacy of Narsoplimab, a Novel MASP-2 Inhibitor for the Treatment of IgA Nephropathy. *Kidney Int. Rep.* **2020**, *5*, 2032–2041. [CrossRef]

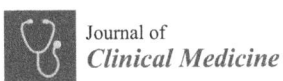

Article

The Role of Complement Component C3 Activation in the Clinical Presentation and Prognosis of IgA Nephropathy—A National Study in Children

Małgorzata Mizerska-Wasiak [1,*,†], Agnieszka Such-Gruchot [1,†], Karolina Cichoń-Kawa [1], Agnieszka Turczyn [1], Jadwiga Małdyk [2], Monika Miklaszewska [3], Dorota Drożdż [3], Agnieszka Firszt-Adamczyk [4], Roman Stankiewicz [4], Agnieszka Rybi-Szumińska [5], Anna Wasilewska [5], Maria Szczepańska [6], Beata Bieniaś [7], Przemysław Sikora [7], Agnieszka Pukajło-Marczyk [8], Danuta Zwolińska [8], Monika Pawlak-Bratkowska [9], Marcin Tkaczyk [9], Jacek Zachwieja [10], Magdalena Drożyńska-Duklas [11], Aleksandra Żurowska [11], Katarzyna Gadomska-Prokop [12], Ryszard Grenda [12] and Małgorzata Pańczyk-Tomaszewska [1]

1 Department of Pediatrics and Nephrology, Medical University of Warsaw, 02-091 Warsaw, Poland; agnieszkasuch.g@gmail.com (A.S.-G.); karolina.cichon@yahoo.com (K.C.-K.); agamosionek@gmail.com (A.T.); mpanczyk1@wum.edu.pl (M.P.-T.)
2 Department of Pathology, Medical University of Warsaw, 02-091 Warsaw, Poland; jagusia.maldyk@wp.pl
3 Department of Pediatric Nephrology and Hypertension, Jagiellonian University Medical College, 30-663 Cracow, Poland; mmiklasz@wp.pl (M.M.); dorota_drozdz@poczta.onet.pl (D.D.)
4 Department of Pediatrics and Nephrology, Ludwik Rydygier Hospital, 87-100 Torun, Poland; afirszt1@wp.pl (A.F.-A.); rstan@wp.pl (R.S.)
5 Department of Pediatrics and Nephrology, Medical University of Bialystok, 15-089 Bialystok, Poland; arybiszuminska@gmail.com (A.R.-S.); annwasil@interia.pl (A.W.)
6 Department of Pediatrics, SMDZ in Zabrze, Silesian Medical University, 41-808 Zabrze, Poland; szczep57@poczta.onet.pl
7 Department of Pediatric Nephrology, Medical University of Lublin, 20-059 Lublin, Poland; beatabienias@umlub.pl (B.B.); sikoraprzem@hotmail.com (P.S.)
8 Department of Pediatric Nephrology, Wroclaw Medical University, 50-367 Wroclaw, Poland; pukajlo@o2.pl (A.P.-M.); danuta.zwolinska@umed.wroc.pl (D.Z.)
9 Department of Pediatrics, Immunology and Nephrology, Polish Mothers Memorial Hospital Research Institute, 93-338 Lodz, Poland; monika.bratkowska@gmail.com (M.P.-B.); marcin.tkaczyk45@gmail.com (M.T.)
10 Department of Pediatric Nephrology and Dialysis, Medical University of Poznan, 61-701 Poznan, Poland; j.zachwieja@mp.pl
11 Department of Pediatrics, Nephrology and Hypertension, Medical University of Gdansk, 80-210 Gdansk, Poland; magdalena.drozynska-duklas@gumed.edu.pl (M.D.-D.); aleksandra.zurowska@gumed.edu.pl (A.Ż.)
12 Department of Nephrology, Kidney Transplantation and Hypertension, Children's Memorial Health Institute, 04-730 Warsaw, Poland; k.gadomska@czd.pl (K.G.-P.); r.grenda@ipczd.pl (R.G.)
* Correspondence: mmizerska@wum.edu.pl
† First author.

Abstract: The aim of the study was to evaluate the influence of the intensity of mesangial C3 deposits in kidney biopsy and the serum C3 level on the clinical course and outcomes of IgAN in children. The study included 148 children from the Polish Pediatric IgAN Registry, diagnosed based on kidney biopsy. Proteinuria, creatinine, IgA, C3 were evaluated twice in the study group, at baseline and the end of follow-up. Kidney biopsy was categorized using the Oxford classification, with a calculation of the MEST-C score. The intensity of IgA and C3 deposits were rated from 0 to +4 in immunofluorescence microscopy. The intensity of mesangial C3 > +1 deposits in kidney biopsy has an effect on renal survival with normal GFR in children with IgAN. A reduced serum C3 level has not been a prognostic factor in children but perhaps this finding should be confirmed in a larger group of children.

Keywords: IgA nephropathy; complement C3; children

1. Introduction

IgA nephropathy (IgAN) or Berger's disease is the most common chronic glomerulonephritis worldwide [1].

In Europe, it is diagnosed in 20% of kidney biopsies performed in childhood [2]. The condition is one of the major causes of end-stage renal disease (ESRD) which develops in 20–40% of patients at 20 years after the diagnosis [3].

The clinical presentation of IgAN may vary, reflecting a wide range of histological findings, from no changes on light microscopy to severe necrotizing lesions with crescents [4]. Clinically, IgAN manifests with persistent or periodic erythrocyturia, either isolated or with concomitant proteinuria of varying severity, sometimes accompanied by hypertension.

The gold standard for the diagnosis of IgAN is the evaluation of a kidney biopsy specimen. The disease is diagnosed based on the predominant IgA deposits on histopathological evaluation. The deposits may also include immunoglobulins M or G. In 90% of cases, the complement component C3 is also identified in the kidney biopsy specimen [3,5]. The Oxford classification (MEST-C) used to evaluate kidney biopsies allows the assessment of risk factors for future renal failure [6].

Proteinuria, reduction of the glomerular filtration rate (GFR), hypertension, old age, male sex and the absence of macroscopic hematuria are independent predictors of a poor outcome of the disease [7–11].

The pathophysiology of the disease is not entirely understood. According to the "four-hits" theory, the initial underlying insult is overproduction of abnormal, galactose-deficient immunoglobulin A1 (GdIgA1) which forms polymers (first hit). Then, specific IgA and/or IgG antibodies against the abnormal IgA1 are produced (second hit), combining and forming circulating immune complexes (third hit). These complexes accumulate in the renal mesangium, inducing a chronic inflammatory response by increased cytokine and growth factor production, which leads to cellular proliferation and mesangial matrix expansion (fourth hit) [2,12,13]. Chronic inflammation results in renal parenchymal fibrosis and progressive renal failure.

A key role in the pathogenesis and progression of IgAN is played by the complement system activation [3,14,15]. IgAN-associated processes involve the alternative and lectin pathways. The processes associated with complement activation likely occur systemically, in the circulating IgA-containing immune complexes and the glomeruli [16].

In the immune system, the ultimate effect of the complement system activation is the formation of C5b-9 sequence (membrane attacking complex, MAC) which perforates the cell membranes of pathogens. Mesangial MAC deposits are commonly observed in IgAN, and its presence is identified by the detection of C9 neoantigen corresponding to the C5b-9. Urinary excretion of the soluble form of MAC was found to be increased in patients with IgAN, likely due to complement activation in the urinary space [16].

The aim of the study was to evaluate the influence of the severity of mesangial C3 deposits in kidney biopsy specimens and the serum C3 level on the clinical course and outcomes of IgAN in children.

2. Material and Methods

The study included 148 children (91 boys and 56 girls) from the 166 patients included in the Polish Pediatric IgAN Registry. The patients included in the study fulfilled the following inclusion criteria: IgAN diagnosed based on kidney biopsy with evaluation by light microscopy and immunofluorescence. Patients without complete clinical and histopathological data, with the glomerular number < 8, with secondary IgAN and IgA vasculitis nephritis (IgAVN, Henoch-Schönlein nephritis) were excluded from the study.

Proteinuria and serum levels of albumin, creatinine, IgA, C3 and C4 were evaluated twice in the study group, at baseline and the end of follow-up.

Nephrotic range proteinuria was defined as ≥ 50 mg/kg/d, and non-nephrotic range proteinuria as <50 mg/kg/d, and urinary protein was measured by the Exton method. Serum creatinine level, expressed in mg/dL, was measured by the dry chemistry method

(Vitro, Ortho Clinical Diagnostic). GFR (mL/min/1.73 m^2) was estimated using the Schwartz formula. Immunoglobulin A and complement component C3 and C4 serum levels were measured by the nephelometric method in 5 centers and by the turbidimetric method in 3 centers. The use of two different methods for assaying immunoglobulin A and C3 and C4 were related to the retrospective nature of the study conducted in various centers. Referring to studies by Denham et al. which indicate good agreement between methods in determining protein levels, including IgA and C3, we considered it as a limitation of the study, but the age-related reference ranges did not differ significantly between the centers [17].

A diagnostic kidney biopsy was performed on all children in the study group.

The specimens from each kidney biopsy were routinely evaluated using light microscopy, immunofluorescence and electron microscopy by at least two pathologists.

Kidney biopsy specimens were routinely evaluated by light microscopy and immunofluorescence, and categorized using the Oxford classification, with a calculation of the MEST-C score (1—present, 0—absent; M—mesangial hypercellularity; E—endocapillary hypercellularity; S—segmental sclerosis/adhesion; T—tubular atrophy/interstitial fibrosis T0 0–25%, T1 26–50%, T2 > 50%; C—crescents, C0 0%, C1 0–25%, C2 > 25%; with the overall score calculated as the sum of M, E, S, T and C).

When evaluated by immunofluorescence microscopy, the intensity of IgA and C3 deposits were rated from 0 to +4.

The patients received renoprotective therapy (angiotensin-converting enzyme inhibitor [ACEI]/angiotensin receptor blocker [ARB]), glucocorticosteroids (Encorton) or immunosuppressive drugs such as azathioprine, cyclophosphamide, cyclosporin A and mycophenolate mofetil. Drug treatment was categorized as I—immunosuppression, S—steroids, R—renoprotection.

The study endpoint was an abnormal glomerular filtration rate (eGFR <90 mL/min).

The study was approved by the Bioethics Committee at the Medical University of Warsaw (No. KB/147/2017). Informed consent for study participation was obtained from the legal guardians of the study participants.

Flow diagram of the study is shown in Figure 1.

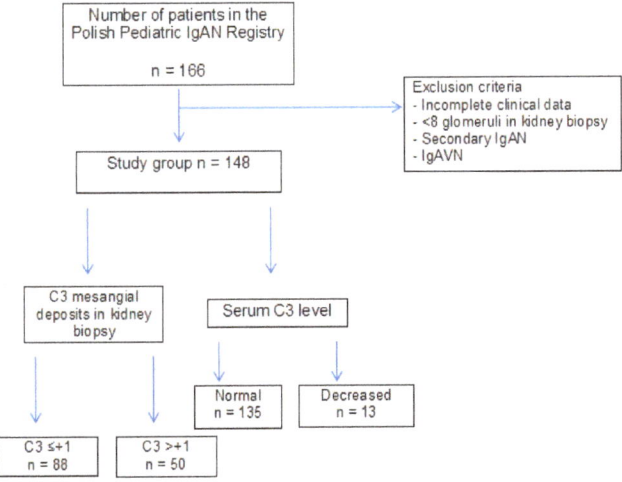

Figure 1. Flow diagram of the study.

Statistical Analysis

Statistical analysis was performed using the Dell Statistica 13.0 PL software. The results were expressed as the mean values and standard deviation for normally distributed variables and as the median and range for non-normally distributed variables. The normality of distributions was evaluated using the Lilliefors and Shapiro-Wilk tests. The significance of differences between the mean values was evaluated using the ANOVA for normally distributed variables and the Kruskal-Wallis test for non-normally distributed variables. The significance of differences between groups was determined using the Student t-test (for normally distributed variables) and the Mann-Whitney test (for non-normally distributed variables). To evaluate differences between baseline and follow-up values, the Student t- test and the Wilcoxon test were used (for normally and non-normally distributed variables, respectively). $p < 0.05$ was considered statistically significant. The Kaplan-Meier and Cox regression analyses were performed to calculate renal survival.

3. Results

The characteristics of the study group are shown in Table 1.

Table 1. Characteristics of the study group.

Parameter	IgAN (n = 148)
Age at disease onset (years)	11.6 ± 4.29
Gender (M/F)	91/57
Time to biopsy (years)	1.2 ± 1.77
Proteinuria (mg/kg/d)	14.0 (0.0–967.0)
GFR (mL/min/1.73 m^2)	95.75 ± 33.56
Creatinine (mg/dL)	0.73 ± 0.33
Albumin (mg/dL)	3.84 ± 0.86
IgA (mg/dL)	275.91 ± 134.45
C3 (mg/dL)	118.12 ± 29.54
C4 (mg/dL)	23.55 ± 8.25
IgA deposits in kidney biopsy/number of patients (n%)	148 (100%)
C3 deposits in kidney biopsy (n%)	98 (66.2%)
Duration of follow-up (years)	3.75 ± 2.90
Age at FU (years)	15.26 ± 3.84
Proteinuria at FU (mg/kg/d)	0.0 (0–370.0)
GFR at FU (mL/min/1.73 m^2)	100.65 ± 22.86
Creatinine at FU (mg/dL)	0.71 ± 0.22
Albumin at FU (mg/dL)	4.3 ± 0.48
IgA at FU (mg/dL)	257.26 ± 122.38
C3 at FU (mg/dL)	106.61 ± 24.87
C4 at FU (mg/dL)	22.61 ± 14.67
Treatment:	
ACEI/ARB/none	43.24% (n = 64)
Glucocorticosteroids alone	29.73% (n = 44)
Immunosuppression + glucocorticosteroids	16.21% (n = 24)

ACEI—angiotensin-converting enzyme inhibitor; ARB—angiotensin receptor blocker; FU—end of follow-up; n—number of patients.

The mean age at the diagnosis of IgAN was 11 ± 4.29 years. Boys and girls comprised 61.47% and 38.53% of the study group, respectively. A kidney biopsy was performed on average 1.2 ± 1.77 years since the initial symptoms, and the mean duration of follow-up was 45 ± 30.75 months.

At baseline, the mean proteinuria was 44.57 ± 120.04 mg/kg/d, creatinine level was 0.73 ± 0.33 mg/dL, and GFR was 96.75 ± 33.56 mL/min/1.73 m^2. At the end of follow-up, the mean proteinuria was 10.11 ± 35.84 mg/kg/d, creatinine level was 0.71 ± 0.22 mg/dL and GFR was 100.65 ± 22.86 mL/min/1.73 m^2.

At baseline, an elevated IgA level was noted in 73 patients (49.32%), and reduced C3 and C4 levels in 13 (8.78%) and 17 patients (11.49%), respectively. At the end of follow-up, an elevated IgA level was noted in 47 patients (31.76%), reduced C3 level in 12 (8.10%) and reduced C4 level in 26 patients (17.57%).

GFR was <90 mL/min in 58 (39.19%) children at baseline and in 46 (31.08%) children at the end of follow-up.

Regarding to the evaluation by the Oxford classification, mesangial hypercellularity (M1) was present in 81.76% of patients in the study group, endocapillary hypercellularity (E1) in 23.65%, segmental sclerosis (S1) in 28.39%, interstitial fibrosis/tubular atrophy (T1/2) in 18.24% and cellular/fibrocellular crescents (C1/2) in 27.7%.

The study group was categorized based on the presence of C3 deposits in kidney biopsy specimens. Low severity of C3 deposits was defined as C3 ≤ +1, and high severity as C3 > +1. Depending on the presence of C3 deposits in kidney biopsy specimens, the patients were divided into two groups: group A—C3 ≤ 1, group B—C3 > 1. The duration of follow-up was 4.19 ± 3.05 years in group A, and 2.91 ± 2.46 years in group B.

The clinical characteristics of the study patients divided into two groups based on the severity of C3 deposits are shown in Table 2.

Table 2. Clinical characteristics of the patient groups based on the severity of C3 deposits.

	Group A (n = 98) C3 ≤ +1	Group B (n = 50) C3 > +1	p
Age at diagnosis (years)	11.26 ± 4.39	12.34 ± 4.06	NS
Proteinuria at baseline (mg/kg/d)	14.0 (0–968)	15.0 (0–202)	NS
Creatinine at baseline (mg/dL)	0.72 ± 0.36	0.76 ± 0.25	NS
GFR at baseline (mL/min)	96.45 ± 35.26	94.44 ± 30.96	NS
Time to biopsy (years)	1.33 ± 1.96 median 0.52	0.92 ± 13.31 median 0.31	NS ($p = 0.06$)
Intensity of IgA deposits (n%)			
+1	47 46.5 %	1 2.0 %	
+2	23 23.2	6 12.0	$p < 0.00001$
+3	20 20.2	23 46.0	
+4	9 9.1	20 40.0	
Overall MEST-C score	1.61 ± 1.08	1.67 ± 1.04	NS
M1 n (%)	79 (80.6%)	42 (84.0%)	
E1 n (%)	25 (25.5%)	10 (20.0%)	
S1 n (%)	24 (24.5%)	18 (36.0%)	
T1-2 n (%)	17 (17.4%)	10 (20.0%)	
C1-2 n (%)	28 (28.6%)	13 (26.0%)	
Duration of follow-up (years)	4.19 ± 3.05	2.91 ± 2.46	$p < 0.05$
Proteinuria at FU (mg/kg/d)	0.0 (0–370)	0.0 (0–84)	NS
Creatinine at FU (mg/dL)	0.71 ± 0.21	0.7 ± 0.16	NS
GFR at FU (mL/min)	101.0 ± 24.45	100.62 ± 20.13	NS
Treatment:			
ACEI/ARB/none	59.2% (n = 58)	42.0% (n = 21)	$p < 0.05$
Glucocorticosteroids alone	13.3% (n = 13)	22.0% (n = 11)	NS
Immunosuppression + glucocorticosteroids	27.6% (n = 27)	34.0% (n = 17)	NS

ACEI—angiotensin-converting enzyme inhibitor; ARB—angiotensin receptor blocker; FU—end of follow-up; n—number of patients.

No differences between group A (n = 98) and group B (n = 50) were found regarding to proteinuria and GFR at baseline and the end of follow-up. Serum creatinine level and severity of IgA and C3 deposits in kidney biopsy were significantly higher in group B ($p < 0.01$).

There were no significant differences between the two groups regarding to the overall MEST-C score.

Renoprotective treatment was used in 58 (59.2%) patients in group A and 21 (42.0%) patients in group B. Glucocorticosteroids were used in 13 (13.3%) patients in group A and 11 (22.0%) patients in group B. Immunosuppressive therapy was administered in 27 (27.6%) patients in group A and 17 (34.0%) patients in group B. Regarding to the drug treatment used, there was a significant difference only in renoprotective treatment between the two groups, there were no significant differences in glucocorticosteroids and immunosuppressive therapy.

There was no difference in the mean GFR at the end of follow-up between patients in groups A and B, as well the percentages of patients with GFR >90 and <90 mL/min ($p = 0.08$).

Survival curve analysis using the Cox proportional hazard model showed a shorter duration of renal survival with normal GFR in children in group B (C3 >1 in kidney biopsy) compared to group A (C3 $\leq$ 1) (Figure 2). In the survival curve analysis, factors affecting longer renal survival with normal GFR included female gender (F > M, Figure 3), older age at the diagnosis and normal GFR at the onset of the disease (Figure 4).

The study group was also divided regarding to the MEST-C score (group I—MEST-C score $\leq$ 1, group II—MEST-C score > 1). The clinical characteristics of patients in these two groups are shown in Table 3. There were no significant differences between groups I and II regarding to albumin, C3 and C4 levels at baseline and the end of follow-up, and the severity of IgA, IgG and IgM deposits in kidney biopsy. Serum creatinine level at baseline was significantly higher in group II ($p < 0.001$), as was IgA level ($p < 0.01$). A significant difference was also found in GFR at baseline (group I > II; $p < 0.01$). At the end of follow-up, a significant difference was noted only for proteinuria which was higher in group II ($p < 0.05$).

Table 3. Clinical characteristics of the patient groups based on the MEST-C score.

	Group I MEST-C $\leq$ 1	Group II MEST-C > 1	p
Age at diagnosis (years)	11.05 ± 4.14	12.52 ± 4.15	NS
Proteinuria at baseline (mg/kg/d)	12.8 (0–920)	16.4 (0–967)	NS
Creatinine at baseline (mg/dL)	0.64 ± 0.18	0.84 ± 0.42	$p < 0.001$
GFR at baseline (mL/min)	104.96 ± 37.32	86.5 ± 30.63	$p < 0.01$
Albumin (mg/dL)	3.99 ± 0.69	3.72 ± 0.91	NS
IgA (mg/dL)	251.04 ± 125.97	309.61 ± 139.45	$p < 0.01$
C3 (mg/dL)	122.83 ± 30.43	116.58 ± 28.3	NS
C4 (mg/dL)	23.21 ± 7.54	24.78 ± 9.1	NS
Intensity of IgA deposits (n%)			
+1	18 (24.3%)	25 (35.7%)	
+2	15 (20.3%)	14 (20.0%)	NS
+3	22 (29.7%)	21 (30.0%)	
+4	19 (25.7%)	10 (14.3%)	
Duration of follow-up (years)	4.27 ± 3.21	3.41 ± 2.53	NS
Proteinuria at FU (mg/kg/d)	0.0 (0–68)	0.0 (0–97)	$p < 0.05$
Creatinine at FU (mg/dL)	0.73 ± 0.19	0.71 ± 0.22	NS
GFR at FU (mL/min)	97.98 ± 20.72	99.37 ± 22.42	NS
Albumin (mg/dL)	4.37 ± 0.47	4.32 ± 0.36	NS
IgA (mg/dL)	248 ± 102.34	285.16 ± 138.75	NS
C3 (mg/dL)	106.13 ± 24.71	105.32 ± 25.59	NS
C4 (mg/dL)	19.86 ± 6.35	25.21 ± 18.97	NS

FU—end of follow-up.

The study group was also divided based on serum C3 level (Group 1—serum C3 level below the reference range, Group 2—serum C3 level within the reference range). The clinical characteristics of patients in these two groups are shown in Table 4. No significant differences between Groups 1 and 2 were found regarding to the severity of proteinuria, GFR and creatinine, albumin and IgA levels at baseline and at the end of follow-up, as well as the intensity of IgA deposits in renal biopsy. Serum C4 level at baseline was significantly higher in Group 2 ($p = 0.01$) but no significant difference in C4 level was found between the groups at the end of follow-up.

Table 4. Clinical characteristics of the patient groups based on serum C3 level.

	Group 1 (*n* = 13) C3 below Reference Range	Group 2 (*n* = 135) C3 within Reference Range	*p*
Age at diagnosis (years)	10.97 ± 3.95	11.65 ± 4.29	NS
Proteinuria at baseline (mg/kg/d)	15.0 (0–967)	14.46 (0–920)	NS
Creatinine at baseline (mg/dL)	0.61 ± 0.22	0.76 ± 0.35	NS, $p = 0.06$
GFR at baseline (mL/min)	104.73 ± 43.32	95.54 ± 31.71	
Albumin (mg/dL)	3.99 ± 0.69	3.72 ± 0.91	NS
IgA (mg/dL)	232.13 ± 64.38	282.2 ± 140.54	NS
C4 (mg/dL)	18.27 ± 4.43	24.07 ± 8.37	$p = 0.01$
Intensity of IgA deposits (*n*%)			
+1	31 (26.0%)	3 (23.0%)	
+2	24 (20.2%)	4 (30.8%)	NS
+3	38 (31.9%)	3 (23.1%)	
+4	26 (21.9%)	3 (23.1%)	
Duration of follow-up (years)	4.11 ± 2.57	3.63 ± 2.94	NS
Proteinuria at FU (mg/kg/d)	0.0 (0–11.4)	0.0 (0–370)	NS
Creatinine at FU (mg/dL)	0.63 ± 0.11	0.72 ± 0.22	NS
GFR at FU (mL/min)	109.57 ± 14.89	100.13 ± 23.0	NS, $p = 0.07$
Albumin (mg/dL)	4.21 ± 0.36	4.33 ± 0.44	NS
IgA (mg/dL)	206.59 ± 60.0	264.63 ± 129.37	NS
C4 (mg/dL)	23.8 ± 17.58	21.95 ± 14.26	NS

FU—end of follow-up.

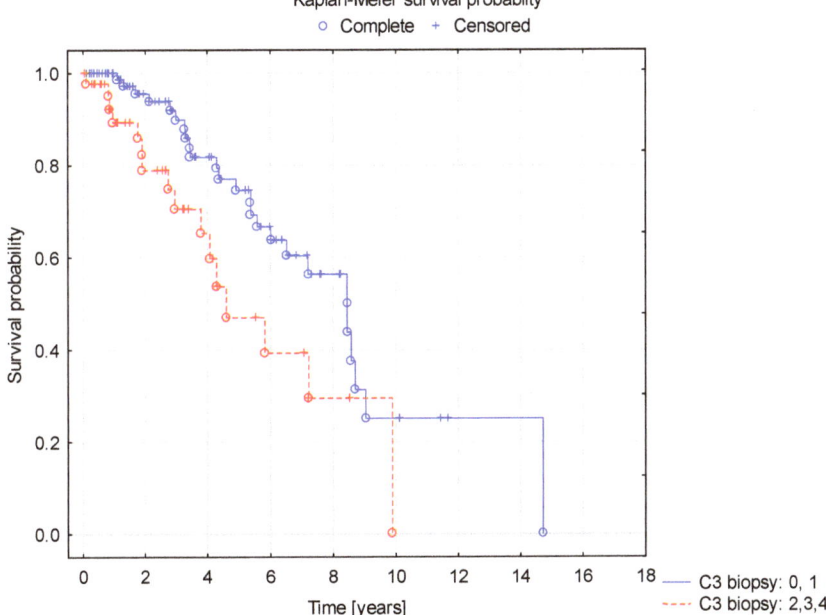

Figure 2. Shorter renal survival with normal GFR in Group B (intensity of C3 deposits = +2, +3, +4) vs. Group A (intensity of C3 deposits = 0, +1).

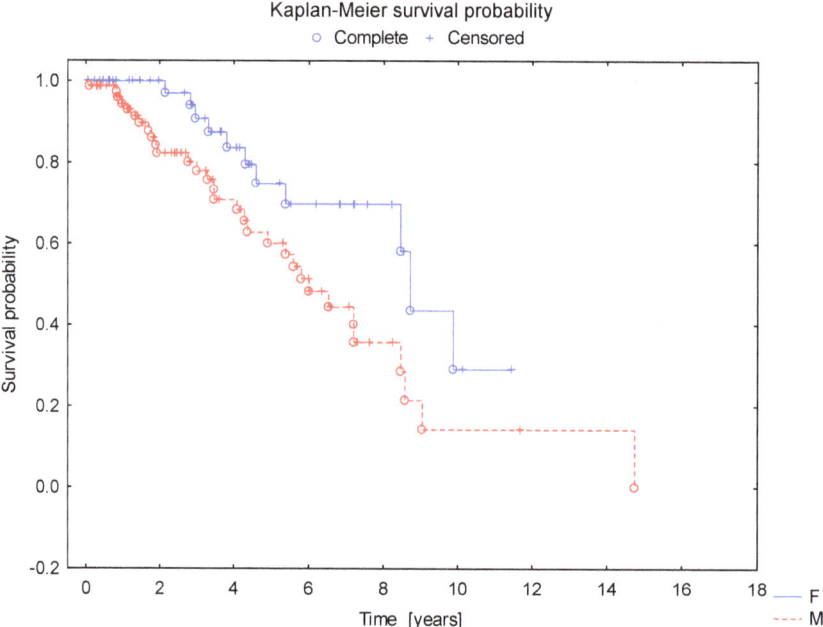

Figure 3. Shorter renal survival with normal GFR in males vs. females.

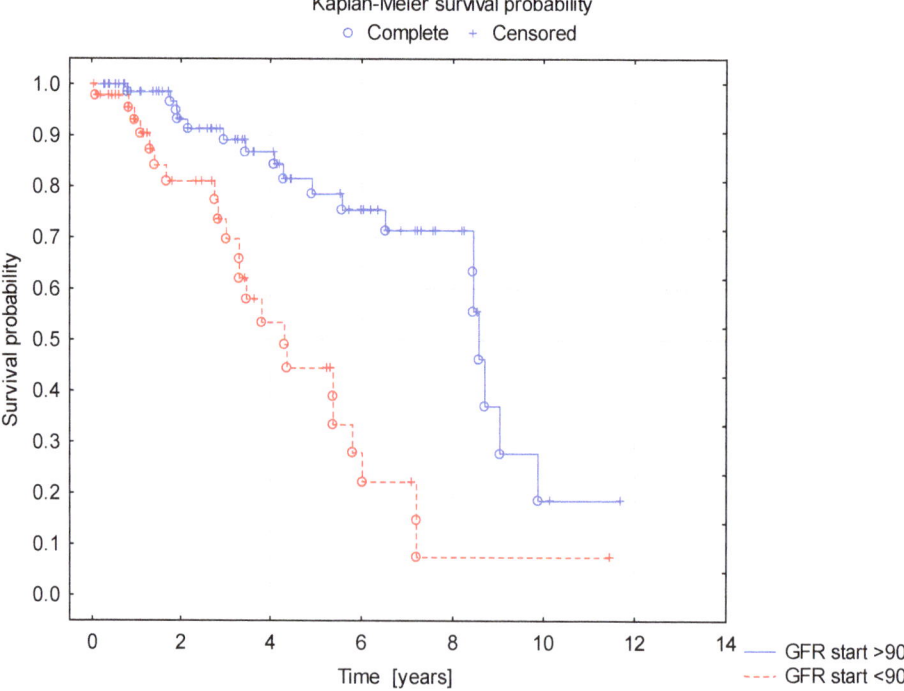

Figure 4. Shorter renal survival with normal GFR in patients with reduced GFR (<90 mL/min) at the time of the diagnosis.

Survival curve analysis using the Cox proportional hazard model showed no difference in renal survival with normal GFR between groups with normal and reduced serum C3 levels at baseline.

4. Discussion

In this retrospective study, we performed a detailed evaluation of the importance of C3 in kidney biopsy specimens and serum for the outcomes of IgAN in children. We found that the presence of >+1 C3 deposits in kidney biopsy is a predictor of worsening renal function (GFR < 90 mL/min) in this group of children, which is the first such study in a large sample collected throughout a European country. However, we did not show similar importance of a reduced serum C3 level at the onset of the disease.

In the study population, C3 deposits in kidney biopsy, mostly rated at +1 or +2, were identified in 66% of patients, which is a rate similar to that reported in an adult population studied by Wu et al. [18].

In patients with IgAN, immune complexes may activate the alternative and lectin pathways of the complement system and initiate inflammation [13,15,19]. Recent studies in adult patients show that the severity of C3 deposits in kidney biopsy and reduced serum C3 level may affect long-term renal outcomes [3,20–22].

In our study from 2015, we evaluated the usefulness of serum Immunoglobulin A/complement factor 3 (IgA/C3) ratio for predicting the severity of histological lesions in kidney biopsy children with IgA nephropathy. We found positive correlations between the IgA/C3 ratio and proteinuria, serum creatinine and serum IgA level. We also determined that the higher the MEST score the higher the IgA/C3 ratio. We also determined the optimal cutoff values of IgA/C3 serum ratio for specific MEST score [23].

In the study by Caliskan et al. in 111 adult patients with IgAN, C3 deposits > +1 were found to be a prognostic factor for the development of chronic kidney disease (CKD) stage G5 or reduction in GFR by ≥50% compared to the baseline [20].

We also confirmed the importance of C3 standing > +1 as an adverse prognostic factor for renal survival in children but in our study, the endpoint was GFR < 90 mL/min, and thus we demonstrated the prognostic significance of C3 deposits for CKD from stage G2 onwards, which is a novel finding, and these observations were made in children, which also contrasts to the conclusions from the studies in adult patients with IgAN [20].

In the study by Kim and Koo in 66 adult patients with IgAN, a prognostically adverse effect of C3 deposits > +1 for the development of ESRD or doubling of serum creatinine level was also shown, and this study also showed an effect of reduced serum C3 level on the renal outcomes, although its predictive value was lower than that of the urinary protein to creatinine ratio [22]. In our study, we were unable to confirm the effect of reduced serum C3 level on renal survival with normal GFR but this may have been related to a low number of children (n = 13, or 8.78%) with reduced serum C3 level at baseline. This finding needs to be replicated in a larger patient sample.

An additional, though already previously known finding of our study is confirmation of an adverse effect of male gender and reduced GFR at baseline on long-term renal outcomes [8–11].

Among children with C3 deposits > +1 and those with a reduced serum C3 level at baseline, we did not find significant differences in the MEST-C score, similarly to the study by Kim et al. who did not find significant differences in the rates of M, E, S and T between groups with C3 deposits > +1 and ≤ +1 [22].

In addition, we found a reduced serum C3 level at the end of follow-up in 10 patients, of whom 3 showed a reduced serum C3 level at baseline. Of these, only one patient had GFR < 90 mL/min at the end of follow-up, which might also confirm no prognostic significance of a reduced serum C3 level at baseline in children, but again, these patient groups were too small to allow any definitive conclusions.

5. Conclusions

The severity of mesangial C3 deposits in kidney biopsy rated > +1 has an effect on renal survival with normal GFR in children with IgAN. A reduced serum C3 level has not been a prognostic factor in this group of children but perhaps this finding should be confirmed in a larger group of children.

Author Contributions: Conceptualization, M.M.-W., A.S.-G. and K.C.-K.; methodology, M.M.-W.; validation, M.M.-W., A.S.-G. and A.T.; formal analysis, M.M.-W. and A.S.-G.; investigation, M.M.-W., A.S.-G. and K.C.-K.; resources, M.M.-W., A.S.-G., K.C.-K., A.T., J.M., M.M., D.D., A.F.-A., R.S., A.R.-S., A.W., M.S., B.B., P.S., A.P.-M., D.Z., M.P.-B., M.T., J.Z., M.D.-D., A.Ż., K.G.-P. and R.G.; data curation, M.M.-W., A.S.-G., K.C.-K., A.T., J.M., M.M., D.D., A.F.-A., R.S., A.R.-S., A.W., M.S., B.B., P.S., A.P.-M., D.Z., M.P.-B., M.T., J.Z., M.D.-D., A.Ż., K.G.-P. and R.G.; writing—M.M.-W. and A.S.-G.; writing—review and editing, M.M.-W., A.S.-G., K.C.-K. and M.P.-T.; supervision M.P.-T. All authors have read and agreed to the published version of the manuscript.

Funding: This research received no external funding.

Institutional Review Board Statement: The study was conducted according to the guidelines of the Declaration of Helsinki, and approved by the Bioethics Committee at the Medical University of Warsaw (No. KB/147/2017).

Informed Consent Statement: Informed consent for study participation was obtained from the legal guardians of the study participants.

Data Availability Statement: The data analyzed in this study are available from the corresponding author on reasonable request.

Conflicts of Interest: The authors declare no conflict of interest.

References

1. Berthoux, F.C.; Mohey, H.; Afiani, A. Natural history of primary IgA nephropathy. *Semin. Nephrol.* **2008**, *28*, 4–9. [CrossRef] [PubMed]
2. Coppo, R.; Robert, T. IgA nephropathy in children and in adults: Two separate entities or the same disease? *J. Nephrol.* **2020**, *33*, 1219–1229. [CrossRef] [PubMed]
3. Rizk, D.V.; Maillard, N.; Julian, B.A.; Knoppova, B.; Green, T.J.; Novak, J.; Wyatt, R.J. The Emerging Role of Complement Proteins as a Target for Therapy of IgA Nephropathy. *Front. Immunol.* **2019**, *10*, 504. [CrossRef]
4. Bellur, S.S.; Troyanov, S.; Cook, H.T.; Roberts, I.S.D.; Working Group of the International IgA Nephropathy Network and the Renal Pathology Society. Immunostaining findings in IgA nephropathy: Correlation with histology and clinical outcome in the Oxford classification patient cohort. *Nephrol. Dial. Transplant.* **2011**, *26*, 2533–2536. [CrossRef]
5. Jenette, J.C. The immunohistology of IgA nephropathy. *Am. J. Kidney Dis.* **1988**, *12*, 348–352. [CrossRef]
6. Trimarchi, H.; Barratt, J.; Cattran, D.C. Oxford Classification of IgA nephropathy 2016: An update from the IgA Nephropathy Classification Working Group. *Kidney Int.* **2017**, *91*, 1014–1021. [CrossRef]
7. Coppo, R. Pediatric IgA Nephropathy in Europe. *Kidney Dis.* **2019**, *5*, 182–188. [CrossRef]
8. Caliskan, Y.; Kiryluk, K. Novel Biomarkers in Glomerular Disease. *Adv. Chronic Kidney Dis.* **2014**, *21*, 205–216. [CrossRef]
9. Tan, M.; Li, W.; Zou, G.; Zhang, C.; Fang, J. Clinicopathological Features and Outcomes of IgA Nephropathy with Hematuria and/or Minimal Proteinuria. *Kidney Blood Press. Res.* **2015**, *40*, 200–206. [CrossRef]
10. Goto, M.; Wakai, K.; Kawamura, T.; Ando, M.; Endoh, M.; Tomino, Y. A scoring system to predict renal outcome in IgA nephropathy: A nationwide 10-year prospective cohort study. *Nephrol. Dial. Transplant.* **2009**, *24*, 3068–3074. [CrossRef]
11. Maixnerova, D.; Neprasova, M.; Skibova, J.; Mokrisova, J.; Rysava, R.; Reiterova, J.; Jancova, E.; Merta, M.; Zadrazil, J.; Honsova, E. Tesar V: IgA nephropathy in Czech patients—Are we able reliably predict the outcome? *Kidney Blood Press. Res.* **2014**, *39*, 555–562. [CrossRef]
12. Suzuki, H. Biomarkers for IgA nephropathy on the basis of multi-hit pathogenesis. *Clin. Exp. Nephrol.* **2019**, *23*, 26–31. [CrossRef]
13. Al Hussain, T.; Hussein, M.H.; Al Mana, H.; Akhtar, M. Pathophysiology of IgA Nephropathy. *Adv. Anat. Pathol.* **2017**, *24*, 56–62. [CrossRef] [PubMed]
14. Daha, M.R.; van Kooten, C. Role of complement in IgA nephropathy. *J. Nephrol.* **2016**, *29*, 14. [CrossRef]
15. Seelen, M.A.J.; Roos, A.; Daha, M.R. Role of complement in innate and autoimmunity. *J. Nephrol.* **2005**, *18*, 642–653. [PubMed]
16. Mailiard, N.; Wyatt, N.J.; Julian, B.A. Current Understanding of the Role of Complement in IgA Nephropathy. *J. Am. Soc. Nephrol.* **2015**, *26*, 1503–1512. [CrossRef] [PubMed]
17. Denham, E.; Mohn, B.; Tucker, L.; Lun, A.; Cleave, P.; Boswell, D.R. Evaluation of immunoturbidimetric specific protein methods using the Architect ci8200: Comparison with immunonephelometry. *Ann. Clin. Biochem.* **2007**, *44*, 529–536. [CrossRef] [PubMed]

18. Wu, L.; Liu, D.; Xia, M.; Chen, G.; Liu, Y.; Zhu, X.; Liu, H. Immunofluorescence deposits in the mesangial area and glomerular capillary loops did not affect the prognosis of immunoglobulin a nephropathy except C1q: A single-center retrospective study. *BMC Nephrol.* **2021**, *22*, 43. [CrossRef]
19. Roos, A.; Bouwman, L.H.; Van Gijlswijk-Janssen, D.J.; Faber-Krol, M.C.; Stahl, G.; Daha, M.R. Human IgA Activates the Complement System Via the Mannan-Binding Lectin Pathway. *J. Immunol.* **2001**, *167*, 2861–2868. [CrossRef]
20. Caliskan, Y.; Ozluk, Y.; Celik, D.; Oztop, N.; Aksoy, A.; Ucar, A.S.; Yazici, H.; Kilicaslan, I.; Sever, M.S. The Clinical Significance of Uric Acid and Complement Activation in the Progression of IgA Nephropathy. *Kidney Blood Press. Res.* **2016**, *41*, 148–157. [CrossRef]
21. Nam, K.H.; Joo, Y.S.; Lee, C.; Lee, S.; Kim, J.; Yun, H.-R.; Park, J.T.; Chang, T.I.; Ryu, D.-R.; Yoo, T.-H.; et al. Predictive value of mesangial C3 and C4d deposition in IgA nephropathy. *Clin. Immunol.* **2020**, *211*, 108331. [CrossRef] [PubMed]
22. Kim, S.J.; Koo, H.M.; Lim, B.J.; Oh, H.J.; Yoo, D.E.; Shin, D.H.; Lee, M.J.; Doh, F.M.; Park, J.T.; Yoo, T.-H.; et al. Decreased Circulating C3 Levels and Mesangial C3 Deposition Predict Renal Outcome in Patients with IgA Nephropathy. *PLoS ONE* **2012**, *7*, e40495. [CrossRef] [PubMed]
23. Mizerska-Wasiak, M.; Małdyk, J.; Rybi-Szuminska, A.; Wasilewska, A.; Miklaszewska, M.; Pietrzyk, J.; Firszt-Adamczyk, A.; Stankiewicz, R.; Bieniaś, B.; Zajączkowska, M.; et al. Relationship between serum IgA/C3 ratio and severity of histological lesions using the Oxford classification in children with IgA nephropathy. *Pediatr. Nephrol.* **2015**, *30*, 1113–1120. [CrossRef] [PubMed]

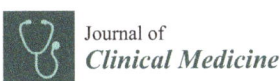

Review

IgA Vasculitis and IgA Nephropathy: Same Disease?

Evangeline Pillebout [1,2]

[1] Nephrology Unit, Saint-Louis Hospital, 75010 Paris, France; evangeline.pillebout@aphp.fr
[2] INSERM 1149, Center of Research on Inflammation, 75870 Paris, France

Abstract: Many authors suggested that IgA Vasculitis (IgAV) and IgA Nephropathy (IgAN) would be two clinical manifestations of the same disease; in particular, that IgAV would be the systemic form of the IgAN. A limited number of studies have included sufficient children or adults with IgAN or IgAV (with or without nephropathy) and followed long enough to conclude on differences or similarities in terms of clinical, biological or histological presentation, physiopathology, genetics or prognosis. All therapeutic trials available on IgAN excluded patients with vasculitis. IgAV and IgAN could represent different extremities of a continuous spectrum of the same disease. Due to skin rash, patients with IgAV are diagnosed precociously. Conversely, because of the absence of any clinical signs, a renal biopsy is practiced for patients with an IgAN to confirm nephropathy at any time of the evolution of the disease, which could explain the frequent chronic lesions at diagnosis. Nevertheless, the question that remains unsolved is why do patients with IgAN not have skin lesions and some patients with IgAV not have nephropathy? Larger clinical studies are needed, including both diseases, with a common histological classification, and stratified on age and genetic background to assess renal prognosis and therapeutic strategies.

Keywords: IgA Vasculitis; IgA Nephropathy; adults; children; presentation; physiopathology; genetics; prognosis; treatment

---

Citation: Pillebout, E. IgA Vasculitis and IgA Nephropathy: Same Disease?. *J. Clin. Med.* **2021**, *10*, 2310. https://doi.org/10.3390/jcm10112310

Academic Editor: Hitoshi Suzuki

Received: 8 April 2021
Accepted: 19 May 2021
Published: 25 May 2021

Publisher's Note: MDPI stays neutral with regard to jurisdictional claims in published maps and institutional affiliations.

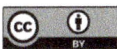

Copyright: © 2021 by the author. Licensee MDPI, Basel, Switzerland. This article is an open access article distributed under the terms and conditions of the Creative Commons Attribution (CC BY) license (https://creativecommons.org/licenses/by/4.0/).

1. Introduction

Since the first descriptions, in the last century, of IgA Nephropathy, at the time called Berger's disease, and IgA vasculitis called Henoch-Schönlein Purpura, the authors suggested that they were two clinical manifestations of the same disease. Recent advances in understanding pathophysiological mechanisms of these two entities have only reinforced this idea. Nevertheless, scientific arguments confirming this hypothesis are scarce.

Many, rather old, clinical cases have been published. They describe episodes of one or the other disease within the same siblings, in particular in homozygous twins [1], simultaneously or successively [2], in a father and son [3], in the same patient at two periods of his life [4–7] and, more recently, recurrences in kidney allograft in one form or another [8–10].

Four rather exhaustive reviews have been published [1,11–13], collecting these cases and gathering data over time to argue in favor of the hypothesis of a common disease. The last review dates from ten years ago. Since then, some clinical studies have been issued, but they are unfortunately too rare.

Indeed, only clinical studies involving patients with IgA vasculitis (IgAV) or IgA Nephropathy (IgAN) within the same cohort would reveal differences or similarities in terms of epidemiology, presentation, prognosis, sensitivity to treatment, physiopathology, biomarkers, and genetics.

2. Epidemiology

Apart from the obvious differences in extra-renal clinical presentation, the main difference between IgAV and IgAN is epidemiological (Table 1). The overall precise prevalence of IgAN or IgAV, in children or adults, is not known, but varies considerably around the world [14].

Table 1. Differences and similarities between IgAN and IgAV.

	IgA Nephropathy	IgA Vasculitis
Age at onset	30 to 39 years	1 to 19 years and 60 to 69 years
Clinical presentation	Only renal	Extra-renal symptoms (skin, gastro-intestinal, joint, neurologic, pulmonary, urologic) ± renal involvement
Renal biopsy	Mesangial IgA1, IgG, IgM, C3 and fibrin on immunofluorescence Mesangial hyper-cellularity with increased mesangial matrix, endo-capillary hyper-cellularity, segmental glomerular sclerosis, cellular crescents on light microscopy	
Outcome	More severe in adults	
Physiopathology	Multi-hit model involving IgA1	

In children, IgAV incidence is about 3 to 26.7/100,000 children per year [15–17]. The risk of progression to end-stage renal disease requiring dialysis in children varies from 2.5% to 25%, but it is on average around 8% [18,19]. In Europe, 3% of children on dialysis are due to IgAV. It is much rarer in adults, where its incidence is around 1.4 to 5.1/100,000 [20–23]. The child/adult ratio would therefore vary from 150 to 205. In adults, the risk of developing chronic renal failure is frequent, from 8 to 68%, on average around 18% within 15 years [24,25].

In children, IgAN incidence varies from 0.03/100,000/year in Venezuela to 9.9/100,000/year in Japan and in adults around 2.5/100,000/year [26,27]. The reported incidence rates are likely to underestimate true rates of IgAN, as this disease can exist sub-clinically and depends on country policy for microscopic hematuria detection in the population and/or renal biopsy indications. The risk of progression to end-stage renal disease (ESRD) is reported from 4% after 4.6 years in Europe [28] to 11% after 15 years of follow-up in Japan [29] and 14% in China [30]. The risk of progression to ESRD requiring dialysis in adults varies from 30% to 40% within 10 to 25 years [31]. In adults, IgAN is the cause of ESRD of 3.6% of newly dialyzed patients [32].

Whatever the studies, there is definitely an age difference between patients with IgAN and those with IgAV. This is particularly demonstrated by this Japanese study [33]: Among 18,967 patients with biopsy-proven disease between July 2007 and December 2012, the authors selected 513 patients with IgAV and 5679 with IgAN from the J-RBR (Japan Renal Biopsy registry) registry. They highlight a bimodal distribution for IgAV with two peaks between 1 to 19 years and 60 to 69 years, whereas for IgAN, the peak is rather between 30 to 39 years.

3. Clinical Presentation and Outcome

Macroscopic hematuria is the most frequent IgAN initial presentation in children, followed by the fortuitous finding of microscopic hematuria accompanied or not by proteinuria. In adults, the diagnosis is often made at the stage of chronic kidney disease (CKD), as if diagnosis in this belated context were made at an advanced stage after missing a pauci-symptomatic form that previously occurred in childhood. By contrast, the diagnosis of IgAV is, in most cases, made much earlier, revealed by the presence of extra-renal signs.

Indeed, by definition, the IgAV is characterized by the combination of cutaneous (palpable purpura), gastrointestinal (colicky pain, bloody stools) and articular (arthralgia) involvement. More rarely, we can observe a neurological, pulmonary or urological involvement [34]. The long-term prognosis of the disease depends on the presence of renal impairment and its evolution. From a histological point of view, it is not possible to distinguish a glomerulonephritis as part of an IgAV from an IgAN. Renal biopsy shows, in the two cases: on immunofluorescence, predominant IgA1 deposits in the mesangium of all glomeruli (Figure 1), with glomerular deposits of IgG, IgM, C3 and fibrin in variable proportions; on light microscopy, mesangial hypercellularity with increased mesangial matrix, endo-capillary hypercellularity, segmental glomerular sclerosis, cellular crescents and tubular atrophy and interstitial fibrosis.

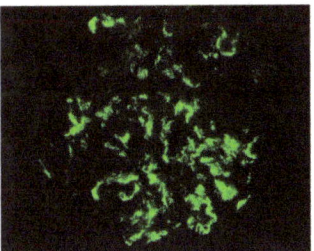

Figure 1. Mesangial and capillary wall IgA deposits (immunofluorescence staining for IgA, original magnification ×400).

IgAV is most common in childhood, but may occur at any age. Macroscopic hematuria is very uncommon after age 40. The importance of asymptomatic urine abnormality as the presentation of IgAN will depend on attitudes to routine urine testing and renal biopsy. It is unclear whether patients referring late, with chronic renal impairment, have a disease distinct from those referring earlier, with macroscopic hematuria (Figure 2: Data from patients presentation in Leicester, UK, 1980–1995 [35]).

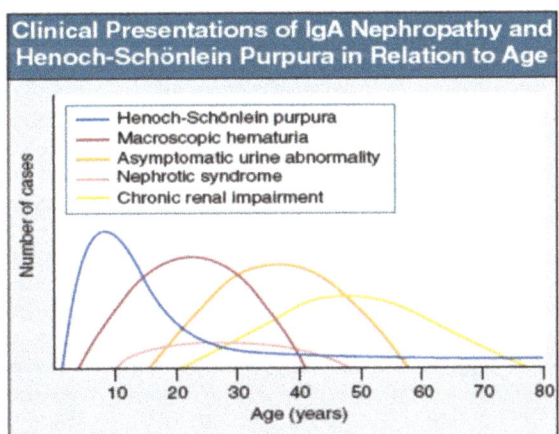

Figure 2. IgAN and IgAV clinical presentation over time from childhood to older age [35]. Reprinted with permission from ref. [35]. Copyright 2000 Rights and Permissions of Elsevier.

Renal involvement occurs in IgAV with a prevalence ranging from 20 to 54% in children and 45 to 85% in adults. Patients with nephritis have hematuria ± proteinuria of varying flow rate. They seem to have a higher frequency of nephritis and rapidly progressive nephritic syndrome at onset, notably in adults, but this is not the case in all published cohorts, as some of them, as we will develop furthermore, even describe the opposite.

Whether or not disease severity at diagnosis and prognosis differs between IgAN and IgAV remains controversial.

With regard to the clinical presentation and prognosis, the results of the few studies comparing the two diseases most frequently show a less favorable evolution for IgAN. Significant differences in the conclusions of the studies from one country to another suggest genetic susceptibility.

A Chinese study [36] compared 31 children with IgA Nephropathy to 120 children with IgA vasculitis and nephropathy, 32 of whom had a renal biopsy. In this pediatric cohort, patients with IgAN were significantly older. Histologically, the kidneys of patients with IgAN were more sclerotic (35.5% versus 3.1%) while there were more endothelial proliferation in those with IgAV (65.6% versus 29%). After 34 months of follow-up, the prognosis seemed better in patients with IgAV, since 72.5% of children from the IgAV group were in complete remission compared with only 19.4% in the IgAN group, in which patients had significantly persistent hematuria and proteinuria.

In another Spanish study [37], 142 patients with IgAV were compared to 61 patients with IgAN, of all ages. Those with IgAV were also younger (mean age at onset 30.6 years (2.9 to 82.7 years), than those with IgAN (37.1 years (14.7 to 78.5 years)). Again, the renal presentation was less severe: a lower rate of renal insufficiency (25% in IgAV vs. 63.4% in IgAN) and nephrotic syndrome (12.5% vs. 43.7%) were reported, while the prognosis, after a median follow-up of 130 months, was better: dialysis (2.9% in IgAV vs. 43.5% in IgAN), renal transplant (0% vs. 36%) and residual chronic renal insufficiency (4.9% vs. 63.8%)

In a Korean study [38], 92 adult patients with kidney biopsy-proven IgAV were compared to 1011 adult patients with kidney biopsy-proven IgAN, 89 and 178, respectively, from each group were matched using a propensity score in order to compare long term renal outcome. Once again patients with nephropathy in the context of IgAV were younger (33.2 ± 15.9 years vs. 37.7 ± 13 years), and less frequently developed renal insufficiency (7.6% vs. 14.4%) and interstitial fibrotic lesions on biopsy: however, these differences disappeared once the propensity score was applied to the subgroup. In addition, while the renal prognosis seemed better in the IgAV group (ESRD 14.1% vs. 22%; remission 28.3% vs. 13.8%), this difference disappeared (ESRD 14.6 vs. 13.5%; remission 28.1% vs. 27.5%) in the cohort of patients matched for clinical, histological and treatment factors. In my opinion, this study is essential, and it is the one that more clearly sheds light on the matter. It substantiates that the worse prognosis ascribed, from the other above-mentioned studies, to IgA Nephropathy, is probably pointed out only because we selected the most severe patients, namely, those who had not recovered spontaneously.

A Chinese pediatric study [39] compared the clinical-histological presentation of 41 patients with IgAN and 137 with IgAV. Patients with IgAV had higher levels of blood white cell, hemoglobin and platelet, and lower levels of hematuria, blood nitrogen and C4, compared to IgAN cases, but without any clinical and histological renal significant difference. The authors did not perform any prospective follow-up.

Another Japanese study [33] compared 513 patients with IgAV and 5679 with IgAN, of all ages, from a renal national biopsy registry. As previously mentioned, the age at diagnosis considerably differed: IgAV peaked at 1 to 19 years and 60 to 69 years, whereas IgAN peaked at 30 to 39 years. In contrast to previous studies, it appears that, regardless of age, patients with IgAV had a more severe clinical presentation with more frequent rapidly progressive renal insufficiency (4.5% vs. 1.4%) and a nephrotic syndrome (10.5% vs. 3%), and biopsies showed more inflammatory lesions including more endocapillary proliferation (6.4% vs. 0.9%) and extra-capillary (6.6% vs. 0.8%) glomerulonephritis. In contrast, patients with IgAN, had significantly more chronic nephritic syndrome (88.5% vs. 61.6%). Unfortunately, this cross-sectional study had no reference to the renal outcomes for any of the patients.

A further Japanese study [40] analyzed cross-sectionally 24 IgAV adult patients with nephritis or 56 adult patients with IgAN, all of whom underwent renal biopsy. The clinical characteristics did not differ between groups. Duration from onset was significantly longer for IgAN (47.6 months vs. 8.8 months). More patients with IgAV received steroid therapy, whereas more patients with IgAN received renin-angiotensin-aldosterone system (RAAS) blockers. Compared to IgAN, the mean rate of global sclerosis or crescent formation were significantly lower in patients with IgAV. Using Oxford classification, IgAV patients had more endothelial injury and IgAN worse mesangial proliferation, crescent formation, and tubulointerstitial injury.

A French retrospective study [41] showed that the risk score of end-stage renal disease or death, including hypertension, proteinuria more than 1 gramme per day and severe pathological lesions (local classification score ≥ 8), validated in a cohort of 1064 patients with an IgAN, was also valid when it was applied to a subgroup of 74 patients with IgAV from this same cohort, after 8.2 years of follow-up.

More recently, the National Institute of Diabetes and Digestive and Kidney Disease (NIDDK) funded the CureGN study to establish a primary glomerular disease consortium with a focus on IgAN and IgAV. Using this longitudinal observational cohort of adults and children with biopsy-proven primary glomerular disease, from all over the world, this first report described the baseline clinical characteristics of the two nosological entities [42]. The next step will be to better predict the long-term follow-up renal outcome, find prognostic biomarkers and identify patients most appropriate for specific therapies. A total of 667 patients were enrolled, including 506 (75.9%) with IgAN and 161 (24.1%) with IgAV, 285 (42.7%) were children. At the moment of biopsy, patients with IgAV were younger, more frequently white, and had a higher estimated glomerular filtration rate and lower serum albumin than those with IgAN. Adults and children with IgAV were similar in terms of proteinuria, hematuria or serum albumin. Patients with IgAV were more likely to be treated with immunosuppressive therapy if compared to those with IgAN, but less likely to receive standard supportive care with RAAS inhibition. No data is available to date about renal histology.

4. Treatment

The Kidney Disease Improving Global Outcome (KDIGO) working group on glomerulonephritis compiled the first evidence-based guidelines for the treatment of IgAN and IgAV in 2012 [43]. Children and adults were treated in the same way.

In adults and children with IgAN, the particular value of RAAS blockers, as angiotensin-converting-enzyme inhibitors [44,45] or angiotensin-receptor blockers [46] in retarding progression of the disease, has been shown in prospective randomized trials. Supportive care is now the first line of treatment, recommended in IgAN and IgAV, as soon as proteinuria is > 1 g per day (in children 0.5 to 1 g/day per 1.73 m^2) with a blood pressure goal < 130/80 mmHg (no BP goals specified for children), and to achieve proteinuria < 1 g per day.

Concerning the use of corticosteroids and other immunosuppressive agents, KDIGO, in 2012 [43], published its guidelines for IgAN and IgAV, in children as in adults, with a quiet low level of proof (no more than 2C) because of the lack of large clinical trials:

The KDIGO practice guidelines have been recently update [47], including several important clinical trials for IgAN published since 2012, either with corticosteroids or other immunosuppressive drugs, mainly mycophenolate mofetil (MMF). Unfortunately, all have excluded patients with IgAV (adult or children) and children with IgAN. No additional recommendation was done for them.

The authors stressed that future guideline recommendations will need to include an assessment of the relative risks and benefits of steroids in individual patients over a broader range of eGFR, with careful consideration of infections and prophylaxis. They emphasize that we must pay particular attention to comorbidities as advanced age, metabolic syndrome, morbid obesity, latent infection as viral hepatitis or HIV, active peptic ulceration or uncontrolled psychiatric illness.

Concerning corticosteroids in adult IgAN, three main clinical studies [48–50] and one meta-analysis [51] are available. They showed that corticosteroids, after optimization supportive treatment (mainly RAAS blockers) and in addition to it, can decrease proteinuria and slow loss of kidney function, particularly in patients with persistent proteinuria more than 1 g/g and preserved renal function (eGFR > 50 mL/min/1.73 m^2). The Supportive Versus Immunosuppressive Therapy for the Treatment of Progressive IgA Nephropathy (STOP-IgAN) study recently published its follow-up data, available for 149 participants, with a median of 7.4 years, which showed no difference of renal outcomes (in terms of serum creatinine, proteinuria, end-stage kidney disease, and death) between the two groups [49,52]. The Therapeutic Evaluation of Steroids in IgA Nephropathy Global Study (TESTING) trial was stopped early after an interim analysis revealed a high risk of infectious serious adverse events including the lethal Pneumocystis Jirovecii pneumonia [50]. Patients with IgAN from the European Validation Study of the Oxford Classification of IgAN (VALIGA) cohort, classified according to the Oxford-MEST classification and medication used, have been retrospectively studied. From the 1147 patients of the cohort, 184 subjects who received corticosteroids and RAAS blockers were matched to 184 patients with a similar risk profile of progression who received only RAAS blockers. Using a propensity score, authors showed that corticosteroids reduced proteinuria and the rate of renal function decline and increased renal survival, even in patients with an eGFR < 50 mL/min per 1.73 m^2 [48].

Although previous studies [53,54] showed that MMF was not effective for treatment of IgAN, recent trials [55,56] add conflicting information. Hou JH and al.'s study reintroduces the possibility that MMF may be useful for IgAN, notably by its steroid-sparing effect.

In adult IgAV, very limited evidence is available regarding the value of corticosteroids, cyclophosphamide or other immunosuppressive agents. Only one RCT is available and shows, in adults with severe IgAV, most of them with nephritis, no additional benefit when cyclophosphamide was added to corticosteroids [57,58]. However, by extrapolating from findings in adults with IgAN, the KDIGO guidelines suggest that a 6-month course of corticosteroid therapy would be effective to treat nephropathy in IgAV, if proteinuria is more than 1 g per day persisting despite RAAS blockade and blood pressure control, whereas it has been shown to be ineffective in IgAN [59], Rituximab seems to be a promising therapy in the management of adults with IgAV [60].

In child IgAV, although earlier studies showed some benefit of corticosteroids, these studies were small and poorly designed. Meta-analyses [61] and more recent randomized controlled trials [62,63] have not clearly shown its benefit and confirm that cyclophosphamide therapy is ineffective in severe renal disease. Despite that, based on the opinions of 16 experts in pediatric rheumatology, systemic vasculitis, and nephrology across Europe, the recent SHARE [64] (Single Hub and Access Point for Paediatric Rheumatology in Europe) initiative recommends corticosteroids to be used for treatment of IgAV nephritis in children, regardless of severity. For severe nephritis, the authors drew on experiences with similar forms of systemic vasculitis to recommend intravenous cyclophosphamide in combination with high-dose steroid therapy to induce remission, followed by azathioprine or MMF in combination with low-dose steroid therapy as a maintenance treatment.

Two randomized placebo-controlled prednisone trials [62,65] and one meta-analysis [61] showed that corticosteroids are ineffective to prevent occurrence of nephritis in children with IgAV. One ongoing study (NCT04008316) will evaluate colchicine in adult patients with IgAV limited to skin to prevent skin relapse (primary endpoint) and occurrence of digestive or kidney involvement (secondary endpoint).

A great quantity of clinical trials concerning IgAN are ongoing (about one hundred registered in ClinicalTrial.gouv), with four molecules particularly attractive (sparsentan, hydrochloroquine, budesonide, glifozine). None of them included IgAV or children. It is therefore not possible to compare the sensitivity to treatment of both diseases in those two populations.

5. Physiopathology

In recent years, considerable progress has been made in understanding the physiopathology of IgAN. The multi-hits hypothesis is now recognized [66]. The first hit comprises the increased level of circulating galactose-deficient (Gd)-IgA1, influenced by both environmental and genetic factors. Second, antibodies (IgA or IgG) recognizing Gd-IgA1 are produced or already present, possibly attributable to molecular mimicry. The formation of Gd-IgA1-containing immune complexes is thirdly mediated by complement factors and IgA receptors as the soluble IgA Fc alpha receptor (FcαR/sCD89), transglutaminase2 (TG2) and transferrin receptor (TfR/CD71) and fourth, Gd-IgA1 containing immune complexes deposit in the mesangium, hereby inducing a proliferation of mesangial cells and an overproduction of extracellular matrix components, cytokines (Interleukins, tumor necrosis factor-alfa (TNF-α), tumor growth factor-beta-1 (TGFβ-1)) and chemokines (monocyte chemotactic protein-1 (MCP-1)), which ultimately leads to renal dysfunction (Figure 3).

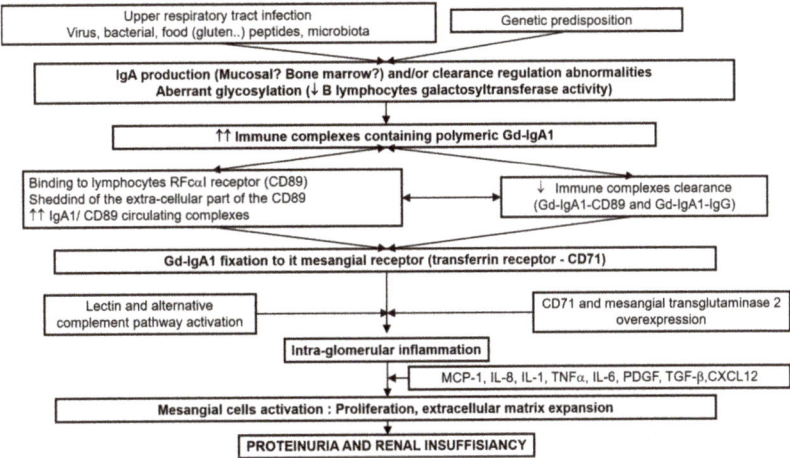

Figure 3. Physiopathology mechanism.

Other pathophysiological pathways are currently being studied, in particular with the aim to develop new treatments. The Toll-like receptors (TLRs) family plays a critical role in the mammalian innate immune system, particularly with regard to the mucosal immunity, which plays a key role in initiating the pathogenic process in IgAN, and it is the first line of host defense against invading pathogens. Activation of TLR-mediated signaling pathways induces gene expression of inflammatory cytokines and type I interferon [67,68]. The complement system, as well, is part of the innate immune system which can enhance the clearance of microorganisms. Skin and mesangial deposits in IgAV and IgAN contain the complement components C3 and C5-C9. Serum levels of activated C3 and mesangial C3 deposition correlate with loss of renal function. The degree of complement activation is also important and have been shown to have prognostic value [69–73].

6. Biomarkers

The search for diagnostic and prognostic biomarkers is based on the above-mentioned physio pathological mechanisms. Finding biomarkers able to identify, at an early stage, patients at risk of renal progression, those who will need treatment, is a challenge.

Most of these studies focused on either IgAN or IgAV, but rarely both in the same study, as shown in Table 2.

Table 2. Potent value of biomarkers correlated to clinical and/or histological activity and outcome evaluated in IgAN and IgAV or both [ref].

	IgAN	IgAV	IgAN + IgAV
GdIgA1	[74,75]	[76–78]	[40,79]
GdIgA1/sCD89	[80]	[77,78]	
GdIgA1/IgG	[81]	[77,78]	
sCD89			[82]
Transglutaminase2			[83]
CD71			[83]
TLR9	[84,85]	[68]	
TLR4			[67,68]
TGF-β1 MCP1			[40]
Complement system	[70,73]	[86]	

Nevertheless, it is now accepted that the aberrantly glycosylated IgA1 (GdIgA1) plays a central role. Several methods are available to highlight and quantify GdIgA1. Mass spectrometry is the reference method, but it is difficult to use in current practice. The Helix aspersa agglutinin (HAA) lectin method is the most commonly used but lacks sensitivity, specificity and reproductivity [87]. Recently, the Japanese Suzuki team has developed a novel lectin-independent method with a specific monoclonal antibody (KM55 mAb) for measuring serum level of GdIgA1, that is clearly more performant and robust [88]. This team first showed that serum IgA, GdIgA1, and immune complexes containing GdIgA1 were increased in patients with IgAN but not in healthy subjects. The IgG anti-GdIgA1 antibody was particularly efficient in this study to make the diagnosis of IgAN since its sensitivity was 89% and its specificity was 92% (compare to the reference test HAA lectin method).

In IgAV, GdIgA1 (measured by HAA lectin method) and immunes complexes containing GdIgA1 are also increased in case of nephritis in children [78] and adults [77]. The team then used their GdIgA1-specific monoclonal antibody KM55 to highlight GdIgA1 in the glomeruli of 48 patients with IgAN and 14 patients with IgAV while it remains undetectable in the glomeruli of 35 with other glomerulopathies in which glomerular IgA deposit is frequent (lupus nephritis, HCV-related nephropathy, mesangio-proliferative glomerulonephritis, membranous nephropathy, hepatic glomerulosclerosis) [74].

Another team analyzed adult patients with renal-biopsy proven IgAN and IgAV. Serum GdIgA1 levels and glomerular GdIgA1 staining, using enzyme-linked immunosorbent essay (ELISA) with the same anti-human GdIgA1 specific monoclonal antibody (KM55), were comparable among patients with IgAN and IgAV [40].

7. Genetics

Familial clustering, ethnic differences, and regional discrepancies suggest a genetic component to IgAN and IgAV.

The genetic influence of GdIgA1 production and expression during IgAN and IgAV is highlighted by a study from Kiryluk et al [89]. Serum GdIgA1 levels (quantified using HAA lectin based ELISA) from 20 children with IgAV and nephritis, and 14 children with IgAN were compared to 51 age- and ethnicity match pediatric controls. Serum level of GdIgA1 were significantly elevated in the 34 children with IgAV or IgAN compare to controls. It was also elevated in a large fraction of 54 first-degree relatives, compared with 141 unrelated healthy adult controls. A unilineal transmission of the trait was found in 17, bilineal transmission in 1, and sporadic occurrence in 5 of 23 families when both parents and the patient were analyzed. There was a significant age-, gender, and household-adjusted heritability of serum GdIgA1 estimated at 76% in pediatric IgAN and at 64% in pediatric IgAV with nephritis.

High heritability of GdIgA1 in IgAN have been previously shown in adults from other ethnic origins: Caucasiens [90], Asians [91], and African Americans [92].

Kiryluk et al. collaborated with many teams around the world to provide insight into why IgAN differs in terms of incidence, presentation and prognosis all over the world, through a huge genome-wide association (GWAS) study to localize five IgAN susceptibility, in 10,775 individuals from Europe, Asia and America [93]. Nevertheless, these studies did not include patients with IgAV. There is only one small genetic study (285 IgAV patients and 1006 healthy controls from Spain genotyped by Illumina HumanCore BeadChips) showing in IgAV, as for IgAN, variations in the loci of the HLA class 2 genes region (HLA-DRB1 position 13 and 11) suggesting the same susceptibilities [94].

8. Discussion and Future Research

After reporting all those studies, can we say that IgA Nephropathy and IgA Vasculitis are two clinical entities of the same disease?

Clinical studies showed that they differentiate clearly in terms of clinical presentation and age at onset.

Concerning outcome, studies are conflicting, but tend to show that if patients are stratified on age and genetic background, IgAN and IgAV have the same renal prognosis. The presence of clinically speaking extra-renal disease makes the diagnosis of IgAV easy at an early stage, whereas in patients whose disease is limited to the kidney, the diagnosis is inevitably belated and therefore more advanced. It is not said, moreover, that these patients had, some years before, some unnoticed purpuric lesions. Therefore, the real question is: Why do some patients with IgAV have no renal involvement, and why do patients with IgAN have no skin lesions?

Physiopathological mechanisms and their related biomarkers are similar, each time they have been evaluated in the same study, none of which have been identified, to date, as having a strong prognostic value, either in IgAN and IgAV. It is thus most essential to identify early diagnostic and prognostic markers, which could be able to detect patients who will not spontaneously heal and require specific treatment (yet to be defined). Working together to set up new clinical studies appears necessary. It will be crucial for those future trials:

- To include both diseases;
- To agree on a common histological classification. Thus far, in fact, there is no consensual renal histologic classification for IgAV. Although the International Study of Kidney Disease in Children (ISKDC) classification is widely use in child IgAV, it is more and more questioned because it does not completely correlate with the clinical presentation and long term renal outcome. Few teams have applied to IgAV the Oxford classification widely used now for IgAN and have shown discordant results [95–98]. Its prognostic interest is actually disputed. A large international study, based on the model, which has resulted in the Oxford classification, is currently being developed for the IgAV;
- To stratify the cohorts on age and genetic background, which are, to date, the only prognostic factors so far clearly identified.

9. Conclusions

Since the last reviews, published more than 10 years ago now, several clinical studies, reported here, provide additional arguments that IgAN and IgAV would be the same disease. In the absence of large studies, including adults and children from different geographical part of the world, suffering from IgAN or IgAV with or without renal impairment, it is not yet possible to conclude on their differences or similarity in terms of prognosis and sensitivity to treatment. Answering these questions gives opportunity to future clinical studies.

Funding: This research received no external funding.

Institutional Review Board Statement: Not applicable.

Informed Consent Statement: Not applicable.

Data Availability Statement: Not applicable.

Acknowledgments: I would like to thank my colleague, D. Pievani for his skillful assistance for writing and text editing, J. Verine for the renal biopsy picture, and J. Barrat for providing Figure 2.

Conflicts of Interest: No conflicts of interest to declare.

References

1. Meadow, S.R.; Scott, D.G. Berger Disease: Henoch-Schönlein Syndrome without the Rash. *J. Pediatr.* **1985**, *106*, 27–32. [CrossRef]
2. Nicoara, O.; Twombley, K. Immunoglobulin A Nephropathy and Immunoglobulin A Vasculitis. *Pediatr. Clin. N. Am.* **2019**, *66*, 101–110. [CrossRef]
3. Montoliu, J.; Lens, X.M.; Torras, A.; Revert, L. Henoch-Schönlein Purpura and IgA Nephropathy in Father and Son. *Nephron* **1990**, *54*, 77–79. [CrossRef]
4. Hughes, F.J.; Wolfish, N.M.; McLaine, P.N. Henoch-Schönlein Syndrome and IgA Nephropathy: A case report suggesting a common pathogenesis. *Pediatr. Nephrol.* **1988**, *2*, 389–392. [CrossRef]
5. Araque, A.; Sánchez, R.; Alamo, C.; Torres, N.; Praga, M. Evolution of Immunoglobulin a Nephropathy into Henoch-Schönlein Purpura in an Adult Patient. *Am. J. Kidney Dis.* **1995**, *25*, 340–342. [CrossRef]
6. Ravelli, A.; Carnevale-Maffè, G.; Ruperto, N.; Ascari, E.; Martini, A. IgA Nephropathy and Henoch-Schönlein Syndrome Occurring in the Same Patient. *Nephron* **1996**, *72*, 111–112. [CrossRef]
7. Kamei, K.; Ogura, M.; Sato, M.; Ito, S.; Ishikura, K. Evolution of IgA Nephropathy into Anaphylactoid Purpura in Six Cases—Further Evidence That IgA Nephropathy and Henoch–Schönlein Purpura Nephritis Share Common Pathogenesis. *Pediatr. Nephrol.* **2016**, *31*, 779–785. [CrossRef]
8. Bachman, U.; Biava, C.; Amend, W.; Feduska, N.; Melzer, J.; Salvatierra, O.; Vincenti, F. The clincial course of IgA-nephropathy and henoch-schönlein purpura following renal transplantation. *Transplantation* **1986**, *42*, 511–514. [CrossRef]
9. Sotoodian, B.; Robert, J.; Mahmood, M.N.; Yacyshyn, E. IgA Cutaneous Purpura Post–Renal Transplantation in a Patient With Long-Standing IgA Nephropathy: Case Report and Literature Review. *J. Cutan. Med. Surg.* **2015**, *19*, 498–503. [CrossRef]
10. McNally, A.; McGregor, D.; Searle, M.; Irvine, J.; Cross, N. Henoch-Schonlein Purpura in a Renal Transplant Recipient with Prior IgA Nephropathy Following Influenza Vaccination. *Clin. Kidney J.* **2013**, *6*, 313–315. [CrossRef]
11. Waldo, F.B. Is Henoch-Schonlein Purpura the Systemic Form of IgA Nephropathy? *Am. J. Kidney Dis.* **1988**, *12*, 373–377. [CrossRef]
12. Davin, J.C. Henoch-Schonlein Purpura Nephritis: Pathophysiology, Treatment, and Future Strategy. *Clin. J. Am. Soc. Nephrol.* **2011**, *6*, 679–689. [CrossRef] [PubMed]
13. Sanders, J.T.; Wyatt, R.J. IgA Nephropathy and Henoch–Schönlein Purpura Nephritis. *Curr. Opin. Pediatr.* **2008**, *20*, 163–170. [CrossRef] [PubMed]
14. O'Shaughnessy, M.M.; Hogan, S.L.; Thompson, B.D.; Coppo, R.; Fogo, A.B.; Jennette, J.C. Glomerular Disease Frequencies by Race, Sex and Region: Results from the International Kidney Biopsy Survey. *Nephrol. Dial. Transplantat.* **2018**, *33*, 661–669. [CrossRef] [PubMed]
15. Gardner-Medwin, J.M.; Dolezalova, P.; Cummins, C.; Southwood, T.R. Incidence of Henoch-Schonlein Purpura, Kawasaki Disease, and Rare Vasculitides in Children of Different Ethnic Origins. *Lancet* **2002**, *360*, 1197–1202. [CrossRef]
16. Piram, M.; Maldini, C.; Biscardi, S.; De Suremain, N.; Orzechowski, C.; Georget, E.; Regnard, D.; Koné-Paut, I.; Mahr, A. Incidence of IgA vasculitis in children estimated by four-source capture–recapture analysis: A population-based study. *Rheumatology* **2017**, *56*, 1358–1366. [CrossRef] [PubMed]
17. Mossberg, M.; Segelmark, M.; Kahn, R.; Englund, M.; Mohammad, A. Epidemiology of Primary Systemic Vasculitis in Children: A Population-Based Study from Southern Sweden. *Scand. J. Rheumatol.* **2018**, *47*, 295–302. [CrossRef] [PubMed]
18. Yang, Y.H.; Hung, C.F.; Hsu, C.R.; Wang, L.C.; Chuang, Y.H.; Lin, Y.T.; Chiang, B.L. A Nationwide Survey on Epidemiological Characteristics of Childhood Henoch-Schonlein Purpura in Taiwan. *Rheumatology* **2005**, *44*, 618–622. [CrossRef]
19. Okubo, Y.; Nochioka, K.; Sakakibara, H.; Hataya, H.; Terakawa, T.; Testa, M.; Sundel, R.P. Nationwide epidemiological survey of childhood IgA vasculitis associated hospitalization in the USA. *Clin. Rheumatol.* **2016**, *35*, 2749–2756. [CrossRef]
20. Watts, R.A.; Lane, S.; Scott, D.G. What is known about the epidemiology of the vasculitides? *Best Pract. Res. Clin. Rheumatol.* **2005**, *19*, 191–207. [CrossRef]
21. Penny, K.; Fleming, M.; Kazmierczak, D.; Thomas, A. An epidemiological study of henoch-schonlein purpura. *Paediatr. Nurs.* **2010**, *22*, 30–35. [CrossRef]
22. Romero-Gómez, C.; Aguilar-García, J.A.; García-de-Lucas, M.D.; Cotos-Canca, R.; Olalla-Sierra, J.; García-Alegría, J.J.; Hernández-Rodríguez, J. Epidemiological study of primary systemic vasculitides among adults in southern spain and review of the main epidemiological studies. *Clin. Exp. Rheumatol.* **2015**, *33*, S-11–S-18.

23. Hočevar, A.; Rotar, Z.; Ostrovršnik, J.; Jurčić, V.; Vizjak, A.; Dolenc Voljč, M.; Lindič, J.; Tomšič, M. Incidence of IgA Vasculitis in the Adult Slovenian Population. *Br. J. Dermatol.* **2014**, *171*, 524–527. [CrossRef]
24. Pillebout, E.; Thervet, E.; Hill, G.; Alberti, C.; Vanhille, P.; Nochy, D. Henoch-schonlein purpura in adults: Outcome and prognostic factors. *J. Am. Soc. Nephrol.* **2002**, *13*, 1271–1278. [CrossRef] [PubMed]
25. Huang, X.; Wu, X.; Le, W.; Hao, Y.; Wu, J.; Zeng, C.; Liu, Z.; Tang, Z. Renal prognosis and related risk factors for henoch-schönlein purpura nephritis: A Chinese adult patient cohort. *Sci. Rep.* **2018**, *8*, 5585. [CrossRef]
26. McGrogan, A.; Franssen, C.F.M.; de Vries, C.S. The incidence of primary glomerulonephritis worldwide: A systematic review of the literature. *Nephrol. Dial. Transplantat.* **2011**, *26*, 414–430. [CrossRef]
27. Shibano, T.; Takagi, N.; Maekawa, K.; Mae, H.; Hattori, M.; Takeshima, Y.; Tanizawa, T. Epidemiological Survey and Clinical Investigation of Pediatric IgA Nephropathy. *Clin. Exp. Nephrol.* **2016**, *20*, 111–117. [CrossRef]
28. Coppo, R. Pediatric IgA Nephropathy in Europe. *Kidney Dis.* **2019**, *5*, 182–188. [CrossRef]
29. Yoshikawa, N.; Tanaka, R.; Iijima, K. Pathophysiology and Treatment of IgA Nephropathy in Children. *Pediatr. Nephrol.* **2001**, *16*, 446–457. [CrossRef] [PubMed]
30. Wu, H.; Fang, X.; Xia, Z.; Gao, C.; Peng, Y.; Li, X.; Zhang, P.; Kuang, Q.; Wang, R.; Wang, M. Long-term renal survival and undetected risk factors of IgA nephropathy in Chinese Children—A Retrospective 1243 cases analysis from single centre experience. *J. Nephrol.* **2020**, *33*, 1263–1273. [CrossRef]
31. Magistroni, R.; D'Agati, V.; Appel, G.; Kiryluk, K. New developments in the genetics, pathogenesis, and therapy of IgA Nephropathy. *Kidney Int.* **2015**, *88*, 974–989. [CrossRef]
32. Lassalle, M.; Couchoud, C.; Prada-Bordenave, E.; Jacquelinet, C. Éditorial. *Néphrol. Thér.* **2013**, *9*, S1. [CrossRef]
33. Komatsu, H.; Fujimoto, S.; Yoshikawa, N.; Kitamura, H.; Sugiyama, H.; Yokoyama, H. Clinical manifestations of henoch-schonlein purpura nephritis and iga nephropathy: Comparative analysis of data from the Japan Renal Biopsy Registry (J-RBR). *Clin. Exp. Nephrol.* **2016**, *20*, 552–560. [CrossRef]
34. Ozen, S.; Pistorio, A.; Iusan, S.M.; Bakkaloglu, A.; Herlin, T.; Brik, R.; Buoncompagni, A.; Lazar, C.; Bilge, I.; Uziel, Y.; et al. EULAR/PRINTO/PRES criteria for henoch-schonlein purpura, childhood polyarteritis nodosa, childhood wegener granulomatosis and childhood takayasu arteritis: Ankara 2008. Part II: Final classification criteria. *Ann. Rheum. Dis.* **2010**, *69*, 798–806. [CrossRef]
35. *Comprehensive Clinical Nephrology*, 6th ed.; Feehally, J. (Ed.) Elsevier: Edinburgh, UK ; New York, NY, USA, 2019; ISBN 978-0-323-47909-7.
36. Zhou, J.; Huang, A.; Liu, T.; Kuang, Y. A clinico-pathological study comparing Henoch-Schonlein purpura nephritis with IgA nephropathy in children. *Zhonghua Er Ke Za Zhi* **2003**, *41*, 808–812.
37. Calvo-Rio, V.; Loricera, J.; Martin, L.; Ortiz-Sanjuan, F.; Alvarez, L.; Gonzalez-Vela, M.C.; Gonzalez-Lamuno, D.; Mata, C.; Gortazar, P.; Rueda-Gotor, J.; et al. Henoch-schonlein purpura nephritis and IgA nephropathy: A comparative clinical study. *Clin. Exp. Rheumatol.* **2013**, *31*, S45–S51.
38. Oh, H.J.; Ahn, S.V.; Yoo, D.E.; Kim, S.J.; Shin, D.H.; Lee, M.J.; Kim, H.R.; Park, J.T.; Yoo, T.H.; Kang, S.W.; et al. Clinical outcomes, when matched at presentation, do not vary between adult-onset henoch-schonlein purpura nephritis and IgA nephropathy. *Kidney Int.* **2012**, *82*, 1304–1312. [CrossRef] [PubMed]
39. Mao, S.; Xuan, X.; Sha, Y.; Zhao, S.; Zhu, C.; Zhang, A.; Huang, S. Clinico-pathological association of henoch-schoenlein purpura nephritis and IgA nephropathy in children. *Int. J. Clin. Exp. Pathol.* **2015**, *8*, 2334–2342. [PubMed]
40. Sugiyama, M.; Wada, Y.; Kanazawa, N.; Tachibana, S.; Suzuki, T.; Matsumoto, K.; Iyoda, M.; Honda, H.; Shibata, T. A cross-sectional analysis of clinicopathologic similarities and differences between henoch-schönlein purpura nephritis and IgA nephropathy. *PLoS ONE* **2020**, *15*, e0232194. [CrossRef] [PubMed]
41. Mohey, H.; Laurent, B.; Mariat, C.; Berthoux, F. Validation of the absolute renal risk of dialysis/death in adults with IgA nephropathy secondary to henoch-schönlein purpura: A monocentric cohort study. *BMC Nephrol.* **2013**, *14*, 169. [CrossRef]
42. Selewski, D.T.; Ambruzs, J.M.; Appel, G.B.; Bomback, A.S.; Matar, R.B.; Cai, Y.; Cattran, D.C.; Chishti, A.S.; D'Agati, V.D.; D'Alessandri-Silva, C.J.; et al. Clinical characteristics and treatment patterns of children and adults with IgA nephropathy or IgA vasculitis: Findings from the cureGN study. *Kidney Int. Rep.* **2018**, *3*, 1373–1384. [CrossRef] [PubMed]
43. Radhakrishnan, J.; Cattran, D.C. The KDIGO practice guideline on glomerulonephritis: Reading between the (guide)lines-Application to the individual Patient. *Kidney Int.* **2012**, *82*, 840–856. [CrossRef] [PubMed]
44. Praga, M.; Gutierrez, E.; Gonzalez, E.; Morales, E.; Hernandez, E. Treatment of IgA Nephropathy with ACE Inhibitors: A randomized and controlled trial. *J. Am. Soc. Nephrol.* **2003**, *14*, 1578–1583. [CrossRef] [PubMed]
45. Coppo, R.; Peruzzi, L.; Amore, A.; Piccoli, A.; Cochat, P.; Stone, R.; Kirschstein, M.; Linne, T. IgACE: A placebo-controlled, randomized trial of angiotensin-converting enzyme inhibitors in children and young people with IgA nephropathy and moderate proteinuria. *J. Am. Soc. Nephrol.* **2007**, *18*, 1880–1888. [CrossRef]
46. Li, P.K.; Leung, C.B.; Chow, K.M.; Cheng, Y.L.; Fung, S.K.; Mak, S.K.; Tang, A.W.; Wong, T.Y.; Yung, C.Y.; Yung, J.C.; et al. Hong Kong study using valsartan in IgA nephropathy (HKVIN): A double-blind, randomized, placebo-controlled study. *Am. J. Kidney Dis.* **2006**, *47*, 751–760. [CrossRef] [PubMed]
47. Floege, J.; Barbour, S.J.; Cattran, D.C.; Hogan, J.J.; Nachman, P.H.; Tang, S.C.W.; Wetzels, J.F.M.; Cheung, M.; Wheeler, D.C.; Winkelmayer, W.C.; et al. Management and treatment of glomerular diseases (Part 1): Conclusions from a kidney disease: Improving Global Outcomes (KDIGO) controversies conference. *Kidney Int.* **2019**, *95*, 268–280. [CrossRef]

48. Tesar, V.; Troyanov, S.; Bellur, S.; Verhave, J.C.; Cook, H.T.; Feehally, J.; Roberts, I.S.; Cattran, D.; Coppo, R. Corticosteroids in IgA nephropathy: A retrospective analysis from the VALIGA study. *J. Am. Soc. Nephrol.* **2015**, *26*, 2248–2258. [CrossRef]
49. Rauen, T.; Eitner, F.; Fitzner, C.; Sommerer, C.; Zeier, M.; Otte, B.; Panzer, U.; Peters, H.; Benck, U.; Mertens, P.R.; et al. Intensive supportive care plus immunosuppression in IgA nephropathy. *N. Engl. J. Med.* **2015**, *373*, 2225–2236. [CrossRef]
50. Lv, J.; Zhang, H.; Wong, M.G.; Jardine, M.J.; Hladunewich, M.; Jha, V.; Monaghan, H.; Zhao, M.; Barbour, S.; Reich, H.; et al. Effect of oral methylprednisolone on clinical outcomes in patients with IgA nephropathy: The TESTING randomized clinical trial. *JAMA* **2017**, *318*, 432–442. [CrossRef]
51. Natale, P.; Palmer, S.C.; Ruospo, M.; Saglimbene, V.M.; Craig, J.C.; Vecchio, M.; Samuels, J.A.; Molony, D.A.; Schena, F.P.; Strippoli, G.F. Immunosuppressive agents for treating IgA nephropathy. *Cochrane Database Syst. Rev.* **2020**. [CrossRef]
52. Rauen, T.; Wied, S.; Fitzner, C.; Eitner, F.; Sommerer, C.; Zeier, M.; Otte, B.; Panzer, U.; Budde, K.; Benck, U.; et al. After Ten Years of Follow-up, No Difference between Supportive Care plus Immunosuppression and Supportive Care Alone in IgA Nephropathy. *Kidney Int.* **2020**, *98*, 1044–1052. [CrossRef] [PubMed]
53. Maes, B.D.; Oyen, R.; Claes, K.; Evenepoel, P.; Kuypers, D.; Vanwalleghem, J.; Van Damme, B.; Vanrenterghem, Y.F. Mycophenolate mofetil in IgA nephropathy: Results of a 3-year prospective placebo-controlled randomized study. *Kidney Int.* **2004**, *65*, 1842–1849. [CrossRef] [PubMed]
54. Frisch, G.; Lin, J.; Rosenstock, J.; Markowitz, G.; D'Agati, V.; Radhakrishnan, J.; Preddie, D.; Crew, J.; Valeri, A.; Appel, G. Mycophenolate Mofetil (MMF) vs placebo in patients with moderately advanced IgA nephropathy: A double-blind randomized controlled trial. *Nephrol. Dial. Transplant.* **2005**, *20*, 2139–2145. [CrossRef] [PubMed]
55. Hogg, R.J.; Bay, R.C.; Jennette, J.C.; Sibley, R.; Kumar, S.; Fervenza, F.C.; Appel, G.; Cattran, D.; Fischer, D.; Hurley, R.M.; et al. Randomized controlled trial of mycophenolate mofetil in children, adolescents, and adults with IgA nephropathy. *Am. J. Kidney Dis.* **2015**, *66*, 783–791. [CrossRef]
56. Hou, J.H.; Le, W.B.; Chen, N.; Wang, W.M.; Liu, Z.S.; Liu, D.; Chen, J.H.; Tian, J.; Fu, P.; Hu, Z.X.; et al. Mycophenolate mofetil combined with prednisone versus full-dose prednisone in IgA nephropathy with active proliferative lesions: A randomized controlled trial. *Am. J. Kidney Dis.* **2017**, *69*, 788–795. [CrossRef]
57. Pillebout, E.; Alberti, C.; Guillevin, L.; Ouslimani, A.; Thervet, E. Addition of cyclophosphamide to steroids provides no benefit compared with steroids alone in treating adult patients with severe henoch schonlein purpura. *Kidney Int.* **2010**, *78*, 495–502. [CrossRef]
58. Audemard-Verger, A.; Terrier, B.; Dechartres, A.; Chanal, J.; Amoura, Z.; Le Gouellec, N.; Cacoub, P.; Jourde-Chiche, N.; Urbanski, G.; Augusto, J.F.; et al. Characteristics and management of IgA vasculitis (henoch-schonlein) in adults: Data from 260 patients included in a french multicenter retrospective survey. *Arthritis Rheumatol.* **2017**, *69*, 1862–1870. [CrossRef]
59. Lafayette, R.A.; Canetta, P.A.; Rovin, B.H.; Appel, G.B.; Novak, J.; Nath, K.A.; Sethi, S.; Tumlin, J.A.; Mehta, K.; Hogan, M.; et al. A Randomized, controlled trial of Rituximab in IgA nephropathy with proteinuria and renal dysfunction. *J. Am. Soc. Nephrol.* **2017**, *28*, 1306–1313. [CrossRef]
60. Maritati, F.; Fenoglio, R.; Pillebout, E.; Emmi, G.; Urban, M.L.; Rocco, R.; Nicastro, M.; Incerti, M.; Goldoni, M.; Trivioli, G.; et al. Brief report: Rituximab for the treatment of adult-onset iga vasculitis (henoch-schonlein). *Arthritis Rheumatol.* **2017**, *70*, 109–114. [CrossRef]
61. Hahn, D.; Hodson, E.; Willis, N.; Craig, J.C. Interventions for preventing and treating kidney disease in henoch-schonlein purpura (HSP) (Review). *Cochrane Libr.* **2015**, *8*. [CrossRef]
62. Dudley, J.; Smith, G.; Llewelyn-Edwards, A.; Bayliss, K.; Pike, K.; Tizard, J.; Tuthill, D.; Millar-Jones, L.; Bowler, I.; Williams, T.; et al. Randomised, double-blind, placebo-controlled trial to determine whether steroids reduce the incidence and severity of nephropathy in Henoch-Schonlein Purpura (HSP). *Arch. Dis. Child.* **2013**, *98*, 756–763. [CrossRef]
63. Ronkainen, J.; Koskimies, O.; Ala-Houhala, M.; Antikainen, M.; Merenmies, J.; Rajantie, J.; Ormala, T.; Turtinen, J.; Nuutinen, M. Early prednisone therapy in henoch-schonlein purpura: A Randomized, double-blind, placebo-controlled trial. *J. Pediatr.* **2006**, *149*, 241–247. [CrossRef]
64. Ozen, S.; Marks, S.D.; Brogan, P.; Groot, N.; de Graeff, N.; Avcin, T.; Bader-Meunier, B.; Dolezalova, P.; Feldman, B.M.; Kone-Paut, I.; et al. European consensus-based recommendations for diagnosis and treatment of immunoglobulin a vasculitis—the SHARE Initiative. *Rheumatology* **2019**, *58*, 1607–1616. [CrossRef] [PubMed]
65. Jauhola, O.; Ronkainen, J.; Koskimies, O.; Ala-Houhala, M.; Arikoski, P.; Holtta, T.; Jahnukainen, T.; Rajantie, J.; Ormala, T.; Nuutinen, M. Outcome of Henoch-Schonlein Purpura 8 years after treatment with a placebo or prednisone at disease onset. *Pediatr. Nephrol.* **2012**, *27*, 933–939. [CrossRef] [PubMed]
66. Novak, J.; Rizk, D.; Takahashi, K.; Zhang, X.; Bian, Q.; Ueda, H.; Ueda, Y.; Reily, C.; Lai, L.Y.; Hao, C.; et al. New insights into the pathogenesis of IgA nephropathy. *Kidney Dis.* **2015**, *1*, 8–18. [CrossRef] [PubMed]
67. Donadio, M.E.; Loiacono, E.; Peruzzi, L.; Amore, A.; Camilla, R.; Chiale, F.; Vergano, L.; Boido, A.; Conrieri, M.; Bianciotto, M.; et al. Toll-like receptors, immunoproteasome and regulatory t cells in children with henoch-schonlein purpura and primary IgA nephropathy. *Pediatr. Nephrol.* **2014**, *29*, 1545–1551. [CrossRef]
68. Saito, A.; Komatsuda, A.; Kaga, H.; Sato, R.; Togashi, M.; Okuyama, S.; Wakui, H.; Takahashi, N. Different expression patterns of toll-like receptor MRNAs in blood mononuclear cells of IgA nephropathy and IgA vasculitis with nephritis. *Tohoku J. Exp. Med.* **2016**, *240*, 199–208. [CrossRef]

69. Yang, Y.-H.; Tsai, I.-J.; Chang, C.-J.; Chuang, Y.-H.; Hsu, H.-Y.; Chiang, B.-L. The interaction between circulating complement proteins and cutaneous microvascular endothelial cells in the development of childhood henoch-schönlein purpura. *PLoS ONE* **2015**, *10*, e0120411. [CrossRef]
70. Maillard, N.; Wyatt, R.J.; Julian, B.A.; Kiryluk, K.; Gharavi, A.; Fremeaux-Bacchi, V.; Novak, J. Current understanding of the role of complement in IgA nephropathy. *J. Am. Soc. Nephrol.* **2015**, *26*, 1503–1512. [CrossRef]
71. Medjeral-Thomas, N.R.; Lomax-Browne, H.J.; Beckwith, H.; Willicombe, M.; McLean, A.G.; Brookes, P.; Pusey, C.D.; Falchi, M.; Cook, H.T.; Pickering, M.C. Circulating complement factor h-related proteins 1 and 5 correlate with disease activity in IgA nephropathy. *Kidney Int.* **2017**, *92*, 942–952. [CrossRef]
72. Kawasaki, Y.; Maeda, R.; Ohara, S.; Suyama, K.; Hosoya, M. Serum IgA/C3 and Glomerular C3 Staining Predict Severity of IgA Nephropathy. *Pediatr. Int.* **2018**, *60*, 162–167. [CrossRef] [PubMed]
73. Rizk, D.V.; Maillard, N.; Julian, B.A.; Knoppova, B.; Green, T.J.; Novak, J.; Wyatt, R.J. The emerging role of complement proteins as a target for therapy of IgA nephropathy. *Front. Immunol.* **2019**, *10*, 504. [CrossRef] [PubMed]
74. Suzuki, H. Biomarkers for IgA nephropathy on the basis of multi-hit pathogenesis. *Clin. Exp. Nephrol.* **2018**, *23*, 26–31. [CrossRef] [PubMed]
75. Wada, Y.; Matsumoto, K.; Suzuki, T.; Saito, T.; Kanazawa, N.; Tachibana, S.; Iseri, K.; Sugiyama, M.; Iyoda, M.; Shibata, T. Clinical significance of serum and mesangial galactose-deficient IgA1 in patients with IgA nephropathy. *PLoS ONE* **2018**, *13*, e0206865. [CrossRef] [PubMed]
76. Allen, A.C.; Willis, F.R.; Beattie, T.J.; Feehally, J. Abnormal IgA Glycosylation in henoch-schonlein purpura restricted to patients with clinical nephritis. *Nephrol. Dial. Transplant.* **1998**, *13*, 930–934. [CrossRef]
77. Berthelot, L.; Jamin, A.; Viglietti, D.; Chemouny, J.M.; Ayari, H.; Pierre, M.; Housset, P.; Sauvaget, V.; Hurtado-Nedelec, M.; Vrtovsnik, F.; et al. Value of biomarkers for predicting immunoglobulin a vasculitis nephritis outcome in an adult prospective cohort. *Nephrol. Dial. Transplant.* **2017**, *33*, 1579–1590. [CrossRef]
78. Pillebout, E.; Jamin, A.; Ayari, H.; Housset, P.; Pierre, M.; Sauvaget, V.; Viglietti, D.; Deschenes, G.; Monteiro, R.C.; Berthelot, L. Biomarkers of IgA vasculitis nephritis in children. *PLoS ONE* **2017**, *12*, e0188718. [CrossRef]
79. Lau, K.K.; Wyatt, R.J.; Moldoveanu, Z.; Tomana, M.; Julian, B.A.; Hogg, R.J.; Lee, J.Y.; Huang, W.Q.; Mestecky, J.; Novak, J. Serum levels of galactose-deficient IgA in children with IgA nephropathy and henoch-schonlein purpura. *Pediatr Nephrol* **2007**, *22*, 2067–2072. [CrossRef]
80. Esteve Cols, C.; Graterol Torres, F.-A.; Quirant Sánchez, B.; Marco Rusiñol, H.; Navarro Díaz, M.I.; Ara del Rey, J.; Martínez Cáceres, E.M. Immunological pattern in IgA nephropathy. *Int. J. Mol. Sci.* **2020**, *21*, 1389. [CrossRef]
81. Suzuki, H.; Moldoveanu, Z.; Julian, B.A.; Wyatt, R.J.; Novak, J. Autoantibodies specific for galactose-deficient IgA1 in IgA vasculitis with nephritis. *Kidney Int. Rep.* **2019**, *4*, 1717–1724. [CrossRef]
82. Moresco, R.N.; Speeckaert, M.M.; Zmonarski, S.C.; Krajewska, M.; Komuda-Leszek, E.; Perkowska-Ptasinska, A.; Gesualdo, L.; Rocchetti, M.T.; Delanghe, S.E.; Vanholder, R.; et al. Urinary myeloid IgA Fc alpha receptor (CD89) and Transglutaminase-2 as new biomarkers for active IgA Nephropathy and henoch-schonlein purpura nephritis. *BBA Clin.* **2016**, *5*, 79–84. [CrossRef] [PubMed]
83. Delanghe, S.E.; Speeckaert, M.M.; Segers, H.; Desmet, K.; Vande Walle, J.; Laecke, S.V.; Vanholder, R.; Delanghe, J.R. Soluble transferrin receptor in urine, a new biomarker for IgA nephropathy and henoch-schonlein purpura nephritis. *Clin. Biochem.* **2013**, *46*, 591–597. [CrossRef] [PubMed]
84. Suzuki, H.; Suzuki, Y.; Narita, I.; Aizawa, M.; Kihara, M.; Yamanaka, T.; Kanou, T.; Tsukaguchi, H.; Novak, J.; Horikoshi, S.; et al. Toll-like receptor 9 affects severity of IgA nephropathy. *J. Am. Soc. Nephrol.* **2008**, *19*, 2384–2395. [CrossRef]
85. Sato, D.; Suzuki, Y.; Kano, T.; Suzuki, H.; Matsuoka, J.; Yokoi, H.; Horikoshi, S.; Ikeda, K.; Tomino, Y. Tonsillar TLR9 expression and efficacy of tonsillectomy with steroid pulse therapy in IgA nephropathy patients. *Nephrol. Dial. Transplant.* **2012**, *27*, 1090–1097. [CrossRef] [PubMed]
86. Jia, M.; Zhu, L.; Zhai, Y.; Chen, P.; Xu, B.; Guo, W.; Shi, S.; Liu, L.; Lv, J.; Zhang, H. Variation in complement factor H affects complement activation in immunoglobulin A vasculitis with nephritis. *Nephrology* **2020**, *25*, 40–47. [CrossRef] [PubMed]
87. Moldoveanu, Z.; Wyatt, R.J.; Lee, J.Y.; Tomana, M.; Julian, B.A.; Mestecky, J.; Huang, W.-Q.; Anreddy, S.R.; Hall, S.; Hastings, M.C.; et al. Patients with IgA nephropathy have increased serum galactose-deficient IgA1 levels. *Kidney Int.* **2007**, *71*, 1148–1154. [CrossRef]
88. Yasutake, J.; Suzuki, Y.; Suzuki, H.; Hiura, N.; Yanagawa, H.; Makita, Y.; Kaneko, E.; Tomino, Y. Novel lectin-independent approach to detect galactose-deficient IgA1 in IgA nephropathy. *Nephrol. Dial. Transplant.* **2015**, *30*, 1315–1321. [CrossRef]
89. Kiryluk, K.; Moldoveanu, Z.; Sanders, J.T.; Eison, T.M.; Suzuki, H.; Julian, B.A.; Novak, J.; Gharavi, A.G.; Wyatt, R.J. Aberrant glycosylation of IgA1 is inherited in both pediatric IgA nephropathy and henoch-schonlein purpura nephritis. *Kidney Int.* **2011**, *80*, 79–87. [CrossRef]
90. Gharavi, A.G.; Moldoveanu, Z.; Wyatt, R.J.; Barker, C.V.; Woodford, S.Y.; Lifton, R.P.; Mestecky, J.; Novak, J.; Julian, B.A. Aberrant IgA1 glycosylation is inherited in familial and sporadic IgA nephropathy. *JASN* **2008**, *19*, 1008–1014. [CrossRef]
91. Lin, X.; Ding, J.; Zhu, L.; Shi, S.; Jiang, L.; Zhao, M.; Zhang, H. Aberrant galactosylation of IgA1 is involved in the genetic susceptibility of chinese patients with IgA nephropathy. *Nephrol. Dial. Transplant.* **2009**, *24*, 3372–3375. [CrossRef]
92. Hastings, M.C.; Moldoveanu, Z.; Julian, B.A.; Novak, J.; Sanders, J.T.; McGlothan, K.R.; Gharavi, A.G.; Wyatt, R.J. Galactose-deficient IgA1 in African Americans with IgA nephropathy: Serum levels and heritability. *CJASN* **2010**, *5*, 2069–2074. [CrossRef]

93. Kiryluk, K.; Li, Y.; Sanna-Cherchi, S.; Rohanizadegan, M.; Suzuki, H.; Eitner, F.; Snyder, H.J.; Choi, M.; Hou, P.; Scolari, F.; et al. Geographic differences in genetic susceptibility to IgA nephropathy: GWAS replication study and geospatial risk analysis. *PLoS Genet.* **2012**, *8*, e1002765. [CrossRef] [PubMed]
94. López-Mejías, R.; Castañeda, S.; Genre, F.; Remuzgo-Martínez, S.; Carmona, F.D.; Llorca, J.; Blanco, R.; Martín, J.; González-Gay, M.A. Genetics of immunoglobulin-A vasculitis (Henoch-Schönlein Purpura): An updated review. *Autoimmun. Rev.* **2018**, *17*, 301–315. [CrossRef] [PubMed]
95. Kim, C.H.; Lim, B.J.; Bae, Y.S.; Kwon, Y.E.; Kim, Y.L.; Nam, K.H.; Park, K.S.; An, S.Y.; Koo, H.M.; Doh, F.M.; et al. Using the Oxford classification of IgA Nephropathy to predict long-term outcomes of henoch-schonlein purpura nephritis in adults. *Mod. Pathol.* **2014**, *27*, 972–982. [CrossRef] [PubMed]
96. Inagaki, K.; Kaihan, A.B.; Hachiya, A.; Ozeki, T.; Ando, M.; Kato, S.; Yasuda, Y.; Maruyama, S. Clinical impact of endocapillary proliferation according to the Oxford classification among adults with henoch-schönlein purpura nephritis: A multicenter retrospective cohort study. *BMC Nephrol.* **2018**, *19*, 208. [CrossRef]
97. Xu, K.; Zhang, L.; Ding, J.; Wang, S.; Su, B.; Xiao, H.; Wang, F.; Zhong, X.; Li, Y. Value of the Oxford classification of IgA nephropathy in children with henoch–schönlein purpura nephritis. *J. Nephrol.* **2018**, *31*, 279–286. [CrossRef]
98. Li, X.; Tang, M.; Yao, X.; Zhang, N.; Fan, J.; Zhou, N.; Sun, Q.; Chen, Z.; Meng, Q.; Lei, L.; et al. A clinicopathological comparison between IgA nephropathy and henoch–schönlein purpura nephritis in children: Use of the Oxford classification. *Clin. Exp. Nephrol.* **2019**, *23*, 1382–1390. [CrossRef]

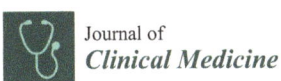

Article

IgA Vasculitis with Nephritis in Adults: Histological and Clinical Assessment

Lingyun Lai [1,2], Shaojun Liu [1], Maria Azrad [3], Stacy Hall [2], Chuanming Hao [1], Jan Novak [2], Bruce A. Julian [4] and Lea Novak [5,*]

1. Division of Nephrology, Fudan University Huashan Hospital, Shanghai 200040, China; lailingyun@fudan.edu.cn (L.L.); liushaojun@fudan.edu.cn (S.L.); chuanminghao@fudan.edu.cn (C.H.)
2. Department of Microbiology, University of Alabama at Birmingham, Birmingham, AL 35294, USA; shall@uab.edu (S.H.); jannovak@uab.edu (J.N.)
3. Department of Nutrition, University of Alabama at Birmingham, Birmingham, AL 35294, USA; mazrad@ches.ua.edu
4. Department of Medicine, University of Alabama at Birmingham, Birmingham, AL 35294, USA; bjulian@uabmc.edu
5. Department of Pathology, University of Alabama at Birmingham, Birmingham, AL 35294, USA
* Correspondence: lnovakpath@gmail.com

Abstract: Patients with IgA vasculitis (IgAV), an immune complex-mediated disease, may exhibit kidney involvement—IgAV with nephritis (IgAVN). The kidney-biopsy histopathologic features of IgAVN are similar to those of IgA nephropathy, but little is known about histopathologic disease severity based on the interval between purpura onset and diagnostic kidney biopsy. We assessed kidney histopathology and clinical and laboratory data in a cohort of adult patients with IgAVN (n = 110). The cases were grouped based on the interval between the onset of purpura and kidney biopsy: Group 1 (G1, <1 month, n = 14), Group 2 (G2, 1–6 months, n = 58), and Group 3 (G3, >6 months, n = 38). Glomerular leukocytes were more common in G1 than in the other groups ($p = 0.0008$). The proportion of neutrophils among peripheral-blood leukocytes was the highest in the patients biopsied within a month after onset of purpura (G1: 71 ± 8%). In the patients with an interval >6 months, the neutrophil proportion was lower, 60%. Moreover, the glomerular mesangial proliferation score correlated with the serum total IgA concentration ($p = 0.0056$). In conclusion, IgAVN patients biopsied <1 month from purpura onset showed an elevated percentage of blood neutrophils and glomerular leukocytes, consistent with an acute-onset inflammatory reaction. In all IgAVN patients, the mesangial proliferation score correlated with the serum IgA level.

Keywords: IgA vasculitis; nephritis; kidney biopsy

1. Introduction

IgA vasculitis (IgAV), formerly known as Henoch–Schönlein purpura, is a systemic immune complex-mediated, small-vessel leukocytoclastic vasculitis. It is characterized by nonthrombocytopenic palpable purpura and/or arthritis, and abdominal pain [1]. IgAV, the most common vasculitis in children, is often a self-limiting and benign disease that spontaneously resolves.

A minority of pediatric IgAV patients exhibits kidney involvement—IgAV with nephritis (IgAVN)—usually 4–6 weeks after the onset of purpura [2–5]. The kidney-biopsy histopathologic features of IgAVN are similar to those of IgA nephropathy (IgAN), including glomerular IgA1-containing immunodeposits [1,2,4,6–11].

IgAV in adults has a more severe course and poor outcome due to the high frequency of glomerulonephritis, i.e., IgAVN—the most serious complication of this vasculitis. However, there is limited information about the histopathologic disease severity as related to disease onset.

In this study, we assessed the kidney histopathology and clinical and laboratory data in a large cohort of adult patients with IgAVN whose diagnostic kidney biopsies had been performed at different intervals after the onset of purpura.

2. Materials and Methods

2.1. IgAVN Patients

This is a retrospective study of 110 adult patients with IgAVN. All patients underwent a diagnostic kidney biopsy between 2002 and 2013 at the Department of Nephrology, Huashan Hospital, Fudan University, Shanghai, China. The diagnosis of IgAVN was based on the documented hematuria and proteinuria associated with a characteristic purpuric eruption, or abdominal or joint pain. IgA as the predominant mesangial immunoglobulin as per immunofluorescence microscopy in kidney biopsy specimens was required for inclusion in the study. We excluded patients whose biopsies contained <8 glomeruli, a number considered inadequate for appropriate histopathologic scoring (12), as detailed below.

The appearance of purpura defined the onset of IgAV. The 110 patients were divided into three groups based on the interval between purpura onset and diagnostic kidney biopsy: Group 1, <1 month (n = 14); Group 2, 1–6 months (n = 58); and Group 3, >6 months (n = 38; mostly >1 year, with the longest interval 13 years). All biopsies were performed for subjects who exhibited proteinuria in an outpatient setting (>0.5 g/24 h or urinary albumin/creatinine ratio >300 mg/g). The clinical features, laboratory data from the time of biopsy, and histopathologic findings in the biopsy specimens were retrospectively compiled for each group. However, no data from the outpatient follow-up visits since the onset of purpura or after kidney biopsy were available for this study. No personal identification information was collected. The study was approved by the ethics board of Huashan Hospital, Fudan University, Shanghai, China.

2.2. Clinical and Demographic Data

All clinical, laboratory, and demographic data were collected at the time of the kidney biopsy. The demographic data included age, gender, and comorbidities such as hypertension, diabetes mellitus, and cardiovascular disease. The characteristics of IgAVN included skin rash, gastrointestinal and joint manifestations, and kidney involvement. Proteinuria was evaluated by a 24-h urine measurement, hematuria was defined as 22 or more red blood cells (RBC) per microliter of urine (microscopic), or visible hematuria (macroscopic). The serum albumin, creatinine, urea nitrogen, uric acid, complement C3, and total IgA levels were measured at the time of kidney biopsy in the central clinical laboratory of Huashan Hospital. The number of urinary RBC had been determined by using a Sysmex UF-1000i analyzer (Siemens, Germany). Peripheral blood cell profiling was performed using a Sysmex xn-2000 analyzer (Siemens, Germany) and expressed as the total number of leukocytes and relative proportions of neutrophils and eosinophils (as % of total leukocytes).

2.3. Kidney Pathology

Two pathologists examined and graded the histopathological changes. To evaluate the glomerular mesangial-cell proliferation, the cellularity of each glomerulus was graded as per the Oxford classification [12] (<4 mesangial cells/mesangial area = 0; 4–5 mesangial cells/mesangial area = 1; 6–7 mesangial cells/mesangial area = 2; >8 mesangial cells/mesangial area = 3), and a mean mesangial score was calculated for each biopsy. Mesangial Score: sum of grades divided by number of glomeruli (excluding globally sclerotic glomeruli). Crescents (%): number of glomeruli with crescents divided by number of glomeruli × 100. Leukocyte infiltration of glomeruli was considered significant when five or more polymorphonuclear and mononuclear cells per glomerulus were observed using the periodic-acid Schiff-stained tissue sections [11,12] (Figure 1).

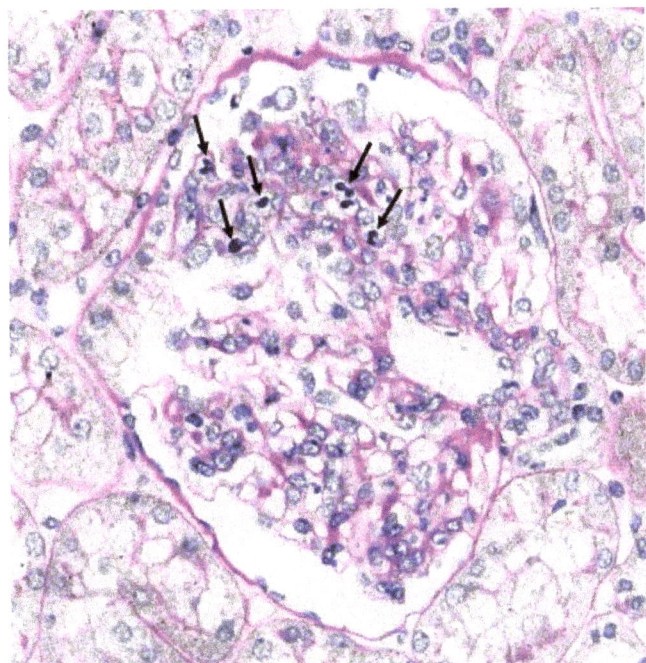

Figure 1. Example of a glomerulus of a patient with IgAVN exhibiting mesangial proliferation and glomerular leukocytes. Representative leukocytes are marked by arrows. PAS stain, magnification 400×.

2.4. Statistical Analyses

Normally distributed variables are expressed as the mean ± standard deviation (SD) and were compared using one-way analysis of variance (ANOVA) or Student's *t*-test. Nonnormally distributed variables are expressed as the median with interquartile range and were compared using the rank sum test. Categorical variables are expressed as percentages and compared using Pearson's chi-square test or Fisher's exact test. All tests were two-tailed, and statistical significance was defined as $p < 0.05$. The SPSS statistical software program (version 15.0, SPSS Inc., Chicago, IL, USA) was used for all analyses.

3. Results

3.1. Baseline Clinical Data at the Time of Kidney Biopsy

IgAVN patients (n = 110) in this study had a mean age of 36.5 ± 16.0 years at the time of kidney biopsy and consisted of 50 males and 60 females (Table 1). All patients presented with cutaneous purpura on at least one occasion; purpura was associated with arthralgia in 30 cases (26%) and with arthralgia and abdominal pain in 31 cases (27%). At the time of kidney biopsy, proteinuria ≥0.30 g/24 h was detected in 105 patients (92%) and 73 patients had proteinuria ≥1 g/24 h (64%). Five patients with proteinuria ≥0.5 g/24 h originally measured in the outpatient clinic had proteinuria <0.30 g/24 h later on admission to the hospital for kidney biopsy, likely due to prior treatment with an angiotensin-converting enzyme inhibitor (ACEi) and/or angiotensin receptor blocker (ARB).

Microscopic hematuria was observed in 86 patients (78%). Hypertension was present in 23 patients (21%) and 4 patients (4%) had diabetes mellitus (DM). Seven patients (6%) had reduced kidney clearance function, with an eGFR <60 mL/min/1.73 m^2 as per the MDRD formula. Twenty-seven patients (25%) had received an ACEi and/or an ARB before kidney biopsy.

Table 1. Clinical characteristics of 110 patients with IgAVN.

Characteristics	Values
Age (years, mean ± SD)	36.5 ± 16.0
Males (%)	50 (45)
Subjects with hypertension (%)	23 (21)
Subjects with diabetes mellitus (%)	4 (4)
Serum creatinine (mg/dL) mean (95% CI)	0.85 (0.78, 0.92)
eGFR (mL/min/1.73 m^2, mean ± SD)	110 ± 43
Subjects on ACEi/ARB before kidney biopsy (%)	27 (25)

Abbreviations: SD, standard deviation; CI, confidence interval; eGFR, estimated glomerular filtration rate; ACEi, angiotensin-converting enzyme inhibitor; ARB, angiotensin receptor blocker.

3.2. Kidney Histopathology and Kidney Function

The light-microscopic features for this cohort are summarized in Table 2. The patients had a mean mesangial score of 1.1 (range 0.3–2.4); 18% exhibited segmental sclerosis; 3%, global sclerosis; 25%, glomerular adhesion; 20%, glomerular leukocytes; 43%, tubular atrophy; 40%, interstitial fibrosis; 39%, interstitial leukocytes; and 9%, crescents. Kidney function was worse in the subjects with crescents than in those without crescents (serum creatinine: 0.91 ± 0.43 mg/dL vs. 0.76 ± 0.20 mg/dL, p = 0.038; eGFR: 93 ± 32 mL/min/1.73 m^2 vs. 109 ± 28 mL/min/1.73 m^2, p = 0.009).

Table 2. Summary of the kidney pathology findings for 110 patients with IgA vasculitis with nephritis.

Characteristics	Values
Mesangial score: mean (95% CI)	1.1 (1.02–1.17)
Segmental sclerosis (%)	18
Global sclerosis (%)	4
Glomerular adhesion (%)	26
Glomerular leukocytes (%)	20
Tubular atrophy (%)	43
Interstitial fibrosis (%)	40
Interstitial leukocytes (%)	39
Crescents (%)	9

Abbreviations: CI, confidence interval.

3.3. Histopathology of Kidney Biopsy Specimens with Different Intervals between Purpura Onset and Diagnostic Kidney Biopsy

We next assessed whether the kidney pathology findings differed based on the interval between purpura onset and diagnostic kidney biopsy. The MEST-C scores (12) were calculated (Table 3). Using ANOVA and Student's t-test, the only significant difference between the groups was for M1 between Group 2 and Group 3 (p = 0.006). Furthermore, glomerular leukocytes were more common in Group 1 (57%) compared to Group 2 and Group 3 (p = 0.0008) (Table 3). Thus, IgAVN patients with kidney biopsy less than one month after purpura onset more frequently had leukocytes in the glomeruli. Furthermore, M1 was more common in Group 3 than in Group 2.

3.4. Neutrophils in Peripheral Blood in Patients with Different Intervals between Purpura Onset and Diagnostic Kidney Biopsy

Patients in Groups 1, 2, and 3 had a similar age, gender representation, mean 24-h proteinuria, hematuria, mean eGFR, and frequency of ACEi/ARB treatment. However, the percentage of neutrophils in the circulating leukocytes differed between groups (Group 1: 71 ± 8%; Group 2: 68 ± 11%; and Group 3: 60 ± 12%; p = 0.001), being the highest in patients biopsied within a month after onset of purpura (Table 3). When we evaluated the neutrophils to lymphocytes ratio (NLR), there was no significant difference for any comparison of the groups (Table 3).

Table 3. Characteristics of 110 patients with IgAVN grouped based on the interval between purpura onset and diagnostic kidney biopsy.

Characteristics	Group 1 [a] (n = 14)	Group 2 (n = 58)	Group 3 (n = 38)	p Value
Age (yr) [c], (mean ± SD)	40.5 ± 19.3	36.8 ± 16.0	34.5 ± 14.9	0.47 [b]
Male gender (% male)	6 (43)	28 (48)	16 (42)	0.82
Hypertension (%)	4 (29)	12 (21)	7 (18)	0.73
Diabetes mellitus (%)	2 (14)	1 (2)	1 (3)	0.07
ACEi/ARB before biopsy (%)	10 (19)	6 (32)	11 (28)	0.74
Proteinuria (g/24 h) (range)	2.23 (1.11, 4.68)	1.39 (0.87, 2.29)	1.13 (0.59, 1.93)	0.08
Urinary RBC (number/μL; mean ± SD)	667 ± 885	369 ± 602	405 ± 660	0.29
SCr (mg/dL; mean ± SD)	0.97 ± 0.34	0.83 ± 0.40	0.83 ± 0.29	0.42
eGFR (mL/min/1.73 m^2; mean ± SD)	91 ± 29	113 ± 49	112 ± 36	0.28
WBC (×10^9/L; mean ± SD)	11.1 ± 7.0	9.3 ± 3.6	8.5 ± 3.4	0.13
Neutrophils (% of WBC; mean ± SD)	71 ± 8	68 ± 11	60 ± 12	1 vs. 2 = 0.3067; 1 vs. 3 = 0.0039; 2 vs. 3 = 0.0008
Eosinophils (% of total WBC; mean ± SD)	2 ± 4	1 ± 2	2 ± 3	0.40
Serum albumin (g/dL; mean ± SD)	3.3 ± 0.6	3.5 ± 0.6	3.7 ± 0.5	0.14
Serum total IgA (g/L; mean ± SD)	3.1 ± 1.2	3.0 ± 1.3	2.9 ± 1.0	0.86
Serum C3 (g/L; mean ± SD)	1.17 ± 0.30	1.09 ± 0.24	1.10 ± 0.25	0.57
Glomeruli with leukocytes (%)	8 (57)	6 (10)	8 (21)	0.0008 [b]
NLR (mean ± SD) c	2.7 ± 0.8	2.6 ± 1.5	2.1 ± 1.4	0.09 [b]
MEST-C score				
M1 (%)	71	68	95	0.0075 [b]; 2 vs. 3 = 0.006
E1 (%)	14	42	30	0.106 [b]
S1 (%)	21	14	24	0.397 [b]
T1/T2 (%)	7	5	14	0.344 [b]
C1/C2 (%)	57	49	60	0.598 [b]

[a] 110 cases were divided into three groups: Group 1, <1 month; Group 2, 1–6 months; and Group 3, >6 months. [b] Fisher's Exact for proportions. [c] Abbreviations: yr, years; SD, standard deviation; SCr, serum creatinine; CI, confidence interval; eGFR, estimated glomerular filtration rate; ACEi, angiotensin-converting enzyme inhibitor; ARB, angiotensin receptor blocker; NLR, neutrophils to lymphocytes ratio; RBC, red blood cells; WBC, white blood cells (leukocytes) in peripheral blood. MEST-C scores were determined as described previously (12). M: mesangial hypercellularity; E: endocapillary hypercellularity; S: segmental glomerulosclerosis; T: tubular atrophy/interstitial fibrosis; C: cellular/fibrocellular crescents.

3.5. Association of Serum Total IgA Concentration and Mesangial Proliferation

The serum total IgA concentration positively correlated with the glomerular mesangial-proliferation score (p = 0.0056) (Figure 2).

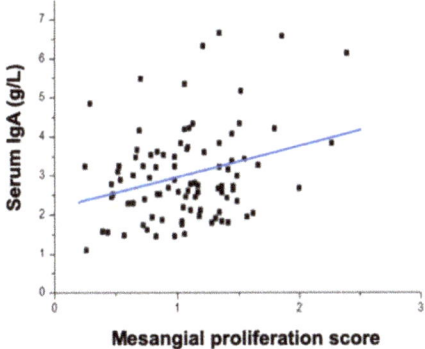

Figure 2. Glomerular mesangial proliferation correlates with serum total IgA level. Serum total IgA levels correlate with the mesangial proliferation score in patients with IgAVN. The line shows a linear fit (p = 0.0056).

4. Discussion

IgAV is the most common vasculitis in children but it can also occur in adults. IgAV spontaneously resolves in about 94% of children and 89% of adults [13], although some IgAV patients exhibit kidney involvement (IgAVN). The disease mechanisms of IgAVN and IgAN are thought to be closely related [6,9]. Both diseases exhibit glomerular IgA immunodeposits with co-deposits of complement C3 [13–18]. The IgA immunodeposits are of the IgA1 subclass [18–20].

Pathogenesis of both IgAN and IgAVN is thought to occur through a multi-hit process [5]. This process includes the production of galactose-deficient IgA1 (Gd-IgA1) [21–29], generation of circulating IgG autoantibodies specific for Gd-IgA1 [29–34], formation of pathogenic Gd-IgA1-containing immune complexes [30,35–43], and the subsequent mesangial deposition of these immune complexes resulting in glomerular injury [34,44]. These conclusions are supported by multiple lines of evidence. For example, serum levels of Gd-IgA1 and the corresponding IgG autoantibodies are associated with a faster decline in kidney function in patients with IgAN [45–47]. Moreover, IgA-containing glomerular immunodeposits are enriched for Gd-IgA1 glycoforms [48,49] and the corresponding IgG autoantibodies [33]. In both IgAN and IgAVN, Gd-IgA1 is produced by IgA1-secreting cells due to dysregulation of key glycosyltransferases [29,50,51].

Circulating levels of Gd-IgA1 and Gd-IgA1-specific IgG autoantibodies are elevated in patients with IgAVN but not in patients with IgAV [29], supporting the hypothesis that IgAVN and IgAN share pathogenetic components. IgAVN patients have the onset of disease defined by purpura, with kidney involvement developing with 4–6 weeks later [5,13,17]. However, there is a limited information about histopathologic disease severity in relation to disease onset.

In this study of 110 adult patients with IgAVN, we assessed histopathologic disease severity based on interval between purpura onset and diagnostic kidney biopsy and correlated the findings with clinical and laboratory data. IgAVN patients biopsied <1 month since the onset of purpura more commonly had glomerular leukocytes and had the highest percentage of neutrophils among peripheral-blood leukocytes. These findings are consistent with an acute-onset inflammatory reaction in patients with IgAVN who were biopsied <1 month after the onset of purpura. Moreover, serum total IgA concentration correlated with the glomerular mesangial proliferation score.

A limitation of this study is the relatively small number of patients from a single center who were of single ethnicity. The patients were followed regularly for up to 6 months after the appearance of purpura at their respective local-area hospitals. However, these data were not been available for this study. This limitation implies that these findings need to be assessed in other cohorts and different ethnic groups, ideally with regular follow-up after the onset of purpura until biopsy as well as after biopsy.

Our study demonstrates a chronological association between leukocytic infiltration and glomeruloproliferative responses in IgAVN patients. These findings raise a question whether patients with IgAV should be followed frequently after the onset of purpura to detect nephritis in the early stages and whether assessment of biomarkers, such as Gd-IgA1- and Gd-IgA1-specific IgG autoantibodies, should be included.

Author Contributions: Conceptualization, L.L., C.H., J.N., B.A.J. and L.N.; data generation, L.L., S.L. and L.N.; statistical analyses, L.L., M.A., S.H. and L.N.; writing—original draft manuscript, L.L. and L.N.; writing—review and editing, L.L., J.N., B.A.J. and L.N. All authors have read and agreed to the published version of the manuscript.

Funding: Supported by NIH grants DK078244 and DK082753 and a gift from the IGA Nephropathy Foundation of America.

Institutional Review Board Statement: The study was conducted according to the guidelines of the Declaration of Helsinki, and was approved by ethics board of Huashan Hospital, Fudan University, Shanghai, China.

Informed Consent Statement: Not Applicable.

Data Availability Statement: Not Applicable.

Conflicts of Interest: B.A.J. and J.N. are co-inventors on US patent application 14/318,082 (assigned to UAB Research Foundation). B.A.J. and J.N. are co-founders and co-owners of and consultants for Reliant Glycosciences, LLC.

References

1. Saulsbury, F.T. Henoch-Schönlein purpura. *Curr. Opin. Rheumatol.* **2010**, *22*, 598–602. [CrossRef]
2. Davin, J.-C. Henoch-Schönlein purpura nephritis: Pathophysiology, treatment, and future strategy. *Clin. J. Am. Soc. Nephrol.* **2011**, *6*, 679–689. [CrossRef] [PubMed]
3. Davin, J.C.; Coppo, R. Henoch-Schönlein purpura nephritis in children. *Nat. Rev. Nephrol.* **2014**, *10*, 563–573. [CrossRef]
4. Haas, M. IgA nephropathy and Henoch-Schönlein purpura nephritis. In *Heptinstall's Pathology of the Kidney*; Jennette, J.C., Olson, J.L., Schwartz, M.M., Silva, F.G., Eds.; Lippincott, Williams and Wilkins: Philadelphia, PA, USA, 2007; pp. 423–486.
5. Hastings, M.C.; Rizk, D.V.; Kiryluk, K.; Nelson, R.; Zahr, R.S.; Novak, J.; Wyatt, R.J. IgA vasculitis with nephritis: Update of pathogenesis with clinical implications. *Pediatr. Nephrol.* **2021**, 1–15. [CrossRef]
6. Davin, J.C.; Ten Berge, I.J.; Weening, J.J. What is the difference between IgA nephropathy and Henoch-Schönlein purpura nephritis? *Kidney Int.* **2001**, *59*, 823–834. [CrossRef]
7. Emancipator, S.N. IgA nephropathy and Henoch-Schönlein syndrome. In *Heptinstall's Pathology of the Kidney*; Jennette, J.C., Olson, J.L., Schwartz, M.M., Silva, F.G., Eds.; Lippincott-Raven Publishers: Philadelphia, PA, USA, 1998; pp. 479–539.
8. Fervenza, F.C. Henoch-Schönlein purpura nephritis. *Int. J. Dermatol.* **2003**, *42*, 170–177. [CrossRef] [PubMed]
9. Waldo, F.B. Is Henoch-Schönlein purpura the systemic form of IgA nephropathy? *Am. J. Kidney Dis.* **1988**, *12*, 373–377. [CrossRef]
10. Wyatt, R.J.; Novak, J.; Gaber, L.W.; Lau, K.K. IgA nephropathy and Henoch-Schönlein purpura nephritis. In *Clinical Pediatric Nephrology*, 2nd ed.; Kher, K.K., Schnapper, H.W., Makker, S.P., Eds.; Informa UK Ltd.: London, UK, 2006; pp. 213–222.
11. Szeto, C.C.; Choi, P.C.L.; To, K.F.; Li, P.K.T.; Hui, J.; Chow, K.M.; Leung, C.B.; Lui, S.F.; Lai, F.M.-M. Grading of acute and chronic renal lesions in Henoch-Schönlein purpura. *Mod. Pathol.* **2001**, *14*, 635–640. [CrossRef]
12. Roberts, I.S.; Cook, H.T.; Troyanov, S.; Alpers, C.E.; Amore, A.; Barratt, J.; Berthoux, F.; Bonsib, S.; Bruijn, J.A. The Oxford classification of IgA nephropathy: Pathology definitions, correlations, and reproducibility. *Kidney Int.* **2009**, *76*, 546–556. [CrossRef]
13. Reamy, B.V.; Servey, J.T.; Williams, P.M. Henoch-Schönlein purpura (IgA vasculitis): Rapid evidence review. *Am. Fam. Physician* **2020**, *102*, 229–233.
14. Urizar, R.E.; Michael, A.; Sisson, S.; Vernier, R.L. Anaphylactoid purpura. II. Immunofluorescent and electron microscopic studies of the glomerular lesions. *Lab. Investig.* **1968**, *19*, 437–450. [PubMed]
15. Berger, J. IgA glomerular deposits in renal disease. *Transplant. Proc.* **1969**, *1*, 939–944. [PubMed]
16. Evans, D.J.; Williams, D.G.; Peters, D.K.; Sissons, J.G.P.; Boulton-Jones, J.M.; Ogg, C.S.; Cameron, J.S.; Hoffbrand, B.I. Glomerular deposition of properdin in Henoch-Schönlein syndrome and idiopathic focal nephritis. *Br. Med. J.* **1973**, *3*, 326–328. [CrossRef] [PubMed]
17. Selewski, D.T.; Ambruzs, J.M.; Appel, G.B.; Bomback, A.S.; Matar, R.B.; Cai, Y.; Cattran, D.C.; Chishti, A.S.; D'Agati, V.D.; D'Alessandri-Silva, C.J.; et al. Clinical characteristics and treatment patterns of children and adults with IgA nephropathy or IgA vasculitis: Findings from the CureGN study. *Kidney Int. Rep.* **2018**, *3*, 1373–1384. [CrossRef] [PubMed]
18. Pillebout, E.; Jamin, A.; Ayari, H.; Housset, P.; Pierre, M.; Sauvaget, V.; Viglietti, D.; Deschenes, G.; Monteiro, R.C.; Berthelot, L.; et al. Biomarkers of IgA vasculitis nephritis in children. *PLoS ONE* **2017**, *12*, e0188718. [CrossRef] [PubMed]
19. Conley, E.M.; Cooper, M.; Michael, A.F. Selective deposition of immunoglobulin A1 in immunoglobulin A nephropathy, anaphylactoid purpura nephritis, and systemic lupus erythematosus. *J. Clin. Investig.* **1980**, *66*, 1432–1436. [CrossRef]
20. Suzuki, H.; Yasutake, J.; Makita, Y.; Tanbo, Y.; Yamasaki, K.; Sofue, T.; Kano, T.; Suzuki, Y. IgA nephropathy and IgA vasculitis with nephritis have a shared feature involving galactose-deficient IgA1-oriented pathogenesis. *Kidney Int.* **2018**, *93*, 700–705. [CrossRef] [PubMed]
21. Saulsbury, F.T. Alterations in the O-linked glycosylation of IgA1 in children with Henoch-Schönlein purpura. *J. Rheumatol.* **1997**, *24*, 2246–2249.
22. Allen, A.C.; Willis, F.R.; Beattie, T.J.; Feehally, J. Abnormal IgA glycosylation in Henoch-Schönlein purpura restricted to pa-tients with clinical nephritis. *Nephrol Dial Transplant.* **1998**, *13*, 930–934. [CrossRef]
23. Lau, K.K.; Wyatt, R.J.; Moldoveanu, Z.; Tomana, M.; Julian, B.J.; Hogg, R.J.; Lee, J.Y.; Huang, W.-Q.; Mestecky, J.; Novak, J. Serum levels of galactose-deficient IgA in children with IgA nephropathy and Henoch-Schoenlein purpura. *Ped. Nephrol.* **2007**, *22*, 2067–2072. [CrossRef]
24. Mizerska-Wasiak, M.; Gajewski, Ł.; Cichoń-Kawa, K.; Małdyk, J.; Dziedzic-Jankowska, K.; Leszczyńska, B.; Szuminska, A.A.R.; Wasilewska, A.; Pukajło-Marczyk, A.; Zwolińska, D.; et al. Serum GDIgA1 levels in children with IgA nephropathy and Henoch-Schönlein nephritis. *Cent. Eur. J. Immunol.* **2018**, *43*, 162–167. [CrossRef] [PubMed]

25. Nakazawa, S.; Imamura, R.; Kawamura, M.; Kato, T.; Abe, T.; Iwatani, H.; Yamanaka, K.; Uemura, M.; Kishikawa, H.; Nishimura, K.; et al. Evaluation of IgA1 O-glycosylation in Henoch-Schönlein purpura nephritis using mass spectrometry. *Transplant. Proc.* **2019**, *51*, 1481–1487. [CrossRef]
26. Novak, J.; Moldoveanu, Z.; Renfrow, M.B.; Yanagihara, T.; Suzuki, H.; Raska, M.; Hall, S.; Brown, R.; Huang, W.-Q.; Goepfert, A.; et al. IgA nephropathy and Henoch-Schoenlein purpura nephritis: Aberrant glycosylation of IgA1, formation of IgA1-containing immune complexes, and activation of mesangial cells. *Contrib. Nephrol.* **2007**, *157*, 134–138. [CrossRef] [PubMed]
27. Moldoveanu, Z.; Wyatt, R.J.; Lee, J.Y.; Tomana, M.; Julian, B.A.; Mestecky, J.; Huang, W.-Q.; Anreddy, S.R.; Hall, S.; Hastings, M.C.; et al. Patients with IgA nephropathy have increased serum galactose-deficient IgA1 levels. *Kidney Int.* **2007**, *71*, 1148–1154. [CrossRef]
28. Kiryluk, K.; Moldoveanu, Z.; Sanders, J.T.; Eison, T.M.; Suzuki, H.; Julian, B.A.; Novak, J.; Gharavi, A.G.; Wyatt, R.J. Aberrant glycosylation of IgA1 is inherited in both pediatric IgA nephropathy and Henoch-Schönlein purpura nephritis. *Kidney Int.* **2011**, *80*, 79–87. [CrossRef] [PubMed]
29. Suzuki, H.; Moldoveanu, Z.; Julian, B.A.; Wyatt, R.J.; Novak, J. Autoantibodies specific for galactose-deficient IgA1 in IgA vasculitis with nephritis. *Kidney Int. Rep.* **2019**, *4*, 1717–1724. [CrossRef]
30. Tomana, M.; Novak, J.; Julian, B.A.; Matousovic, K.; Konecny, K.; Mestecky, J. Circulating immune complexes in IgA nephropathy consist of IgA1 with galactose-deficient hinge region and antiglycan antibodies. *J. Clin. Investig.* **1999**, *104*, 73–81. [CrossRef]
31. Suzuki, H.; Fan, R.; Zhang, Z.; Brown, R.; Hall, S.; Julian, B.A.; Chatham, W.W.; Suzuki, Y.; Wyatt, R.J.; Moldoveanu, Z.; et al. Aberrantly glycosylated IgA1 in IgA nephropathy patients is recognized by IgG antibodies with restricted heterogeneity. *J. Clin. Investig.* **2009**, *119*, 1668–1677. [CrossRef]
32. Huang, Z.Q.; Raska, M.; Stewart, T.J.; Reily, C.; King, R.G.; Crossman, D.K.; Crowley, M.R.; Hargett, A.; Zhang, Z.; Suzuki, H.; et al. Somatic mutations modulate autoantibodies against galactose-deficient IgA1 in IgA nephropathy. *J. Am. Soc. Nephrol.* **2016**, *27*, 3278–3284. [CrossRef] [PubMed]
33. Rizk, D.V.; Saha, M.K.; Hall, S.; Novak, L.; Brown, R.; Huang, Z.-Q.; Fatima, H.; Julian, B.A.; Novak, J. Glomerular immunodeposits of patients with IgA nephropathy are enriched for IgG autoantibodies specific for galactose-deficient IgA1. *J. Am. Soc. Nephrol.* **2019**, *30*, 2017–2026. [CrossRef]
34. Moldoveanu, Z.; Suzuki, H.; Reily, C.; Satake, K.; Novak, L.; Xu, N.; Huang, Z.-Q.; Knoppova, B.; Khan, A.; Hall, S.; et al. Experimental evidence of pathogenic role of IgG autoantibodies in IgA nephropathy. *J. Autoimmun.* **2021**, *118*, 102593. [CrossRef] [PubMed]
35. Novak, J.; Tomana, M.; Brown, R.; Hall, S.; Novak, L.; Julian, B.A.; Wyatt, R.J.; Mestecky, J.; Matousovic, K. IgA1-containing immune complexes in IgA nephropathy differentially affect proliferation of mesangial cells. *Kidney Int.* **2005**, *67*, 504–513. [CrossRef] [PubMed]
36. Novak, J.; Kafkova, L.R.; Suzuki, H.; Tomana, M.; Matousovic, K.; Brown, R.; Hall, S.; Sanders, J.T.; Eison, T.M.; Moldoveanu, Z.; et al. IgA immune complexes from pediatric patients with IgA nephropathy activate cultured human mesangial cells. *Nephrol. Dial. Transplant.* **2011**, *26*, 3451–3457. [CrossRef] [PubMed]
37. Moura, I.C.; Arcos-Fajardo, M.; Sadaka, C.; Leroy, V.; Benhamou, M.; Novak, J.; Vrtovsnik, F.; Haddad, E.; Chintalacharuvu, K.R.; Monteiro, R.C. Glycosylation and size of IgA1 are essential for interaction with mesangial transferrin receptor in IgA nephropathy. *J. Am. Soc. Nephrol.* **2004**, *15*, 622–634. [CrossRef] [PubMed]
38. Maillard, N.; Wyatt, R.J.; Julian, B.A.; Kiryluk, K.; Gharavi, A.; Fremeaux-Bacchi, V.; Novak, J. Current Understanding of the role of complement in IgA nephropathy. *J. Am. Soc. Nephrol.* **2015**, *26*, 1503–1512. [CrossRef]
39. Coppo, R.; Andrulli, S.; Amore, A.; Gianoglio, B.; Conti, G.; Peruzzi, L.; Locatelli, F.; Cagnoli, L. Predictors of outcome in Henoch-Schönlein nephritis in children and adults. *Am. J. Kidney Dis.* **2006**, *47*, 993–1003. [CrossRef] [PubMed]
40. Coppo, R.; Basolo, B.; Martina, G.; Rollino, C.; De Marchi, M.; Giacchino, F.; Mazzucco, G.; Messina, M.; Piccoli, G. Circulating immune complexes containing IgA, IgG and IgM in patients with primary IgA nephropathy and with Henoch-Schönlein nephritis. Correlation with clinical and histologic signs of activity. *Clin. Nephrol.* **1982**, *18*, 230–239.
41. Coppo, R.; Basolo, B.; Piccoli, G.; Mazzucco, G.; Bulzomì, M.R.; Roccatello, D.; De Marchi, M.; Carbonara, A.O.; Di Belgiojoso, G.B. IgA1 and IgA2 immune complexes in primary IgA nephropathy and Henoch-Schönlein nephritis. *Clin. Exp. Immunol.* **1984**, *57*, 583–590. [PubMed]
42. Coppo, R.; Mazzucco, G.; Cagnoli, L.; Lupo, A.; Schena, F.P. Long-term prognosis of Henoch-Schönlein nephritis in adults and children. *Nephrol. Dial. Transplant.* **1997**, *12*, 2277–2283. [CrossRef] [PubMed]
43. Counahan, R.; Winterborn, M.H.; White, R.H.; Heaton, J.M.; Meadow, S.R.; Bluett, N.H.; Swetschin, H.; Cameron, J.S.; Chantler, C. Prognosis of Henoch-Schönlein nephritis in children. *BMJ* **1977**, *2*, 11–14. [CrossRef]
44. Suzuki, H.; Kiryluk, K.; Novak, J.; Moldoveanu, Z.; Herr, A.; Renfrow, M.B.; Wyatt, R.; Scolari, F.; Mestecky, J.; Gharavi, A.G.; et al. The pathophysiology of IgA nephropathy. *J. Am. Soc. Nephrol.* **2011**, *22*, 1795–1803. [CrossRef] [PubMed]
45. Zhao, N.; Hou, P.; Lv, J.; Moldoveanu, Z.; Li, Y.; Kiryluk, K.; Gharavi, A.G.; Novak, J.; Zhang, H. The level of galactose-deficient IgA1 in the sera of patients with IgA nephropathy is associated with disease progression. *Kidney Int.* **2012**, *82*, 790–796. [CrossRef] [PubMed]
46. Berthoux, F.; Suzuki, H.; Thibaudin, L.; Yanagawa, H.; Maillard, N.; Mariat, C.; Tomino, Y.; Julian, B.A.; Novak, J. Autoantibodies targeting galactose-deficient IgA1 associate with progression of IgA nephropathy. *J. Am. Soc. Nephrol.* **2012**, *23*, 1579–1587. [CrossRef]

47. Maixnerová, D.; Ling, C.; Hall, S.; Reily, C.; Brown, R.; Neprasova, M.; Suchanek, M.; Honsova, E.; Zima, T.; Novak, J.; et al. Galactose-deficient IgA1 and the corresponding IgG autoantibodies predict IgA nephropathy progression. *PLoS ONE* **2019**, *14*, e0212254. [CrossRef] [PubMed]
48. Allen, A.C.; Bailey, E.M.; Brenchley, P.; Buck, K.S.; Barratt, J.; Feehally, J. Mesangial IgA1 in IgA nephropathy exhibits aberrant O-glycosylation: Observations in three patients. *Kidney Int.* **2001**, *60*, 969–973. [CrossRef]
49. Hiki, Y.; Odani, H.; Takahashi, M.; Yasuda, Y.; Nishimoto, A.; Iwase, H.; Shinzato, T.; Kobayashi, Y.; Maeda, K. Mass spectrometry proves under-O-glycosylation of glomerular IgA1 in IgA nephropathy. *Kidney Int.* **2001**, *59*, 1077–1085. [CrossRef]
50. Suzuki, H.; Moldoveanu, Z.; Hall, S.; Brown, R.; Vu, H.L.; Novak, L.; Julian, B.A.; Tomana, M.; Wyatt, R.J.; Edberg, J.C.; et al. IgA1-secreting cell lines from patients with IgA nephropathy produce aberrantly glycosylated IgA1. *J. Clin. Investig.* **2008**, *118*, 629–639. [CrossRef]
51. Suzuki, H.; Raska, M.; Yamada, K.; Moldoveanu, Z.; Julian, B.A.; Wyatt, R.J.; Tomino, Y.; Gharavi, A.G.; Novak, J. Cytokines alter IgA1 O-glycosylation by dysregulating C1GalT1 and ST6GalNAc-II enzymes. *J. Biol. Chem.* **2014**, *289*, 5330–5339. [CrossRef] [PubMed]

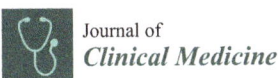

Review

Crescents and IgA Nephropathy: A Delicate Marriage

Hernán Trimarchi [1], Mark Haas [2,*] and Rosanna Coppo [3]

[1] Nephrology Service, Hospital Britanico de Buenos Aires, Buenos Aires C1280 AEB, Argentina; htrimarchi@hotmail.com
[2] Department of Pathology and Laboratory Medicine, Cedars-Sinai Medical Center, Los Angeles, CA 90048, USA
[3] Fondazione Ricerca Molinette, Regina Margherita Hospital, 10126 Turin, Italy; rosanna.coppo@unito.it
* Correspondence: mark.haas@cshs.org; Tel.: +1-310-248-6695; Fax: +1-310-423-5881

Abstract: IgA nephropathy (IgAN) is a progressive disease with great variability in the clinical course. Among the clinical and pathologic features contributing to variable outcomes, the presence of crescents has attracted particular interest as a distinct pathological feature associated with severity. Several uncontrolled observations have led to the general thought that the presence and extent of crescents was a prognostic indicator associated with poor outcomes. However, KDIGO 2021 guidelines concluded that either the presence or the relative number of crescents should not be used to determine the progression of IgAN nor should they suggest the choice of immunosuppression. Our aim is to report and discuss recent data on the debated issue of the value of active (cellular and fibrocellular) crescents in the pathogenesis and clinical progression of IgAN, their predictive value, and the impact of immunosuppression on renal function. We conclude that the value of crescents should not be disregarded, although this feature does not have an independent predictive value for progression in IgAN, particularly when considering immunosuppressed patients. An integrated overall evaluation of crescents with other active MEST scores, clinical data, and novel biomarkers must be considered in achieving a personalized therapeutic approach to IgAN patients.

Keywords: IgA nephropathy; crescents; proteinuria; glomerular filtration rate; Oxford score

1. Introduction

IgA nephropathy (IgAN), defined by prevalent mesangial IgA deposits [1], displays a variable clinical course, ranging from persistent mild microscopic hematuria with or without mild proteinuria and normal renal function to nephrotic syndrome or, rarely, a rapidly progressive course of kidney function loss. Moreover, in approximately 30% of cases, it leads to end-stage kidney disease over a 20-year follow-up period [2]. This variability represents a challenge for the clinician and has elicited the search for clinical and pathologic features predictive of progression [3] but definitively demonstrates that IgAN cannot be considered as a benign condition.

Shortly after the identification of IgAN as a histological pattern of glomerular injury with a variable clinical course, the presence of crescents attracted particular interest as a distinct pathological feature associated with severity. In small but well-described case series, crescents were found to be present in patients with macroscopic hematuria and worse renal function [4] and with a rapid progressive course with loss of renal function in cases with more than 30% of glomeruli involved with crescents [5]. A relationship between crescents and transplanted kidney dysfunction with loss of grafts in patients with recurrent IgAN was also reported [6] and further supported by the observation of an increased recurrence rate of in patients with crescentic forms of IgAN in their native kidneys, despite baseline immunosuppressive therapy [7]. Moreover, the value of crescents to classify children with IgA vasculitis nephritis (IgAVN) established by the International Study for Kidney Disease in Children (ISKDC) [8] suggested a possible similar role for crescents as a histologic marker

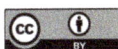

and as a potential tool to assess treatment decisions concerning immunosuppression in primary IgAN, due to the strong similarities between both entities.

These observations have led to the general thought that finding crescents in kidney biopsies of IgAN cases was a prognostic indicator associated with poor outcomes [9]. Furthermore, results from many clinical studies supported the value of crescents as markers of progression that benefited from immunosuppressive approaches [10,11].

Interestingly, the predictive value of crescents was difficult to demonstrate with recent sophisticated statistical approaches on large cohorts enrolling patients with or without corticosteroid-immunosuppressive treatments, since patients with crescents were those most frequently treated [12]. Other reasons that complicate this analysis are the different definitions employed to identify crescents; the inclusion of extra-capillary proliferation with either cellular, fibrocellular, or fibrous components; and the relative number of crescents in relation to the total number of glomeruli encountered in a kidney biopsy. Different prognostication models employing artificial intelligence provided differing conclusions regarding the inclusion of crescents as predictive markers of progression in IgAN [13]. In this regard, the variability of these results led the Kidney Disease Improving Global Outcomes (KDIGO) 2021 guidelines for the management of IgAN to recommend that either the presence or the relative number of crescents should not be used to determine the likely progression of IgAN nor should they suggest the choice of immunosuppression [14]. KDIGO also made the controversial proposal that even the presence of crescents in >50% of glomeruli in a kidney biopsy in the absence of a concomitant change in glomerular filtration rate (GFR) does not constitute a rapidly progressive situation and ought not to bias therapy.

Despite these negative authoritative considerations, for most nephrologists, the value of crescents remains an unsolved conundrum, since it is commonly recognized that cellular crescents are often associated with a rapid progression of kidney disease and clinically severe proteinuria and hematuria in patients with IgAN, particularly when the relative number is high in a kidney biopsy. Unfortunately, the issue of the value of crescents in IgAN cannot be explored in experimental IgAN, since in these models mostly mesangial proliferation and glomerular sclerosis, but not crescents, are reproduced [15].

The aim of this review is to report recent data on the debated issue of the value of active (cellular and fibrocellular) crescents in the pathogenesis and clinical progression of IgAN, their predictive value as a histological marker, and the impact of immunosuppressive treatment on renal function.

2. Molecular Factors Involved in Crescent Formation in IgAN

In IgAN, fibrinogen and fibrin-related molecules are present in crescents (Figure 1). Moreover, components of the glomerular basement membrane, such as collagen types IV and V, laminin, fibronectin, and cytokeratin, are persistently positive within all stages of crescents. Vimentin, usually located in podocytes and parietal epithelial cells as well as in interstitial cells, is also present in all stages of crescents in IgAN, suggesting that at early stages of crescent development in IgAN podocytes may play a key role. In addition, the presence of intrinsic basement membrane constituents is consistent with GBM rupture, likely related at least in part to necrotizing lesions within the glomerular tuft, representing a precursor to crescent formation. Fibrinoid necrosis may be seen in IgAN, most often in cases with active crescentic lesions, although in most studies from Europe and North America, this is relatively uncommon, especially when compared to, for example, anti-neutrophil cytoplasmic antibody (ANCA) glomerulonephritis and vasculitis. Nevertheless, in a French study of 128 adults with IgAN, glomerular necrotizing lesions, which were seen in 9 cases, were significantly associated with development of end-stage kidney disease (ESKD) or the doubling of serum creatinine by univariate (but not multivariable) analysis [16]. In an Italian study, glomerular necrotizing lesions were seen in 35 of 340 IgAN patients and were associated with a greater probability of progression to ESKD only in patients who were not treated with immunosuppression [17]. Notably, glomerular necrotizing lesions tend to be seen more frequently in patients from Asia, perhaps related to more frequent activation of the lectin pathway of complement in these patients (see below). Shen et al. [18] examined 60 Chinese patients with active IgAN who underwent a kidney biopsy, followed by corticosteroid therapy and a follow-up biopsy within 6 months of the initial biopsy. In this cohort, 31 patients had one or more glomerular necrotizing lesions, 51 had one or more cellular or fibrocellular crescents, and 22 had E1 lesions on the initial biopsy. After steroid therapy, necrotizing lesions, active crescents, and E1 lesions were seen on 2, 15, and 5 follow-up biopsies, respectively, and none of these lesions on the initial biopsy were associated with a composite endpoint of ESKD or 30% decline in eGFR [18]. The apparent higher steroid sensitivity of necrotizing lesions compared with crescents is consistent with the former representing an earlier form of a related inflammatory process, although clearly this requires validation.

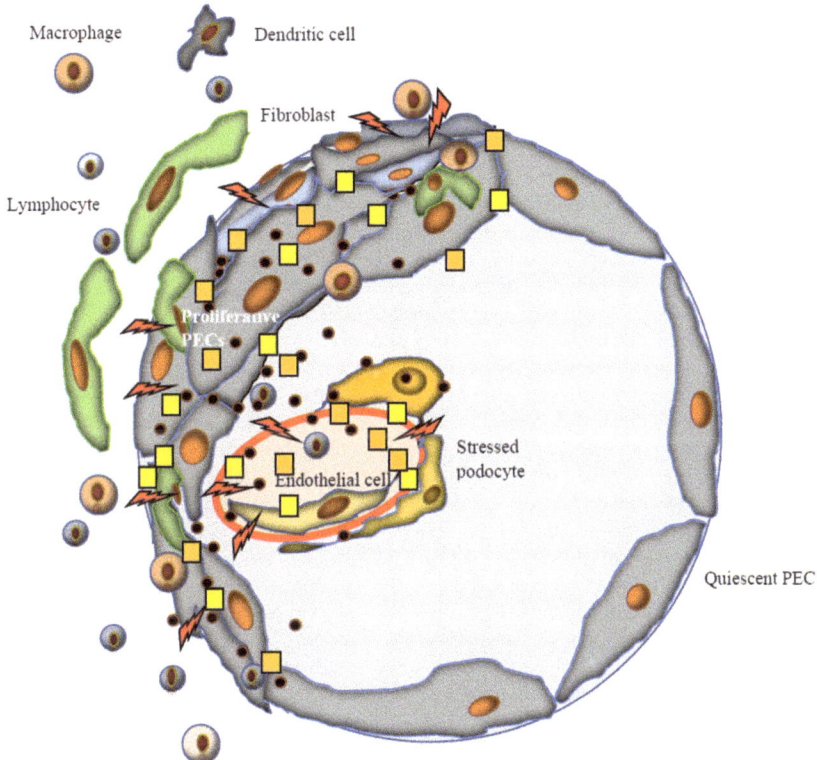

Figure 1. Main cells and molecules involved in crescent development in IgAN. In IgAN, crescent formation could be divided into two steps. First of all, there is an initial damage to the endothelium of the glomerular filtration barrier (rents ⚡)from where podocytes and parietal cells interact within and outside the surrounding glomerulus. The second step is the consequence of this interaction: The development of the crescent itself. Main molecules involved: Fibrinogen and fibrin-related antigens ● , type IV and V collagens, laminin, fibronectin, cytokeratin persistently positive at all stages of crescents, as well as vimentin, distributed in podocytes and parietal epithelial cells (PECs). At early stages of crescent formation in IgAN, podocytes play a key role, while the accumulation of basement membrane components adds to the progression of the crescents (Figure 1). In IgAN, endothelial proliferation associates with crescent appearance. Crescent formation in IgAN is associated with activation of the lectin ▢ and alternative pathways ▢ .

It appears that monocytes and macrophages may not play a critical role in the development of crescents in IgAN, in contrast with what occurs in other glomerular diseases, in which these cells are active players in crescent pathogenesis [19,20]. This characteristic may explain why the appearance of some or occasional crescents in kidney biopsies may not be indicative of severe lesions when compared to other forms of glomerulonephritis with crescents, unless the GBM is not preserved. In IgAN, endocapillary hypercellularity was found more frequently in cases with crescents [18], although numbers of glomerular CD68+ macrophages were found to be associated with endocapillary hypercellularity but not crescents [21]. A possible explanation for this may be the difficulty of accurate histologic diagnosis of endocapillary hypercellularity even by skillful nephropathologists, especially in the presence of segmental glomerulosclerosis that is often associated with fibrocellular crescents [21,22].

Several studies have reported that, in IgAN, complement activation plays a role in crescent formation. Complement components and factors related to complement activation are partly produced by intrinsic glomerular cells including mesangial and endothelial cells [23]. Podocytes also display complement component receptors at their cell surface. It has been reported that there is an increased intensity of properdin and factor B staining in murine IgAN with more severe glomerular injury including crescent formation, indicating the involvement of an activated alternative pathway of complements [24]. IgAN patients with increased glomerular mannose-binding lectin (MBL)-associated serine protease type 1 (MASP-1) deposition presented with higher levels of proteinuria and increased proportions of extracapillary proliferation, glomerular sclerosis, and renal dysfunction [25]. IgAN with crescents has been reported to present with higher levels of tissue C5b-9, MASP 1/3, MASP2, properdin, and factor B than IgAN without crescents, indicating an activation of both the lectin and alternative pathways of complement [26].

Glomerular C4d staining in the absence of C1q deposits is considered a typical sign of lectin pathway activation. C4d-positive IgAN biopsies are associated with a worse prognosis and a trend to develop ESKD [24]. In a cohort of 100 IgAN Chinese patients with various proportions of crescents, signs of complement activation in urine samples were significantly increased in comparison to healthy controls in cases with crescents involving >50% of glomeruli, presenting with high levels of the common complement pathway—C3a, C5a, and C5b-9—as well as markers of an alternative pathway—Bb—and the lectin pathway—C4d and MBL [27]. The levels of urinary C4d showed a highly significant linear association with the number of crescents. In a subgroup of these patients, immunohistochemistry was performed on renal biopsy tissue. Glomerular staining for C4d (>25% of glomeruli) was observed in 20% of cases in the group with crescents <25% of glomeruli, in 70% of cases with 25–49% crescents, and all cases with crescents in ≥50%. Positive glomerular staining was seen predominantly in the mesangial area, very often within the crescents and sclerotic lesions. Glomerular C5b-9 deposition and C3d staining were observed in almost all crescentic cases. These data stress the role of lectin pathway activation in Chinese patients with crescentic IgAN.

3. Turning from MEST to MEST-C Score

In studies of the cohort of 265 patients on which the original Oxford classification was based [28], the presence or absence of cellular/fibrocellular crescents was not a significant predictor of the rate of eGFR decline or a composite outcome of ESKD or a ≥50% decline in eGFR. This was also true in several validation studies [29–32], which like the original Oxford study excluded patients with an eGFR of <30 mL/min at the time of biopsy and/or progression to ESKD within 12 months of the biopsy. However, other studies with less restrictive entry criteria found crescents to be a prognostic indicator of a poor outcome [33–36]. Noteworthily, Katafuchi et al. found similar results to those in the original Oxford study in patients meeting entry criteria for the latter, although in their entire cohort of 702 patients and in those 286 patients not meeting the entry criteria of the original Oxford study, crescents independently predicted the development of ESKD [33].

Twenty studies published between 2009 and 2016 evaluating the association between crescents and kidney outcome involving more than 5000 patients with IgAN were included in a meta-analysis [37]. Nine of these studies [28,30–32,35,38–41] compared measures of kidney function between patients with no crescents or any crescents. Those patients with crescents had lower eGFR levels ($p = 0.023$); higher proteinuria ($p = 0.024$); more frequent M1 ($p = 0.003$), E1 ($p < 0.001$), S1 ($p = 0.016$), and T1/2 ($p < 0.001$) lesions; and received immunosuppressive therapy more frequently ($p < 0.001$) than those without crescents. Pooled results also showed that crescents were associated with progression to ESKD ($p < 0.001$), suggesting that potential inclusion of crescents in the Oxford Classification needed further evaluation.

In addition, two studies of pediatric patients with IgAN from Japan [35] and Sweden [36] without restrictive entry criteria also found cellular or fibrocellular crescents to be predictive of a poor outcome (eGFR <60 mL/min/1.73 m^2 and ESKD or eGFR reduction >50%, respectively) by univariate analysis and by multivariable analysis (including eGFR, mean arterial pressure, and proteinuria at the time of biopsy) in the Japanese cohort.

In response to these findings, a working group of the International IgA Nephropathy Network (IIgANN) performed a multicenter study of the impact of crescents on renal outcomes in over 3000 patients with IgA nephropathy pooled from four previously studied, well-defined cohorts: the European VALIGA study cohort [42], two large Asian cohorts [31,33], and the original Oxford cohort [28] that included patients from four continents. Notably, while each of the three former studies validated the findings of the original Oxford study with regard to the impact of M, S, and T scores on renal outcomes, just one [33] showed crescents to be an independent predictor of a poor outcome (ESKD), although in the VALIGA study [42] an association with eGFR loss was noted only for patients not treated with immunosuppression. The working group study [10] was limited to cellular and fibrocellular (at least 10% cells) crescents, as in the original Oxford study identification of fibrous crescents showed poor inter-observer reproducibility [43]. In this study, one or more crescents were seen in 36% of biopsies (<10% crescents in 61%). The presence of crescents was associated with a faster rate of renal function decline compared to no crescents and a reduced survival from a combined event of ESKD or a ≥ 50% decline in eGFR in a multivariable analysis including eGFR at the time of biopsy and time-averaged proteinuria and mean arterial pressure during follow up [28]. This study also validated the association of the Oxford M, S, and T scores with the combined event in all patients although, in patients treated with corticosteroids and/or other immunosuppressive agents, only the T score remained a significant, independent predictor of increased risk of the combined event. The lack of an impact of crescents in patients treated with immunosuppressive agents is consistent with a repeat biopsy study from China that showed complete resolution of cellular/fibrocellular crescents following immunosuppressive therapy in 36/51 patients having one or more crescents on their initial biopsy [18]. Notably, however, the presence of cellular or fibrocellular crescents in $\geq 1/4$ of the glomeruli was independently associated with a combined event even in patients who received corticosteroids and/or other immunosuppressive agents [18]. Thus, a revised version of the Oxford classification for IgA nephropathy published in 2017 includes a C (crescent) score in addition to the original MEST scores: C0 (no cellular or fibrocellular crescents), C1 (crescents in <25% of glomeruli, suggesting a poor prognosis in patients not receiving immunosuppressive therapy), and C2 (crescents in ≥ 25% of glomeruli) [21].

While the predictive value of crescents on renal outcomes was not evident in the initial VALIGA study [44], Coppo et al. [42] performed a follow-up study of this patient cohort based on a prolonged follow-up period (median 7 years, as compared with 4.7 years in the original study) of up to 35 years. This longer-term analysis of the VALIGA cohort, which included adults and children, showed that, in patients who never received corticosteroids/and or other immunosuppressive treatment, the presence of crescents (C1 + C2) was related to the rate of renal functional decline, independent of the MEST score and other risk factors. There was not a significant effect of crescents on the composite endpoint of

50% loss of eGFR or ESKD, perhaps because the patients enrolled had a modest median annual eGFR loss (1.8 mL/min/year) and the fraction of patients with crescents was only 10.5% (C1 = 8.6%; C2 = 1.9%).

4. Risk Prediction Models for IgAN and Crescents in Adults

In recent years, several models using novel mathematical statistics or artificial intelligence approaches have been developed to predict, at the time of kidney biopsy, the risk of progression of IgAN toward ESKD or 50% decline in eGFR [45]. Variables most commonly included were age, gender, blood pressure, creatinine, eGFR, proteinuria, and renal biopsy lesions according to the Oxford classification. The most recognized, due to the great number of included cases from global multiethnic cohorts, is that developed by the IIgANN, which considered two models with and without ethnicity and used clinical predictors and MEST scores at the time of renal biopsy to predict the risk of 50% decline in eGFR or ESKD at 8 years [45].

This IIgANN prediction tool was validated in external cohorts and was updated for its use also in children [46] and for its employment up to two years from the time of biopsy [47]. This tool, now available for clinical use online in a mobile-app calculator, has been recommended by 2021 KDIGO glomerulonephritis guidelines [14]. Each MEST score component was required to be entered in the prediction formula, but crescents were excluded, as their presence or absence was apparently not associated with clinical outcomes. Crescents were significantly associated with race/ethnicity (more frequent in Japanese ethnicity) and with use of corticosteroid/immunosuppressive therapy after biopsy (56% vs. 36%, $p < 0.001$). In the recently published prediction tool, at time points after renal biopsy, the value of crescents (present or absent) was re-checked, adding this variable in the post-biopsy models, but there was no improvement in in model fit or in calibration indices [47].

Other prediction models generated in different cohorts, reported the effects of crescents in untreated patients. Among 3380 Korean patients, crescents improved the discrimination performance of the prediction model only in patients not receiving corticosteroids/immunosuppressive agents [48]. However, this study did not employ the Oxford classification. A more recent report, using the MEST score, investigated 545 Korean patients to generate a prognostication model that considered C1 (found in 24% of patients) and C2 (found in 1.3%). When adding crescents to their full model with clinical data and MEST score, the predictor was not superior to the full model. However, the prediction performance of crescents was significantly improved after 5 years of follow up in the subgroup of 426 patients not treated with corticosteroid-immunosuppressive drugs ($p < 0.02$) [49].

In recent years, artificial intelligence has arisen in the medical field to assess new prediction models, claiming that machine learning techniques may outperform conventional statistical models, with an improved capability to identify variants relevant to clinical outcome. A prediction model using an artificial intelligence statistical approach developed in 2047 Chinese patients with a median of 10 years of follow up did not include crescents due to non-significance [50]. In a Caucasian cohort mostly involving the VALIGA European patients, the artificial intelligence tool showed a performance value of 0.82 in patients with a follow up of 5 years. Crescents were included, although these were not associated with significantly increased risk to develop ESKD by Cox proportional hazard models [13].

5. Risk Prediction Models for IgAN and Crescents in Children

The IIgANN gathered 1060 pediatric cases of IgAN from various continents. As in adults, crescents were more frequent in patients of East Asian ethnicity (65.9% of Japanese and 45.7% of Chinese versus 25.5% of Caucasians) [46]. Children received steroid therapy in 58% of the cases, more frequently in the presence of crescents (70% of children with crescents versus 48% without crescents). No association of crescents (absent versus present) with the secondary outcome of 30% reduction in eGFR or end-stage kidney disease was found, even after adjusting for immunosuppression. The prediction performance was the same in subgroups of treated versus untreated by immunosuppression. Any prediction improvement associated with crescents is confounded by the effects of other predictor variables already included in the model, such as race/ethnicity. However, the prediction model performed equally well in treated and untreated cases, indicating that the combination of risk factors contained in the models predicted outcome similarly in treated and untreated children.

In a pediatric cohort from Japan, a threshold of 30% of glomeruli with crescents was found to be predictive of development of an eGFR below 60 mL/min/1.73 m^2 by both univariate analysis and a multivariate analysis including MEST scores and proteinuria at the time of biopsy [35].

6. IgAN with Crescents Involving >50% of Glomeruli

Crescentic IgAN, defined as >50% cellular crescentic glomeruli on kidney biopsy, was investigated in 113 Chinese adult patients [11]. At biopsy, the mean serum creatinine level was 4.3 mg/dL, and the mean percentage of crescents was 66%. Kidney survival rate at 5 years after biopsy was 45.8%. Multivariable Cox regression revealed initial serum creatinine as the only independent risk factor for end-stage kidney disease ($p = 0.002$). Notably, the percentage of crescents was not independently associated with ESKD.

A recent report from Japan focused on children with >50% glomeruli with crescents, accounting for 25 cases (4.9% of the whole cohort of 515 Japanese children with IgAN) [51]. No prior history of urinary abnormalities was reported in 16/25 children, who were referred from school screening programs. These children with crescentic IgAN had more frequent gross hematuria (76%), proteinuria ≥ 1 g/day, and shorter duration from clinical onset to renal biopsy, median 4 months versus 8 months. There was a significantly increased frequency of M1 (80%) and E1 (83%) in comparison with the other children, although T > 0 was rare in both groups. At the time of renal biopsy, renal function was actually well preserved (eGFR 120 mL/min) in comparison to the other children (eGFR 104 mL/min). Although eighteen children with crescentic IgA were treated with prednisolone or prednisolone plus other immunosuppressive agents, only 8/25 patients with these lesions had remission of proteinuria (6 of whom received immunosuppression) and 4 (16%) progressed to an endpoint of eGFR < 60 mL/min/1.73 m^2 or ESKD compared to 13 (2.7%) of the remaining 490 patients, the majority of whom had C1 (n = 228) or C2 (n = 40). Children with crescentic IgAN had significantly lower survival from this composite endpoint at 13 years post-biopsy (77.1% vs. 92.6%, $p < 0.0001$). Failure of treatment to induce a remission of proteinuria and a higher percentage of tubular atrophy/interstitial fibrosis were also predictors of an unfavorable outcome [51].

7. Timing of Renal Biopsy and Crescents

A challenge in establishing the value of percentage of crescents as a risk factor for progression in IgAN is represented by the timing of renal biopsy, due to changes which may occur over time [52]. A study in Japanese children with IgAN [53] considered the time elapsed from the diagnosis of urinary abnormalities—mostly detected after school screening programs—and renal biopsy and reported that a shorter time from onset to renal biopsy was associated with higher glomerular percentage of crescents, in addition to higher M and E lesions. This suggests that crescents are associated with disease onset and then likely undergo a healing process into sclerotic lesions, which are commonly detected in biopsies performed years after onset.

8. Treatment and Crescents in IgAN

According to all the data presented in this review, the literature reports showing benefits of corticosteroid/immunosuppressive treatment in patients (adults and children) having IgAN with crescents are uncontrolled and retrospective. The coincidence of other MEST lesions with C, the variable morphology of crescents (cellular or fibrocellular, segmental or global glomerular involvement) and association with other lesions not included in the MEST scores (e.g., necrosis, interstitial inflammation) render the understanding of the role of crescents as an independent feature promoting progression of IgAN very difficult. Moreover, the reports describe patients treated with corticosteroids and other immunosuppressive drugs at varying doses and over varying intervals, with different levels of supportive care (e.g., renin–angiotensin system (RAS) inhibitors).

A recently published Argentinian–Spanish retrospective study assessed the impact of steroids plus mycophenolate in a cohort of 25 patients with progressive IgAN [54]. Progressive IgAN was defined by a decrease in eGFR of at least 10 mL/min in the 12 months prior to the start of treatment and proteinuria $\geq$0.75 g/day despite maximum tolerated doses of RAS blockade, and hematuria ($\geq$5 red blood cells per high power field) at the beginning of treatment. The mean interval between the performance of kidney biopsy and the onset of therapy was 4.5 $\pm$ 11.9 months. Ten patients (47.6%) had C1 scores and three (14.3%) displayed C2 scores (patients with crescents in >50% of glomeruli were excluded). The mean duration of immunosuppression treatment was 24.7 $\pm$ 15.2 months. In the 12 months prior to treatment, the median rate of kidney function decline had been 23 mL/min/year. After the onset of treatment, the median eGFR slope was 5 mL/min/year (p = 0.001 with respect to the 12 months prior to treatment). Proteinuria decreased from 1.8 g/day (range 1.0–2.5) at baseline to 0.6 g/day (range 0.3–1.2) at the end of treatment (p = 0.01), and hematuria disappeared in 40% of patients. There were no serious adverse effects requiring treatment discontinuation. In this study, in which >50% of the population presented with active crescents in their biopsies, the addition of immunosuppression decreased the rate of decline of kidney function plus the degree of proteinuria and hematuria.

There are few data on the predictive impact of MEST-C scores in randomized clinical trial settings. An exploratory analysis was performed in 70 available renal biopsies from 162 randomized STOP-IgAN trial participants and correlated the results with clinical outcomes [55]. Kidney biopsies had been performed from 6.5 to 95 months (median 9.4) prior to randomization. This secondary analysis of STOP-IgAN biopsies indicated that M1, T1/2, and C1/2 scores were associated with worse renal outcomes. In particular, patients with glomerular crescents (C1/2 scores) in their biopsies were more likely to develop ESKD during the 3-year trial phase, but this trend was only significant in patients under supportive care.

As commented previously, consideration of crescents in managing the treatment of IgAN has been strongly discouraged by KDIGO 2021, which does not support the value of MEST score in general as a guide of treatment and, in particular, disregards the value of percentage of crescents as an independent risk factor supporting a more aggressive therapy. According to KDIGO guidelines, the presence of crescents in kidney biopsy, even when involving $\geq$50% of glomeruli, in the absence of a concomitant rise in serum creatinine does not constitute a rapidly progressive form of IgAN, which is instead defined as a >50% decline in eGFR over >3 months, where reversible causes are excluded. KDIGO guidelines suggest repeating renal biopsy in case of insufficient benefits from supportive care, but this is in contrast with the suggestion not to use pathology scores to guide treatment. A few uncontrolled studies have repeated renal biopsies in selected cases [18,56] after corticosteroid or other immunosuppressive drugs had been administered and showed a reduction in crescents in most treated cases. Notably, in one repeat-biopsy study, it was found that, in patients with crescents on their original biopsy, those who continued to have crescents on their repeated biopsy were significantly more likely to develop ESKD than those whose second biopsy showed resolution of crescents [56].

Recently, a single-center Chinese study investigated 140 patients enrolled between 2008 and 2016 with C1 and proteinuria <1 g/day who received supportive care (n = 52) or steroid-based immunosuppressive therapy (n = 88) [57]. The primary outcome was the rate of renal function decline. Baseline data showed a population with mild renal disease, median proteinuria of 0.6 g/day, and a median fraction of crescents of 7% (5–12%), with a follow-up time of 69 months. The rate of renal function decline was slower in the steroid-based immunosuppressive therapy group than in the supportive care group.

Multivariable linear regression analyses showed that steroid-based immunosuppressive therapy significantly slowed the rate of renal function decline ($p = 0.013$) after adjusting for age, sex, mean arterial blood pressure, proteinuria, eGFR, M1, E1, S1, T1-2, the fraction of crescents, and use of RAS inhibitors. Similar findings were seen in 66 patients (33 from each group) who were matched for baseline demographic, clinical, and pathologic findings. In the matched cohort, the rate of renal function decline was also slower in the steroid-based immunosuppressive therapy group. The conclusion was that steroid-based immunosuppressive therapy may slow down the rate of renal function decline of IgAN patients with C1 and proteinuria ≤ 1 g/day.

Novel therapies are under evaluation for the treatment of IgAN (Table 1). These drugs are presently targeting persistent proteinuria despite several months of optimized supportive care, but the perspective is that at least some of them could be of benefit in the control of the most active and progressive cases such as those with high presence of crescents.

Table 1. New drugs under evaluation for treatment of IgA nephropathy: selected from studies published in the U.S. National Library of Medicine Clinical Trials.gov.

Agent	Activity/Target	Registered Trial N (NCT)
B cell immunomodulators		
Atacicept	BLyS-APRIL inhibitor	02808429
BION-1301	APRIL inhibitor	03945318
VIS-649 Sibeprenlimab	APRIL inhibitor	04287985
RC-18	BLyS receptor inhibitor	04291782
Complement inhibitors		
LNP-023 Iptacopan	Factor B inhibitor	04578834
FB-LRx	Anti-sense factor B inhibitor	04014335
OMS-721 Narsoplimab	MASP inhibitor	03608033
ALN-CC5-Cemdisarin	C5 inhibitor	03841448
CCX-168 Avacopan	C5a receptor inhibitor	02384317
Ravulizumab	C5 inhibitor	04564339
APL-2	C3 inhibitor	04564339
Various		
CHK-01 Atrasentan	Endothelin A receptor inhibitor	04573920
Sparsentan	Endothelin and Angiotensin II receptor inhibitor	03762850
RTA-402 Bardoxolone methyl	Nuclear factor erythroid-derived 2-related factor agonist	03366337

The agents being tested include (a) drugs blocking B cell function and survival by inhibiting B-lymphocyte stimulator (BLyS, also known as B cell activating factor, BAFF) and APRIL (a proliferation-inducing ligand); (b) complement activation inhibitors, targeting the lectin complement pathway (mannose-associated serine protease, MASP), the alternative complement pathway (factor B) or the common complement pathway (C3, C5, and its proinflammatory activation product C3a); and (c) other hemodynamic and inflammatory pathways such as endothelin, angiotensin II, nuclear factor erythroid-derived 2-related factor agonist (Table 1). Future perspectives are expected from the next results of these studies for treating patients with active histological forms of IgAN, including crescentic IgAN, independently from the persistence of proteinuria despite optimal supportive care.

9. Conclusions

Several factors may account for the variable results regarding the impact of crescents on clinical outcomes in IgAN. These include (a) the different patient ethnicities; (b) different timing of the renal biopsy after onset of clinical manifestations; (c) the histologic type of crescents included in each study, either cellular, fibrocellular, or fibrous; (d) the association of crescents with other histopathologic markers of activity, which blunted their independent value; (e) the varying choice of immunosuppressive treatments and dosage regimens; and (f) the different clinical outcomes.

In contrast to the case in some other forms of proliferative glomerulonephritis, the most evident conclusion from the data reported in this review is that crescents do not appear to be an independent predictor of clinical outcomes in patients with IgAN, especially those receiving corticosteroids or other immunosuppressive agents. Although the benefit of such treatment in IgAN with crescents indirectly emerges from this consideration, there is a lack of direct evidence of beneficial effect of corticosteroids or immunosuppressive drugs in every patient with IgAN presenting with crescentic lesions. Over the last decades most severely crescentic cases received corticosteroid-immunosuppressive treatment, and a placebo-controlled RCT in these patients is not conceivable. However, the value of crescents should not be disregarded. An integrated overall consideration including other MEST scores and clinical data and novel biomarkers should be undertaken in achieving a more promising personalized therapeutic approach to IgAN patients.

Author Contributions: All authors have contributed equally to the present manuscript. All authors have read and agreed to the published version of the manuscript.

Funding: This review article received no external funding.

Institutional Review Board Statement: Not applicable.

Informed Consent Statement: Not applicable.

Data Availability Statement: Not applicable.

Conflicts of Interest: The authors declare no conflict of interest.

References

1. Berger, J.; Hinglais, N. Les dépôts intercapillaires d'IgA-IgG [Intercapillary deposits of IgA-IgG]. *J. Urol. Nephrol.* **1968**, *74*, 694–695. (In French)
2. Donadio, J.V.; Grande, J.P. IgA Nephropathy. *N. Engl. J. Med.* **2002**, *347*, 738–748. [CrossRef] [PubMed]
3. Radford, M.G., Jr.; Donadio, J.V., Jr.; Bergstralh, E.J.; Grande, J.P. Predicting renal outcome in IgA nephropathy. *J. Am. Soc. Nephrol.* **1997**, *8*, 199–207. [CrossRef] [PubMed]
4. Abuelo, J.G.; Esparza, A.R.; Matarese, R.A.; Endreny, R.G.; Carvalho, J.S.; Allegra, S.R. Crescentic IgA Nephropathy. *Medicine* **1984**, *63*, 396–406. [CrossRef] [PubMed]
5. Bennett, W.M.; Kincaid-Smith, P. Macroscopic hematuria in mesangial IgA nephropathy: Correlation with glomerular crescents and renal dysfunction. *Kidney Int.* **1983**, *23*, 393–400. [CrossRef] [PubMed]
6. Jeong, H.J.; Kim, Y.S.; Kwon, K.H.; Kim, S.I.; Kim, M.S.; Choi, K.H.; Lee, H.Y.; Han, D.S.; Park, K. Glomerular crescents are responsible for chronic graft dysfunction in post-transplant IgA nephropathy. *Pathol. Int.* **2004**, *54*, 837–842. [CrossRef]
7. Avasare, P.E.; Zaky, Z.S.; Tsapepas, D.S.; Appel, G.B.; Markowitz, G.S.; Bomback, A.S.; Canetta, P.A. Predicting Post-Transplant Recurrence of IgA Nephropathy: The Importance of Crescents. *Am. J. Nephrol.* **2017**, *45*, 99–106. [CrossRef]
8. Counahan, R.; Winterborn, M.H.; White, R.H.; Heaton, J.M.; Meadow, S.R.; Bluett, N.H.; Swetschin, H.; Cameron, J.S.; Chantler, C. Prognosis of Henoch-Schonlein nephritis in children. *BMJ* **1977**, *2*, 11. [CrossRef]
9. Lai, K.N.; Tang, S.C.; Schena, F.P.; Novak, J.; Tomino, Y.; Fogo, A.B.; Glassock, R.J. IgA nephropathy. *Nat. Rev. Dis. Prim.* **2016**, *2*, 16001. [CrossRef]
10. Haas, M.; Verhave, J.C.; Liu, Z.-H.; Alpers, C.E.; Barratt, J.; Becker, J.U.; Cattran, D.; Cook, H.T.; Coppo, R.; Feehally, J.; et al. A Multicenter Study of the Predictive Value of Crescents in IgA Nephropathy. *J. Am. Soc. Nephrol.* **2016**, *28*, 691–701. [CrossRef]
11. Lv, J.; Yang, Y.; Zhang, H.; Chen, W.; Pan, X.; Guo, Z.; Wang, C.; Li, S.; Zhang, J.; Zhang, J.; et al. Prediction of Outcomes in Crescentic IgA Nephropathy in a Multicenter Cohort Study. *J. Am. Soc. Nephrol.* **2013**, *24*, 2118–2125. [CrossRef]
12. Barbour, S.J.; Coppo, R.; Zhang, H.; Liu, Z.-H.; Suzuki, Y.; Matsuzaki, K.; Katafuchi, R.; Er, L.; Espino-Hernandez, G.; Kim, S.J.; et al. Evaluating a New International Risk-Prediction Tool in IgA Nephropathy. *JAMA Intern. Med.* **2019**, *179*, 942–952. [CrossRef]

13. Schena, F.P.; Anelli, V.W.; Trotta, J.; Di Noia, T.; Manno, C.; Tripepi, G.; D'Arrigo, G.; Chesnaye, N.C.; Russo, M.L.; Stangou, M.; et al. Development and testing of an artificial intelligence tool for predicting end-stage kidney disease in patients with immunoglobulin A nephropathy. *Kidney Int.* **2021**, *99*, 1179–1188. [CrossRef] [PubMed]
14. Rovin, B.H.; Adler, S.G.; Barratt, J.; Bridoux, F.; Burdge, K.A.; Chan, T.M.; Cook, H.T.; Fervenza, F.C.; Gibson, K.L.; Glassock, R.J.; et al. Executive summary of the KDIGO 2021 Guideline for the Management of Glomerular Diseases. *Kidney Int.* **2021**, *100*, 753–779. [CrossRef] [PubMed]
15. Monteiro, R.C.; Suzuki, Y. Are there animal models of IgA nephropathy? *Semin. Immunopathol.* **2021**, *43*, 639–648. [CrossRef] [PubMed]
16. El Karoui, K.; Hill, G.S.; Karras, A.; Moulonguet, L.; Caudwell, V.; Loupy, A.; Bruneval, P.; Jacquot, C.; Nochy, D. Focal segmental glomerulosclerosis plays a major role in the progression of IgA nephropathy. II. Light microscopic and clinical studies. *Kidney Int.* **2011**, *79*, 643–654. [CrossRef] [PubMed]
17. D'Amico, G.; Napodano, P.; Ferrario, F.; Rastaldi, M.P.; Arrigo, G. Idiopathic IgA nephropathy with segmental necrotizing lesions of the capillary wall. *Kidney Int.* **2001**, *59*, 682–692. [CrossRef] [PubMed]
18. Shen, X.-H.; Liang, S.-S.; Chen, H.-M.; Le, W.-B.; Jiang, S.; Zeng, C.-H.; Zhou, M.-L.; Zhang, H.-T.; Liu, Z.-H. Reversal of active glomerular lesions after immunosuppressive therapy in patients with IgA nephropathy: A repeat-biopsy based observation. *J. Nephrol.* **2015**, *28*, 441–449. [CrossRef]
19. Yoshioka, K.; Takemura, T.; Akano, N.; Miyamoto, H.; Iseki, T.; Maki, S. Cellular and non-cellular compositions of crescents in human glomerulonephritis. *Kidney Int.* **1987**, *32*, 284–291. [CrossRef]
20. Trimarchi, H. Crescents in primary glomerulonephritis: A pattern of injury with dissimilar actors. A pathophysiologic perspective. *Pediatr. Nephrol.* **2021**, *37*, 1205–1214. [CrossRef]
21. Trimarchi, H.; Barratt, J.; Cattran, D.C.; Cook, H.T.; Coppo, R.; Haas, M.; Liu, Z.-H.; Roberts, I.S.; Yuzawa, Y.; Zhang, H.; et al. Oxford Classification of IgA nephropathy 2016: An update from the IgA Nephropathy Classification Working Group. *Kidney Int.* **2017**, *91*, 1014–1021. [CrossRef] [PubMed]
22. Soares, M.F.; Genitsch, V.; Chakera, A.; Smith, A.; MacEwen, C.; Bellur, S.S.; Alham, N.K.; Roberts, I.S.D. Relationship between renal CD68+ infiltrates and the Oxford Classification of IgA nephropathy. *Histopathology* **2018**, *74*, 629–637. [CrossRef] [PubMed]
23. Itami, H.; Hara, S.; Samejima, K.; Tsushima, H.; Morimoto, K.; Okamoto, K.; Kosugi, T.; Kawano, T.; Fujiki, K.; Kitada, H.; et al. Complement activation is associated with crescent formation in IgA nephropathy. *Virchows Arch.* **2020**, *477*, 565–572. [CrossRef] [PubMed]
24. Roos, A.; Rastaldi, M.P.; Calvaresi, N.; Oortwijn, B.D.; Schlagwein, N.; Van Gijlswijk-Janssen, D.J.; Stahl, G.; Matsushita, M.; Fujita, T.; van Kooten, C.; et al. Glomerular Activation of the Lectin Pathway of Complement in IgA Nephropathy Is Associated with More Severe Renal Disease. *J. Am. Soc. Nephrol.* **2006**, *17*, 1724–1734. [CrossRef]
25. Hashimoto, A.; Suzuki, Y.; Suzuki, H.; Ohsawa, I.; Brown, R.; Hall, S.; Tanaka, Y.; Novak, J.; Ohi, H.; Tomino, Y. Determination of Severity of Murine IgA Nephropathy by Glomerular Complement Activation by Aberrantly Glycosylated IgA and Immune Complexes. *Am. J. Pathol.* **2012**, *181*, 1338–1347. [CrossRef]
26. Daha, M.R.; Van Kooten, C. Is there a role for locally produced complement in renal disease? *Nephrol. Dial. Transplant.* **2000**, *15*, 1506–1509. [CrossRef]
27. Wang, Z.; Xie, X.; Li, J.; Zhang, X.; He, J.; Wang, M.; Lv, J.; Zhang, H. Complement Activation Is Associated with Crescents in IgA Nephropathy. *Front. Immunol.* **2021**, *12*, 676919. [CrossRef]
28. A Working Group of the International IgA Nephropathy Network and the Renal Pathology Society; Cattran, D.C.; Coppo, R.; Cook, H.T.; Feehally, J.; Roberts, I.S.; Troyanov, S.; Alpers, C.E.; Amore, A.; Barratt, J.; et al. The Oxford classification of IgA nephropathy: Rationale, clinicopathological correlations, and classification. *Kidney Int.* **2009**, *76*, 534–545. [CrossRef]
29. Herzenberg, A.M.; Fogo, A.B.; Reich, H.N.; Troyanov, S.; Bavbek, N.; Massat, A.E.; Hunley, T.; Hladunewich, M.A.; Julian, B.A.; Fervenza, F.C.; et al. Validation of the Oxford classification of IgA nephropathy. *Kidney Int.* **2011**, *80*, 310–317. [CrossRef]
30. Le, W.; Zeng, C.-H.; Liu, Z.; Liu, D.; Yang, Q.; Lin, R.-X.; Xia, Z.-K.; Fan, Z.-M.; Zhu, G.; Wu, Y.; et al. Validation of the Oxford classification of IgA nephropathy for pediatric patients from China. *BMC Nephrol.* **2012**, *13*, 158. [CrossRef]
31. Zeng, C.-H.; Le, W.; Ni, Z.; Zhang, M.; Miao, L.; Luo, P.; Wang, R.; Lv, Z.; Chen, J.; Tian, J.; et al. A Multicenter Application and Evaluation of the Oxford Classification of IgA Nephropathy in Adult Chinese Patients. *Am. J. Kidney Dis.* **2012**, *60*, 812–820. [CrossRef] [PubMed]
32. Shi, S.-F.; Wang, S.-X.; Jiang, L.; Lv, J.-C.; Liu, L.-J.; Chen, Y.-Q.; Zhu, S.-N.; Liu, G.; Zou, W.-Z.; Zhang, H.; et al. Pathologic Predictors of Renal Outcome and Therapeutic Efficacy in IgA Nephropathy: Validation of the Oxford Classification. *Clin. J. Am. Soc. Nephrol.* **2011**, *6*, 2175–2184. [CrossRef] [PubMed]
33. Katafuchi, R.; Ninomiya, T.; Nagata, M.; Mitsuiki, K.; Hirakata, H. Validation Study of Oxford Classification of IgA Nephropathy: The Significance of Extracapillary Proliferation. *Clin. J. Am. Soc. Nephrol.* **2011**, *6*, 2806–2813. [CrossRef] [PubMed]
34. Walsh, M.; Sar, A.; Lee, D.; Yilmaz, S.; Benediktsson, H.; Manns, B.; Hemmelgarn, B. Histopathologic Features Aid in Predicting Risk for Progression of IgA Nephropathy. *Clin. J. Am. Soc. Nephrol.* **2010**, *5*, 425–430. [CrossRef] [PubMed]
35. Shima, Y.; Nakanishi, K.; Hama, T.; Mukaiyama, H.; Togawa, H.; Hashimura, Y.; Kaito, H.; Sako, M.; Iijima, K.; Yoshikawa, N. Validity of the Oxford classification of IgA nephropathy in children. *Pediatr. Nephrol.* **2012**, *27*, 783–792. [CrossRef]
36. Halling, S.E.; Söderberg, M.P.; Berg, U.B. Predictors of outcome in paediatric IgA nephropathy with regard to clinical and histopathological variables (Oxford classification). *Nephrol. Dial. Transplant.* **2012**, *27*, 715–722. [CrossRef]

37. Shao, X.; Li, B.; Cao, L.; Liang, L.; Yang, J.; Wang, Y.; Feng, S.; Wang, C.; Weng, C.; Shen, X.; et al. Evaluation of crescent formation as a predictive marker in immunoglobulin A nephropathy: A systematic review and meta-analysis. *Oncotarget* 2017, *8*, 46436–46448. [CrossRef]
38. Lee, M.J.; Kim, S.J.; Oh, H.J.; Ko, K.I.; Koo, H.M.; Kim, C.H.; Doh, F.M.; Yoo, T.-H.; Kang, S.-W.; Choi, K.H.; et al. Clinical implication of crescentic lesions in immunoglobulin A nephropathy. *Nephrol. Dial. Transplant.* 2014, *29*, 356–364. [CrossRef]
39. Kaneko, Y.; Yoshita, K.; Kono, E.; Ito, Y.; Imai, N.; Yamamoto, S.; Goto, S.; Narita, I. Extracapillary proliferation and arteriolar hyalinosis are associated with long-term kidney survival in IgA nephropathy. *Clin. Exp. Nephrol.* 2015, *20*, 569–577. [CrossRef]
40. Bazzi, C.; Rizza, V.; Raimondi, S.; Casellato, D.; Napodano, P.; D'Amico, G. In Crescentic IgA Nephropathy, Fractional Excretion of IgG in Combination with Nephron Loss Is the Best Predictor of Progression and Responsiveness to Immunosuppression. *Clin. J. Am. Soc. Nephrol.* 2009, *4*, 929–935. [CrossRef]
41. Li, J.; Liu, C.H.; Gao, B.; Xu, D.L. Clinical-pathologic significance of CD163 positive macrophage in IgA nephropathy patients with crescents. *Int. J. Clin. Exp. Med.* 2015, *8*, 9299–9305. [PubMed]
42. Coppo, R.; D'Arrigo, G.; Tripepi, G.; Russo, M.L.; Roberts, I.S.D.; Bellur, S.; Cattran, D.; Cook, T.H.; Feehally, J.; Tesar, V.; et al. Is there long-term value of pathology scoring in immunoglobulin A nephropathy? A validation study of the Oxford Classification for IgA Nephropathy (VALIGA) update. *Nephrol. Dial. Transplant.* 2020, *35*, 1002–1009. [CrossRef] [PubMed]
43. A Working Group of the International IgA Nephropathy Network and the Renal Pathology Society; Roberts, I.S.; Cook, H.T.; Troyanov, S.; Alpers, C.E.; Amore, A.; Barratt, J.; Berthoux, F.; Bonsib, S.; Bruijn, J.A.; et al. The Oxford classification of IgA nephropathy: Pathology definitions, correlations, and reproducibility. *Kidney Int.* 2009, *76*, 546–556. [CrossRef] [PubMed]
44. Coppo, R.; Troyanov, S.; Bellur, S.; Cattran, D.; Cook, H.T.; Feehally, J.; Roberts, I.S.; Morando, L.; Camilla, R.; Tesar, V.; et al. Validation of the Oxford classification of IgA nephropathy in cohorts with different presentations and treatments. *Kidney Int.* 2014, *86*, 828–836. [CrossRef] [PubMed]
45. Barbour, S.; Reich, H. An update on predicting renal progression in IgA nephropathy. *Curr. Opin. Nephrol. Hypertens.* 2018, *27*, 214–220. [CrossRef] [PubMed]
46. Barbour, S.J.; Coppo, R.; Er, L.; Russo, M.L.; Liu, Z.-H.; Ding, J.; Katafuchi, R.; Yoshikawa, N.; Xu, H.; Kagami, S.; et al. Updating the International IgA Nephropathy Prediction Tool for use in children. *Kidney Int.* 2021, *99*, 1439–1450. [CrossRef]
47. Barbour, S.J.; Coppo, R.; Zhang, H.; Liu, Z.H.; Suzuki, Y.; Matsuzaki, K.; Er, L.; Reich, H.N.; Barratt, J.; Catrran, D.C.; et al. Application of the International IgA Nephropathy Prediction Tool one or two years post-biopsy. *Kidney Int.* 2022, in press. [CrossRef]
48. Park, S.; Baek, C.H.; Park, S.-K.; Kang, H.G.; Hyun, H.S.; Park, E.; Han, S.H.; Ryu, D.-R.; Kim, D.K.; Oh, K.-H.; et al. Clinical Significance of Crescent Formation in IgA Nephropathy—A Multicenter Validation Study. *Kidney Blood Press. Res.* 2019, *44*, 22–32. [CrossRef]
49. Hwang, D.; Choi, K.; Cho, N.; Park, S.; Yu, B.C.; Gil, H.; Lee, E.Y.; Choi, S.J.; Park, M.Y.; Kim, J.K.; et al. Validation of an international prediction model including the Oxford classification in Korean patients with IgA nephropathy. *Nephrology* 2021, *26*, 594–602. [CrossRef]
50. Chen, T.; Li, X.; Li, Y.; Xia, E.; Qin, Y.; Liang, S.; Xu, F.; Liang, D.; Zeng, C.; Liu, Z. Prediction and Risk Stratification of Kidney Outcomes in IgA Nephropathy. *Am. J. Kidney Dis.* 2019, *74*, 300–309. [CrossRef]
51. Shima, Y.; Nakanishi, K.; Hama, T.; Mukaiyama, H.; Sato, M.; Tanaka, Y.; Tanaka, R.; Kaito, H.; Nozu, K.; Sako, M.; et al. Crescentic IgA nephropathy in children. *Pediatr. Nephrol.* 2020, *35*, 1005–1014. [CrossRef] [PubMed]
52. Coppo, R.; Davin, J.-C. The difficulty in considering modifiable pathology risk factors in children with IgA nephropathy: Crescents and timing of renal biopsy. *Pediatr. Nephrol.* 2015, *30*, 189–192. [CrossRef] [PubMed]
53. Shima, Y.; Nakanishi, K.; Hama, T.; Sato, M.; Mukaiyama, H.; Togawa, H.; Tanaka, R.; Kaito, H.; Nozu, K.; Iijima, K.; et al. Biopsy timing and Oxford classification variables in Childhood/Adolescent IgA nephropathy. *Pediatr. Nephrol.* 2015, *30*, 293–299. [CrossRef] [PubMed]
54. Huerta, A.; Mérida, E.; Medina, L.; Fernandez, M.; Gutierrez, E.; Hernandez, E.; López-Sánchez, P.; Sevillano, A.; Portolés, J.; Trimarchi, H.; et al. Corticosteroids and mycophenolic acid analogues in immunoglobulin A nephropathy with progressive decline in kidney function. *Clin. Kidney J.* 2021, *4*, 771–777. [CrossRef]
55. Schimpf, J.I.; Klein, T.; Fitzner, C.; Eitner, F.; Porubsky, S.; Hilgers, R.-D.; Floege, J.; Groene, H.-J.; Rauen, T. Renal outcomes of STOP-IgAN trial patients in relation to baseline histology (MEST-C scores). *BMC Nephrol.* 2018, *19*, 328. [CrossRef]
56. Jullien, P.; Laurent, B.; Berthoux, F.; Masson, I.; Dinic, M.; Claisse, G.; Thibaudin, D.; Mariat, C.; Alamartine, E.; Maillard, N. Repeat renal biopsy improves the Oxford classification-based prediction of immunoglobulin A nephropathy outcome. *Nephrol. Dial. Transplant.* 2020, *35*, 1179–1186. [CrossRef]
57. Jia, Q.; Ma, F.; Yang, X.; Li, L.; Liu, C.; Sun, R.; Li, R.; Sun, S. Long-term outcomes of IgA nephropathy patients with less than 25% crescents and mild proteinuria. *Clin. Exp. Nephrol.* 2021, *26*, 257–265. [CrossRef]

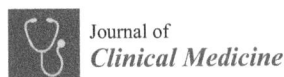

Article

The Impact of Obesity on the Severity of Clinicopathologic Parameters in Patients with IgA Nephropathy

Yu Ah Hong [1], Ji Won Min [2], Myung Ah Ha [2], Eun Sil Koh [3], Hyung Duk Kim [4], Tae Hyun Ban [5], Young Soo Kim [6], Yong Kyun Kim [7], Dongryul Kim [8], Seok Joon Shin [8], Won Jung Choi [1], Yoon Kyung Chang [1], Suk Young Kim [1], Cheol Whee Park [4], Young Ok Kim [6], Chul Woo Yang [4] and Hye Eun Yoon [8],*

1. Department of Internal Medicine, Daejeon St. Mary's Hospital, College of Medicine, The Catholic University of Korea, Daejeon 34943, Korea; amorfati@catholic.ac.kr (Y.A.H.); 1jungchoi@gmail.com (W.J.C.); racer@catholic.ac.kr (Y.K.C.); alterego54@catholic.ac.kr (S.Y.K.)
2. Department of Internal Medicine, Bucheon St. Mary's Hospital, College of Medicine, The Catholic University of Korea, Bucheon 14647, Korea; blueberi12@gmail.com (J.W.M.); hamyunga@naver.com (M.A.H.)
3. Department of Internal Medicine, Yeouido St. Mary's Hospital, College of Medicine, The Catholic University of Korea, Seoul 07345, Korea; fiji79@catholic.ac.kr
4. Department of Internal Medicine, Seoul St. Mary's Hospital, College of Medicine, The Catholic University of Korea, Seoul 06591, Korea; scamph@catholic.ac.kr (H.D.K.); cheolwhee@hanmail.net (C.W.P.); yangch@catholic.ac.kr (C.W.Y.)
5. Department of Internal Medicine, Eunpyeong St. Mary's Hospital, College of Medicine, The Catholic University of Korea, Seoul 03476, Korea; deux0123@catholic.ac.kr
6. Department of Internal Medicine, Uijeongbu St. Mary's Hospital, College of Medicine, The Catholic University of Korea, Uijeongbu 11765, Korea; dr52916@catholic.ac.kr (Y.S.K.); cmckyo@catholic.ac.kr (Y.O.K.)
7. Department of Internal Medicine, St. Vincent's Hospital, College of Medicine, The Catholic University of Korea, Suwon 16247, Korea; drkimyk@catholic.ac.kr
8. Department of Internal Medicine, Incheon St. Mary's Hospital, College of Medicine, The Catholic University of Korea, Incheon 22711, Korea; imndrkim@gmail.com (D.K.); imkidney@catholic.ac.kr (S.J.S.)
* Correspondence: berrynana@catholic.ac.kr; Tel.: +82-32-280-5886

Received: 30 July 2020; Accepted: 15 August 2020; Published: 31 August 2020

Abstract: Several studies reported the effect of obesity on the progression of IgA nephropathy (IgAN). However, the impact of obesity on the clinicopathologic presentation of IgAN remains uncertain. This is a retrospective cross-sectional study from eight university hospitals in South Korea. Patients were categorized into three groups using the Asia-Pacific obesity classification based on body mass index (BMI). Clinical and histopathologic data at the time of renal biopsy were analyzed. Among 537 patients with IgAN, the obese group was more hypertensive and had lower estimated glomerular filtration rate and more proteinuria than other groups. The histologic scores for mesangial matrix expansion (MME), interstitial fibrosis, tubular atrophy, and mesangial C3 deposition differed significantly between the three groups. Among these histopathologic parameters, BMI was independently positively associated with MME score on multivariable linear regression analysis ($p = 0.028$). Using multivariable logistic regression analysis, the obese group was independently associated with higher MME scores compared to the normal weight/overweight group ($p = 0.020$). However, BMI was not independently associated with estimated glomerular filtration rate or proteinuria on multivariable analysis. Obesity was independently associated with severe MME in patients with IgAN. Obesity may play an important pathogenetic role in mesangial lesions seen in IgAN.

Keywords: obesity; mesangial matrix expansion; body mass index; IgA nephropathy

1. Introduction

The prevalence of obesity has been rising regardless of age, sex, and race for the past few decades [1] and is a growing public healthcare concern worldwide [2–4]. Obesity has been implicated in the development of several chronic comorbidities, including type 2 diabetes mellitus, hypertension, cardiovascular disease, stroke, dyslipidemia, obstructive sleep apnea, fatty liver and biliary disease, osteoarthritis, and malignancies, leading to increased cardiovascular and all-cause mortality [5–7]. Obesity is also associated with a significantly increased risk of chronic kidney disease (CKD) progression and development of end-stage renal disease (ESRD) [8,9].

The renal effects of obesity include both structural and functional adaptations. Excessive body weight is related to intrarenal hemodynamic parameters, namely increased renal blood flow and hyperfiltration. Pathologically, this promotes low glomerular density with glomerulomegaly and thickening of the glomerular basement membrane (GBM) [10–12]. These glomerular changes are defined as obesity-related glomerulopathy, a secondary form of focal segmental glomerulosclerosis (FSGS) [13]. Clinically, obesity-related glomerulopathy presents with subnephrotic or nephrotic-range proteinuria without other features of nephrotic syndrome and rapid loss of kidney function [14,15]. In addition to obesity-related glomerulopathy, obesity may be a risk factor for progression of IgA nephropathy (IgAN) [16–21]. Most studies demonstrated that excessive BMI, especially a BMI greater than 25 kg/m^2, was a risk factor for renal disease progression in IgAN patients [16,17]. On the other hand, BMI was not an independent predictor for IgAN progression in some reports [18,22]. Furthermore, recent research showed that underweight, rather than obesity, was an independent risk factor for progression to ESRD, which might be associated with malnutrition status [21]. Therefore, it is difficult to conclude the overall effect of BMI on progression of IgAN with the existing evidence. This may be due to the complex pathophysiological association among obesity, metabolic abnormalities, and renal outcomes.

To date, there are few studies regarding the effect of obesity on histopathological changes in IgAN. Therefore, we conducted a multi-center cohort study using a kidney biopsy registry to elucidate the complex association between obesity and the clinicopathological characteristics of IgAN in Korea. We focused on the impact of obesity on histopathologic and clinical severity at the time of kidney biopsy in IgAN.

2. Materials and Methods

2.1. Study Design and Data Source

This was a cross-sectional study of a multi-center cohort that included patients older than 18 who underwent kidney biopsy at eight university hospitals affiliated with the College of Medicine Catholic University of Korea between January 2015 and November 2019. This study was conducted in accordance with the Declaration of Helsinki and was approved by the Institutional Review Board of the College of Medicine, Catholic University of Korea (XC19OEDI0025). Written informed consent was obtained from patients at the time of biopsy.

We retrospectively collected records from patients with primary IgAN. We excluded 20 out of 557 patients diagnosed with IgAN whose histologic descriptive form was not in accordance with others. A total of 537 patients were finally enrolled in the present study. Patients with Henoch-Schonlein purpura nephritis were ineligible. Patients were divided into three groups according to body mass index (BMI). BMI was calculated as (weight in kilograms)/(height in meters)^2. Subjects were categorized according to the Asia-Pacific obesity classification as follows: underweight (<18.5 kg/m^2), normal weight/overweight (18.5–24.9 kg/m^2), and obese (≥25 kg/m^2) [23]. The BMI cut-offs in the World Health Organization (WHO) classification have categorized BMI 25–29.9 as overweight and ≥30 kg/m^2 as obese [24]. The Asia-Pacific classification of BMI has a lower cut-off for overweight and obese categories compared to the WHO classification. Because the Korean Society for the Study of Obesity defined obesity as BMI ≥ 25 kg/m^2 according to the Asia-Pacific obesity classification [25], we used a cut-off point for BMI of 25 kg/m² in the present study. A flow diagram for patient selection is presented in Figure S1 (Supplementary Materials).

2.2. Data Collection and Definitions

Using the database from the Kidney Biopsy Registry of Catholic Medical Center, all patients were admitted for kidney biopsy and we collected the following data at the time of kidney biopsy. Baseline demographics and clinical data ([including age, sex, height, weight, BMI, co-morbidities, systolic blood pressure (SBP), diastolic blood pressure (DBP), laboratory data, and treatment characteristics) were collected. Blood chemistry data included hemoglobin, high sensitivity-C-reactive protein (hs-CRP), fasting glucose, creatinine, albumin, aspartate aminotransferase (AST), alanine aminotransferase (ALT), uric acid, total cholesterol, triglycerides, low density lipoprotein-cholesterol (LDL-C), high density lipoprotein-cholesterol (HDL-C), serum complement 3 (C3), complement 4 (C4), and serum IgA levels. Proteinuria was assessed by 24 h urine collection. The estimated glomerular filtration rate (eGFR) was calculated from the Chronic Kidney Disease Epidemiology Collaboration (CKD-EPI) equation [26]. The degree of urinary red blood cells (RBC) sediment was scored in five phases, as follows: <3 RBCs/high power field (HPF), 0; 3–5 RBCs/HPF, 1; 5–9 RBCs/HPF, 2; 10–19 RBCs/HPF, 3; and more than 19 RBCs/HPF, 4. We also assessed treatment plans after the diagnosis of IgAN, including use of anti-hypertensive medications, diuretics, lipid-lowering drugs, and immunosuppressive medications.

2.3. Histopathologic Parameters

All kidney tissue specimens were obtained by percutaneous needle biopsy. Pathologic slides were reviewed by expert renal pathologists in each center. On light microscopy, the total number of glomeruli and the percentage of glomerulosclerosis and crescents were assessed quantitatively. Renal histologic findings were scored according to the histologic grading system from our university as follows. The severity of mesangial matrix expansion (MME), mesangial cell proliferation, endocapillary proliferation, interstitial fibrosis (IF), tubular atrophy (TA), arterial intimal hyalinosis, and fibrous vessel wall thickening were semi-quantitatively graded from 0 to 4 as follows: grade 0, absent; grade 1, trace (<20%); grade 2, mild (20%–40%); grade 3, moderate (40%–70%); and grade 4, severe (≥70%). Renal biopsy findings were also assessed according to the Oxford classification (MEST score) [27] or the WHO classification (class I to VI) [28]. On immunofluorescence microscopy, the severity of mesangial deposition of IgA, C3, and C4d were graded as 0 (absent), +1 (trace), +2 (mild), +3 (moderate), and +4 (marked).

2.4. Statistical Analysis

Continuous data were expressed as mean ± standard deviation and were compared using one-way ANOVA followed by Scheffe's post-hoc comparisons (parametric) or Kruskal–Wallis test (non-parametric) as appropriate. Categorical data were expressed as numbers (percentage) and compared using the chi-squared test. Spearman correlation coefficients were calculated for correlations between BMI and clinical/laboratory variables. Linear regression analyses were performed to evaluate the association between BMI and histopathologic parameters and the associations between eGFR and 24 h proteinuria and clinicopathological parameters. Logistic regression analyses were performed to estimate the odds ratios (ORs) and 95% confidence intervals (CIs) for high grades of MME, IF, and TA, and positive mesangial deposition of C3 and IgA according to the BMI groups. High-grade MME, IF, and TA were defined as grades 2–4, and positive mesangial C3 and IgA deposition was defined as scores ≥ +2. A p value of <0.05 was considered statistically significant. The statistical analyses were performed using SPSS version 20.0 software (SPSS, Inc., Chicago, IL, USA).

3. Results

3.1. Baseline Characteristics of the Study Subjects Stratified by BMI

The mean age of the subjects was 41.2 ± 14.7 years, and the mean BMI was 24.1 ± 4.1 kg/m^2. Among 537 patients, 32 patients (5.9%) were underweight, 312 patients (57.8%) were normal weight or overweight, and 193 patients (35.7%) were obese. The baseline clinical characteristics of the study population were compared between the three groups according to BMI classification (Table 1). The obese group was older and had a higher prevalence of hypertension than the underweight and normal weight/overweight groups. SBP and DBP and blood levels of hemoglobin, fasting glucose, liver enzymes, uric acid, total cholesterol, triglycerides, LDL-C, 24-h proteinuria, C3, and C4 were higher in the obese group compared to the other groups, while the eGFR was lower. Figure S2 shows the distribution of BMI according to age and sex categories. For all patients, the BMI distribution peak was shifted to the left. Patients with BMI ≥ 25 kg/m^2 accounted for 35.9% of the total subjects (40.4% in males and 31.8% in females). Patients who had lower BMI tended to be younger, and the distribution of BMI was similar between males and females.

Table 1. Baseline clinical variables of the three BMI groups at the time of renal biopsy.

	BMI			
	<18.5 kg/m^2 (n = 32)	18.5–24.9 kg/m^2 (n = 312)	≥25 kg/m^2 (n = 193)	p
Age (year)	34.3 ± 14.8	40.0 ± 15.2 *	44.1 ± 13.3 *	<0.001
Sex (male, %)	15 (46.9)	140 (44.9)	105 (54.4)	0.112
Alcohol (yes, %)	7 (21.9)	56 (17.9)	39 (20.3)	0.737
Smoking (yes, %)	7 (21.9)	42 (13.5)	35 (18.7)	0.219
Diabetes mellitus (%)	3 (9.4)	14 (4.5)	15 (7.8)	0.218
Hypertension (%)	5 (15.6)	75 (24.0)	74 (38.5)	0.001
BMI (kg/m^2)	17.7 ± 0.7	22.0 ± 1.7 *	28.5 ± 3.1 *,†	<0.001
SBP (mmHg)	115.5 ± 15.5	122.9 ± 16.5 *	127.8 ± 14.5 *	<0.001
DBP (mmHg)	69.8 ± 11.6	75.3 ± 10.0 *	78.8 ± 10.0 *	<0.001
Hemoglobin (g/dL)	12.7 ± 1.9	13.0 ± 2.0 *	13.8 ± 1.8 *	<0.001
hs-CRP (mg/dL)	0.6 ± 0.6	0.7 ± 4.3	0.8 ± 2.4	0.783
Glucose (mg/dL)	96.7 ± 14.5	105.1 ± 29.5	113.3 ± 37.2 *	0.004
Serum creatinine (mg/dL)	1.1 ± 0.9	1.1 ± 1.0	1.1 ± 0.6	0.945
eGFR (mL/min/1.73 m^2)	111.1 ± 38.1	101.7 ± 36.9	93.3 ± 32.1 *	0.006
Serum albumin (g/dL)	4.1 ± 0.5	4.0 ± 0.6	3.9 ± 0.6	0.303
AST (IU/L)	19.6 ± 5.1	22.3 ± 10.9	24.3 ± 10.0 *	0.021
ALT (IU/L)	12.7 ± 6.2	20.2 ± 28.0	25.9 ± 19.6 *	0.003
Serum uric acid (mg/dL)	5.3 ± 1.9	5.9 ± 1.9	6.5 ± 2.0 *	<0.001
Total cholesterol (mg/dL)	169.8 ± 38.5	183.7 ± 48.8	201.0 ± 68.0 *	0.001
Triglyceride (mg/dL)	95.5 ± 49.2	132.8 ± 99.5	209.0 ± 163.3 *,†	<0.001
LDL-C (mg/dL)	94.4 ± 132.8	104.9 ± 37.1	118.0 ± 46.3 *	<0.001
HDL-C (mg/dL)	59.3 ± 17.0	54.1 ± 16.1	48.4 ± 16.9 *	<0.001
24-h proteinuria (g/day)	0.45 ± 0.85	0.93 ± 1.52	1.46 ± 2.71 *	0.007
Urine RBCs (grade)	3.0 ± 1.5	2.8 ± 1.6	2.8 ± 1.6	0.697
Serum C3 (mg/dL)	87.2 ± 17.1	101.1 ± 19.6 *	117.8 ± 20.7 *,†	<0.001
Serum C4 (mg/dL)	22.7 ± 5.4	27.4 ± 9.0 *	31.6 ± 8.9 *,†	<0.001
Serum IgA (mg/dL)	284.0 ± 109.0	316.1 ± 164.3	310.7 ± 147.6	0.475

* ALT, alanine aminotransferase; AST, aspartate aminotransferase; BMI, body mass index; C3, complement 3; C4, complement 4; DBP, diastolic blood pressure; eGFR, estimated glomerular filtration rate; HDL-C, high density lipoprotein-cholesterol; hs-CRP, high sensitivity-C-reactive protein; IgA, immunoglobulin A LDL-C, low density lipoprotein-cholesterol; RBCs, red blood cells; SBP, systolic blood pressure. * $p < 0.05$ vs. BMI < 18.5 kg/m^2 and † $p < 0.05$ vs. BMI 18.5–24.9 kg/m^2 by one-way ANOVA with Scheffe's post-hoc analysis.

3.2. Histopathologic Findings of the Study Subjects Stratified by BMI

We compared histopathologic features between the three BMI groups in Tables 2 and 3 and Figure 1. Total number of glomeruli and the mean mesangial C3 deposition score were lower ($p = 0.003$ and $p < 0.001$, respectively), and the mean MME ($p = 0.042$), IF ($p = 0.046$) and TA ($p = 0.033$) score was higher in the obese group compared to the other groups (Table 2). On light microscopy, the glomeruli, mesangium, tubules, interstitium, vessels, and mesangial IgA deposition score did not differ between the three groups. There was an increasing trend of high grade MME ($p = 0.007$), IF ($p = 0.03$), and TA ($p = 0.039$) as the BMI increased. The distribution of the C3 deposition severity was different among the three groups ($p < 0.001$, Figure 1). The distributions for WHO and Oxford classifications of IgAN were not significantly different between the three BMI groups (Table 3).

Table 2. Histopathological findings of the three BMI groups.

	BMI			
	<18.5 kg/m²	18.5–24.9 kg/m²	≥25 kg/m²	p
Total glomerular number	15.9 ± 8.9	13.9 ± 7.9	12.1 ± 7.1 *,†	0.003
Light microscopy				
Glomerulosclerosis, Total (%)	20.1 ± 27.8	24.3 ± 24.6	26.9 ± 25.1 *	0.101
Global sclerosis (%)	10.2 ± 20.4	16.7 ± 19.4 *	17.8 ± 19.9 *	0.015
Segmental sclerosis (%)	7.3 ± 9.7	8.3 ± 13.0	9.5 ± 14.5	0.731
Mesangial matrix expansion (0–4)	1.7 ± 1.0	2.1 ± 0.9	2.2 ± 0.7 *	0.042
Mesangial cell proliferation (0–4)	1.8 ± 1.1	2.0 ± 0.9	2.1 ± 0.9	0.292
Crescents (%)	1.6 ± 4.7	2.6 ± 8.0	2.0 ± 7.5	0.951
Interstitial fibrosis (0–4)	1.1 ± 1.0	1.3 ± 1.0	1.4 ± 0.9 *	0.046
Tubular atrophy (0–4)	1.3 ± 1.0	1.2 ± 1.0	1.4 ± 0.9 †	0.033
Arterial intimal hyalinosis (0–4)	0.3 ± 0.6	0.2 ± 0.6	0.3 ± 0.8	0.213
Fibrous wall thickening (0–4)	0.3 ± 0.7	0.5 ± 0.9	0.6 ± 1.0	0.269
Immunofluorescence microscopy				
IgA Mesangial deposit (0–4)	2.9 ± 1.2	3.3 ± 0.9	3.2 ± 1.0	0.177
C3 Mesangial deposit (0–4)	2.3 ± 1.3	2.3 ± 1.1	1.8 ± 1.2 *,†	<0.001
C4d Mesangial deposit (0–4)	0.1 ± 0.2	0.2 ± 0.1	0.1 ± 0.4	0.903

* BMI, body mass index; C3, complement 3; C4, complement 4; IgA, immunoglobulin A. * $p < 0.05$ vs. BMI < 18.5 kg/m² and † $p < 0.05$ vs. BMI 18.5–24.9 kg/m² by post-hoc analysis of Kruskal-Wallis test.

Table 3. The distribution of histological classifications according to the three BMI groups.

	BMI			
	<18.5 kg/m²	18.5–24.9 kg/m²	≥25 kg/m²	p
WHO classification (n = 436)	n = 22	n = 255	n = 159	
Grade (1–6)	2.91 ± 0.92	2.93 ± 0.93	2.98 ± 0.86	0.834
Oxford classification (n = 173)	n = 10	n = 95	n = 68	
M0 (%)	4 (40)	51 (53.7)	33 (48.5)	0.630
M1 (%)	6 (60)	44 (46.3)	35 (51.5)	
E0 (%)	6 (60)	73 (76.8)	50 (73.5)	0.492
E1 (%)	4 (40)	22 (23.2)	18 (26.5)	
S0 (%)	3 (30.0)	53 (55.8)	29 (42.6)	0.117
S1 (%)	7 (70.0)	42 (44.2)	39 (57.4)	
T0 (%)	7 (70.0)	72 (75.8)	50 (73.5)	0.778
T1 (%)	3 (30.0)	18 (18.9)	16 (23.5)	
T2 (%)	0 (0)	5 (5.3)	2 (2.9)	

BMI, body mass index; WHO, World Health Organization. Oxford classification: M; mesangial hypercellularity, E; endocapillary proliferation, S; segmental sclerosis, T tubular atrophy/interstitial fibrosis. Statistical analysis was performed by Kruskal-Wallis test in WHO classifications and using the chi-squared test in Oxford classifications.

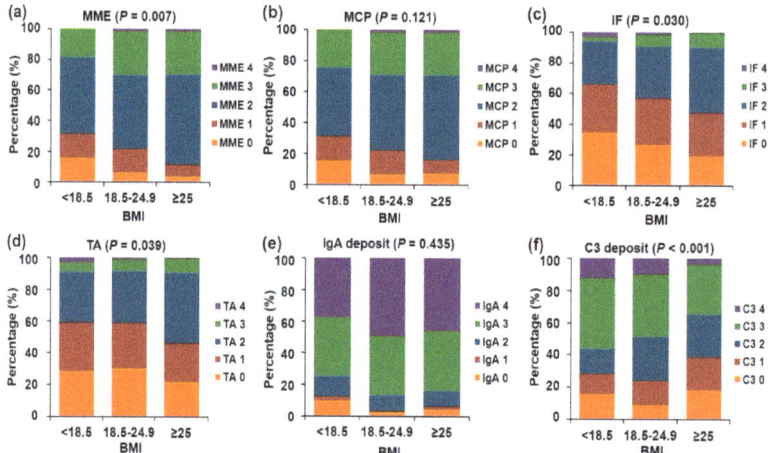

Figure 1. The distribution of histopathologic scores according to the three BMI groups. (**a**) Mesangial matrix expansion (MME). (**b**) Mesangial cell proliferation (MCP). (**c**) Interstitial fibrosis (IF). (**d**) Tubular atrophy (TA). (**e**) IgA mesangial deposition. (**f**) C3 mesangial deposition.

3.3. Association between BMI and Histopathologic Parameters

Univariable linear regression analysis showed that scores for MME, endocapillary proliferation, IF, and TA were positively correlated with BMI, while the number of total glomeruli and the mesangial C3 deposition score were negatively correlated with BMI (Table 4). Multivariable linear regression analysis showed that the MME and mesangial IgA deposition scores were positively associated with BMI ($p = 0.028$; adjusted $R^2 = 0.291$ and $p = 0.041$; adjusted $R^2 = 0.291$, respectively), while total number of glomeruli was negatively associated with BMI ($p = 0.029$; adjusted $R^2 = 0.286$) after adjusting for clinical parameters including age, SBP, hemoglobin, glucose, albumin, AST, ALT, uric acid, total cholesterol, eGFR, 24-h proteinuria, and serum C3, C4, and IgA levels.

Table 4. Linear regression analysis for BMI and the histopathologic parameters.

	BMI					
	Univariable			Multivariable		
	β	t	p	β	t	p
Total glomerular number	−0.162	−3.802	<0.001	−0.092	−2.192	0.029
Mesangial matrix expansion	0.086	2.004	0.046	0.091	2.205	0.028
Mesangial cell proliferation	0.048	1.112	0.266	0.066	1.585	0.114
Segmental sclerosis	0.040	0.934	0.351	0.062	1.428	0.154
Endocapillary proliferation	0.128	2.974	0.003	0.052	1.236	0.217
Interstitial fibrosis	0.087	2.020	0.044	0.028	0.547	0.585
Tubular atrophy	0.099	2.286	0.023	0.036	0.701	0.484
IgA Mesangial Deposit	−0.025	−0.5825	0.561	0.086	2.048	0.041
C3 Mesangial Deposit	−0.151	−3.521	<0.001	0.008	0.187	0.852
C4d Mesangial Deposit	0.026	0.588	0.557	0.004	0.086	0.932

BMI, body mass index, C3, complement 3; C4d, cleavage product of complement 4; IgA, immunoglobulin A. Multivariable analysis was adjusted for each histologic parameter and clinical parameters, including age, systolic blood pressure, hemoglobin, glucose, albumin, AST, ALT, uric acid, total cholesterol, eGFR, 24-h proteinuria, and serum C3, C4 and IgA levels.

Table 5 shows the OR and 95% CI for high MME, IF, TA, and positive mesangial deposition of C3 and IgA for the three BMI groups. Considering the normal weight or overweight group as a reference, the obese group showed higher risks for high MME and TA, and lower risk for mesangial C3 deposition. After adjusting for age, sex, the presence of hypertension and diabetes mellitus, and SBP (Model 1), the obese group exhibited higher risk for severe MME (OR = 2.066, 95% CI 1.227–3.478, p = 0.006) and lower risk for mesangial C3 deposition (OR = 0.544, 95% CI 0.365–0.810, p = 0.003). After adjusting for model 1 with total glomerular number, eGFR, 24-h proteinuria, and blood levels of hemoglobin, glucose, albumin, AST, ALT, uric acid, total cholesterol, C3, C4, and IgA (Model 2), the obese group still had a significantly higher risk for severe MME (OR = 2.060, 95% CI 1.120–3.788, p = 0.020), while the underweight group had a significantly lower risk for severe MME (OR = 0.369, 95% CI 0.150–0.904, p = 0.029) and mesangial IgA deposition (OR = 0.208, 95% CI 0.049–0.889, p = 0.034).

Table 5. Logistic regression analysis for BMI groups and histopathologic parameters.

	Crude OR		Model 1		Model 2	
	OR (95% CI)	p	OR (95% CI)	p	OR (95% CI)	p
	Mesangial matrix expansion					
<18.5	0.595 (0.269–1.318)	0.201	0.586 (0.259–1.327)	0.200	0.369 (0.150–0.904)	0.029
18.5–24.9	1 (Ref.)		1 (Ref.)		1 (Ref.)	
≥25	2.201 (1.249–3.539)	0.005	2.066 (1.227–3.478)	0.006	2.060 (1.120–3.788)	0.020
	Interstitial fibrosis					
<18.5	0.685 (0.319–1.471)	0.332	1.084 (0.475–2.472)	0.848	0.568 (0.157–2.056)	0.389
18.5–24.9	1 (Ref.)		1 (Ref.)		1 (Ref.)	
≥25	1.436 (1.000–2.062)	0.05	1.121 (0.761–1.651)	0.564	1.297 (0.759–2.216)	0.341
	Tubular Atrophy					
<18.5	0.983 (0.468–2.063)	0.964	1.550 (0.282–1.550)	0.282	0.861 (0.252–2.937)	0.811
18.5–24.9	1 (Ref.)		1 (Ref.)		1 (Ref.)	
≥25	1.679 (1.168–2.413)	0.005	1.338 (0.909–1.969)	0.140	1.644 (0.961–2.812)	0.070
	IgA mesangial deposit					
<18.5	0.236 (0.069–0.800)	0.021	0.236 (0.069–0.800)	0.021	0.208 (0.049–0.889)	0.034
18.5–24.9	1 (Ref.)		1 (Ref.)		1 (Ref.)	
≥25	0.508 (0.215–1.199)	0.508	0.553 (0.228–1.344)	0.191	0.871 (0.279–2.714)	0.812
	C3 mesangial deposit					
<18.5	0.812 (0.360–1.831)	0.615	0.533 (0.321–1.800)	0.533	0.516 (0.167–1.599)	0.252
18.5–24.9	1 (Ref.)		1 (Ref.)		1 (Ref.)	
≥25	0.506 (0.343–0.749)	<0.001	0.544 (0.365–0.810)	0.003	0.805 (0.469–1.380)	0.430

BMI, body mass index; C3, complement; IgA, immunoglobulin A. Model 1 was adjusted for age, sex, the presence of hypertension, the presence of diabetes mellitus and systolic blood pressure. Model 2 was adjusted for model 1 + total glomerular number, eGFR, 24-h proteinuria, and blood levels of hemoglobin, glucose, albumin, aspartate aminotransferase, alanine aminotransferase, uric acid, total cholesterol, and serum C3, C4, and serum IgA levels.

To evaluate whether the association between BMI and MME in IgAN is an incidental finding in obese patients, we analyzed subjects with tubulointerstitial disease without glomerular injury (acute tubular necrosis, interstitial nephritis, and pyelonephritis) during the same period in our kidney biopsy cohort (n = 80). There was no significant association between BMI groups and MME in subjects with tubulointerstitial diseases (Table S1 (Supplementary Materials)).

3.4. Association of BMI with Clinical Variables, Renal Function, and Proteinuria

There was a positive relationship between BMI and 24 h proteinuria, total cholesterol, triglycerides, and serum C3 and C4 levels and a negative relationship between BMI and eGFR (Figure 2). The association of BMI with renal function and proteinuria was evaluated by adjusting for clinical and histopathological variables in linear regression analysis (Table 6). BMI was negatively correlated with eGFR in univariable analysis; however, this relationship was not significant on multivariable analysis. Factors significantly associated with eGFR were age, SBP, levels of serum albumin and HDL-C, total number of glomeruli, and the interstitial fibrosis score (adjusted R^2 = 0.460). BMI showed a positive linear association with 24-h proteinuria on univariable analysis, but the association was not significant on multivariable analysis. eGFR and serum levels of albumin and C3 were significantly associated with 24-h proteinuria (adjusted R^2 = 0.260).

Table 6. Linear regression analysis for renal function and 24-h proteinuria.

	eGFR								24-h Proteinuria							
	Univariable				Multivariable				Univariable				Multivariable			
	β	t	p		β	t	p		β	t	p		β	t	p	
Age	−0.438	−11.270	<0.001		−0.273	−7.079	<0.001		0.106	2.283	0.023		-	-	-	
SBP	−0.264	−6.315	<0.001		−0.101	−0.265	0.008		0.167	3.629	<0.001		-	-	-	
DBP	−0.221	5.224	<0.001						0.088	1.878	0.061		-	-	-	
BMI	−0.175	−4.102	<0.001						0.135	2.921	0.004		-	-	-	
Hemoglobin	0.306	7.403	<0.001						−0.015	−0.315	0.753		-	-	-	
Glucose	−0.089	−2.036	0.042						−0.020	−0.414	0.679		-	-	-	
eGFR	-	-	-						−0.272	−6.049	<0.001		−0.120	−2.653	0.008	
Albumin	0.413	10.482	<0.001		0.201	5.260	<0.001		−0.455	−10.933	<0.001		−0.429	−9.454	<0.001	
Total cholesterol	−0.59	−1.351	0.177						0.193	4.206	<0.001		-	-	-	
Triglyceride	−0.125	−2.884	0.004						0.058	1.233	0.218		-	-	-	
LDL-C	−0.083	−1.878	0.061						0.216	4.661	<0.001		-	-	-	
HDL-C	0.197	4.500	<0.001		0.087	2.314	0.021		0.006	0.122	0.903		-	-	-	
Serum C3	0.046	1.035	0.301						0.159	3.390	0.001		0.162	3.851	<0.001	
Serum C4	−0.233	−5.389	<0.001						0.170	3.631	<0.001		-	-	-	
Serum IgA	−0.142	−3.166	0.002						−0.017	−0.353	0.724		-	-	-	
24-h proteinuria	−0.272	−6.049	<0.001						-	-	-		-	-	-	
Total glomerular number	0.103	2.392	0.017		0.109	2.967	0.003		−0.089	−1.909	0.057		-	-	-	
Mesangial matrix expansion	−0.065	−1.495	0.136						0.058	1.246	0.213		-	-	-	
Mesangial cell proliferation	−0.023	−0.532	0.595						0.059	1.263	0.207		-	-	-	
Endocapillary proliferation	−0.108	−2.496	0.013						0.028	0.601	0.548		-	-	-	
Interstitial fibrosis	−0.511	−13.678	<0.001		−0.408	−10.284	<0.001		0.191	4.140	<0.001		-	-	-	
Tubular atrophy	−0.485	−12.759	<0.001						0.192	4.173	<0.001		-	-	-	
Mesangial deposit, IgA	0.104	2.414	0.016						0.012	0.250	0.803		-	-	-	
Mesangial deposit, C3	−0.002	−0.046	0.963						0.007	0.142	0.888		-	-	-	

BMI, body mass index; C3, complement 3; DBP, diastolic blood pressure; eGFR, estimated glomerular filtration rate; HDL-C, high density lipoprotein-cholesterol; IgA, immunoglobulin A; LDL-C, low density lipoprotein-cholesterol; SBP, systolic blood pressure. The variables included in the multivariable linear regression model were statistically significant variables in the univariable linear regression ($p < 0.1$). Dashes indicate that the variable did not enter the multivariable linear regression model.

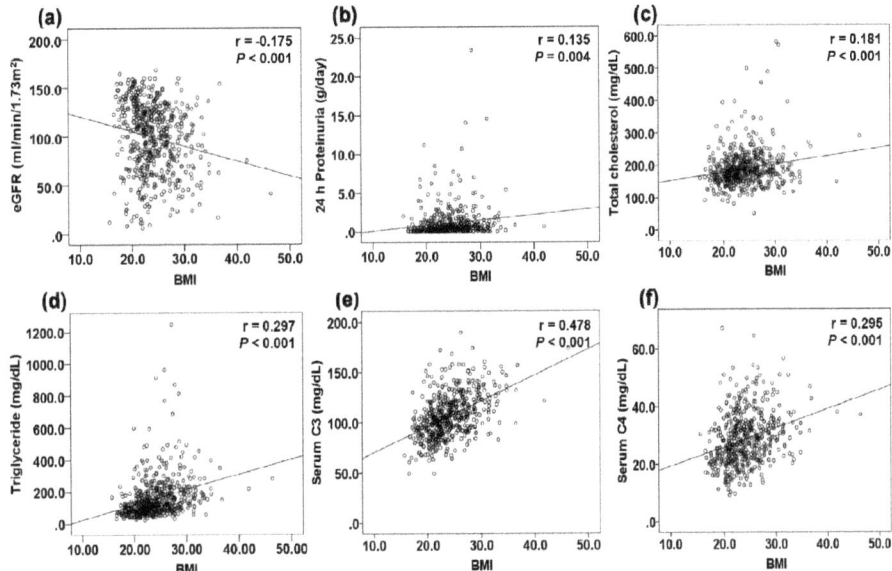

Figure 2. The correlation graphs between BMI and clinical variables. (**a**) CKD-EPI eGFR. (**b**) 24 h proteinuria. (**c**) Total cholesterol level. (**d**) Triglyceride level. (**e**) Serum C3 level. (**f**) Serum C4 level.

3.5. Treatment Patterns of the Study Subjects Stratified by BMI

At the time of kidney biopsy, there was no significant difference in the use of renin-angiotensin-aldosterone system (RAAS) blockers among the three groups ($p = 0.252$); BMI < 18.5 kg/m^2 (n = 13, 40.6%) vs. 18.5–24.9 kg/m^2 (n = 87, 27.9%) vs. ≥ 25 kg/m^2 (n = 51, 26.4%). Several treatment strategies were chosen within 6 months after kidney biopsy and these were compared between the three groups. More patients in the obese group were treated with RAAS blockers, calcium channel blockers (CCBs), β-blockers, thiazide, statins, and corticosteroids compared to the underweight and normal/overweight groups (Table 7).

Table 7. Distribution of treatment after renal biopsy according to the three BMI groups.

	BMI			
	<18.5 kg/m^2	18.5–24.9 kg/m^2	≥25 kg/m^2	p
Anti-hypertensive medications				
RAAS blocker	21 (65.6)	223 (71.5)	157 (81.3)	0.029
CCB	3 (9.4)	41 (13.1)	57 (29.5)	<0.001
B-blocker	1 (3.1)	14 (4.5)	22 (11.4)	0.015
Diuretics				
Thiazide	0 (0.0)	1 (0.3)	7 (3.6)	0.033
Furosemide	2 (6.2)	23 (7.4)	21 (10.9)	0.523
Lipid lowering agents				
Statin	6 (18.8)	74 (23.7)	83 (43.0)	<0.001
Omega-3 fatty acid	3 (9.4)	53 (17.0)	38 (19.7)	0.266
Immunosuppressive agents				
Any immunosuppression	24 (75.0)	210 (67.3)	128 (66.3)	0.248
Steroid	4 (12.5)	84 (26.9)	63 (32.6)	0.036

BMI, body mass index; CCB, calcium channel blocker; RAAS, renin-angiotensin-aldosterone system.

4. Discussion

In this study, we evaluated the histopathological and clinical implications of obesity in patients with IgAN. Intriguingly, multivariable logistic regression demonstrated that a BMI greater than 25 kg/m^2 was independently associated with high MME in patients with IgAN. Patients with elevated BMI were more hypertensive and had increased proteinuria, but the association of BMI with renal function and proteinuria was modest in IgAN.

Only a few studies have investigated the influence of obesity on histological parameters in IgAN. First, Bonnet et al. suggested that vascular, tubular, and interstitial indices were higher in obese patients than non-obese patients using a semi-quantitative classification scheme, but the glomerular index did not differ significantly. A recent cohort analysis of 481 IgAN patients also showed that high BMI was associated with a high risk of IF [22]. These previous studies did not focus and evaluate the association between increased BMI and MME in IgAN. Tanaka et al. [29] also reported that obese patients with IgAN showed significantly increased proteinuria, accompanied by GBM thickening and glomerulomegaly, mimicking obesity-related glomerulopathy. This study showed no significant differences in the severity of mesangial proliferation and matrix expansion between obese and non-obese group, but the number of enrolled patients were very small. Our study is the first study to show an independent association between obesity and MME in IgAN. Moreover, in subjects with tubulointerstitial disease, obesity did not show a significant association with MME, which means that the association between obesity and MME in IgAN is not an incidental finding seen in obese patients. Although the precise mechanism by which obesity causes MME remains unclear, obesity can lead to a rise in the concentration of leptin, which stimulates the expression of transforming growth factor-β1 (TGF-β1). TGF-β1 is known to act as the main driver of extracellular matrix accumulation, mesangial cell proliferation, and progressive glomerulosclerosis [30,31]. These in turn may be responsible for the proliferation of mesangial cells and expanded mesangial matrix. MME has been regarded as a step towards glomerular sclerosis [32]. Although FSGS has long been recognized as the hallmark lesion of obesity-related glomerulopathy [13], Serra et al. [33] also found that increased mesangial matrix, podocyte hypertrophy, and mesangial cell proliferation were more frequent in extremely obese patients compared to normal weight controls. Of note, our study supports these findings in that obesity could independently increase MME after adjustment for confounding factors and strengthens our knowledge of the pathogenic role of obesity in mesangial lesions in IgAN.

Obesity-induced subclinical inflammation is responsible for activation of the complement system [34]. C3 and C4 are expressed and secreted by adipose tissue [35], and serum C3 is strongly associated with components of metabolic syndrome, such as insulin resistance, lipid profile, and BMI [36–38]. Furthermore, weight gain increases C3, which decreases upon weight loss [39]. Therefore, C3 has been linked to the etiology of obesity, and to a wide range of obesity sequelae. In this study, serum C3 and C4 levels were increased in patients with higher BMI. Serum C3 level was positively associated with 24 h proteinuria using multivariable analysis. Consistent with our study, some researchers previously reported that serum C3 and C4 levels were positively correlated with increased BMI and severe proteinuria in IgAN patients [19,21]. High serum C4 level was also associated with severe proteinuria and renal pathological damage in IgAN [40]. Altogether, these findings suggest that obesity may activate the complement system and is related to the severity of renal presentation in patients with IgAN.

In this study, mesangial C3 deposition decreased as BMI increased, but multivariable linear regression and logistic regression analyses showed that mesangial C3 deposition was not independently associated with BMI. Additionally, mesangial C3 deposition was not significantly associated with eGFR or 24 h proteinuria. Therefore, we speculate that the effect of obesity on the activation of the local complement system is modest in IgAN. Previous studies revealed conflicting results, suggesting an important role of local complement activation in the pathogenesis of IgAN. Mesangial C3c deposition was associated with active inflammation in IgAN [41], and mesangial C3 deposition was an independent risk factor for progression of IgAN [42]. A recent study also reported that mesangial C3 deposition was associated with poor outcome in IgAN; however, eGFR or proteinuria at the time of kidney biopsy did not differ according to the degree of mesangial C3 deposition [43]. The implications of mesangial complement deposition may have differential effects on renal presentation and prognosis, and further analysis is needed to clarify the pathologic role of mesangial complement deposition in IgAN.

Another interesting finding is that obesity was not independently associated with clinical parameters such as renal function and proteinuria in IgAN. In this study, obese patients showed decreased eGFR and increased 24 h proteinuria compared to other groups, but there were no significant relationships between BMI and eGFR or 24-h proteinuria in multivariable analysis. In addition, the histologic classification of IgAN, such as the Oxford classification or WHO classification, was not different between the groups. Previous studies demonstrated similar findings to our results. A prospective cohort study of 331 French IgAN patients showed that patients with elevated BMI had worse renal presentations and outcomes, but that obesity, per se, did not directly affect these outcomes [18]. In a study of 481 Chinese IgAN patients, there was no significant difference in clinical parameters or Oxford classification scores among BMI groups [22]. In a study including a small number of IgAN patients, obesity had no significant impact on serum creatinine levels or pathological severity in multiple linear regression models [44]. These findings suggest that obesity may not be independently related to decreased renal function, increased proteinuria, or severe forms of histologic classification in IgAN, although it likely affects histologic damage. Obese patients may simultaneously have multiple unhealthy lifestyle behaviors, such as smoking, increased energy intake, low physical activity, and various medical conditions including hypertension, diabetes mellitus, and dyslipidemia, which are known risk factors for renal disease progression [45]. In this study, we also showed that obese patients with IgAN had more the presence of hypertension and dyslipidemia, and were more actively treated with supportive managements, such as anti-hypertensive medications, thiazide, and statins, as well as corticosteroids, than underweight or normal/overweight patients. Therefore, increased weight alone may not be enough to induce severe renal parameters and histologic classifications. To elucidate a direct association between obesity and long-term kidney damage, we need to perform further studies involving a larger number of patients with IgAN.

This study has several limitations. First, our findings are limited by the cross-sectional and retrospective design, uncertain causality, and possible influence of confounding factors that could not be captured; in addition, there were no longitudinal follow-up data. Therefore, a prospective, multi-center, large scale study with a longer follow-up period is required to define the histopathological impact of BMI more clearly in IgAN. Second, although this study included eight university hospitals, the evaluation of renal biopsy specimens was conducted by expert renal pathologists in each center. Therefore, there may be interobserver variability. However, each hospital shares the same renal biopsy report form, and the pathologists at each hospital were trained by one pathologist. Thus, observer bias in histologic assessment may be relatively small. To compensate for this limitation, the histologic grading and staging of IgAN were described according to both the Oxford and WHO classifications. Third, the inclusion of only Korean patients may limit the generalizability of our findings to other ethnic populations. Current practice guidelines suggested that obesity is typically defined quite simply as excess body weight for height, but this simple definition of obesity cannot reflect the consideration of age or race/ethnicity. Therefore, further studies may be needed to elucidate the association with obesity and clinicopathologic parameters in various ethnic groups of IgAN. Fourth, we did not measure the anthropometric parameters associated with metabolic syndrome, such as waist circumference, skin fold thickness and waist-to-hip ratio, and the index of insulin resistance in this study. Further studies will be required to determine whether these markers may be more reliable measures than BMI in IgAN.

5. Conclusions

In conclusion, our study showed that obesity was independently associated with MME in Korean IgAN patients and these findings suggest that obesity may have an important pathogenetic role in mesangial lesions in IgAN.

Supplementary Materials: The following are available online at http://www.mdpi.com/2077-0383/10/9/2824/s1, Figure S1: Flow chart of study design. Figure S2: Distribution of BMI according to age and sex categories. Bars of the BMI were divided by age (a) and sex categories (b). Table S1: Logistic regression analysis for BMI groups and MME in tubulointerstitial diseases from our kidney biopsy registry cohort (n = 80).

Author Contributions: Conceptualization, Y.A.H. and H.E.Y.; methodology, J.W.M., M.A.H. and E.S.K.; formal analysis, D.K. and W.J.C.; investigation, S.J.S., Y.K.C. and S.Y.K.; data curation, H.D.K., T.H.B., Y.S.K. and Y.K.K.; writing—original draft preparation, Y.A.H.; writing—review and editing, H.E.Y.; supervision, C.W.P., Y.O.K., and C.W.Y. All authors have read and agreed to the published version of the manuscript.

Funding: This work was supported by the National Research Foundation of Korea (NRF) grant funded by the Korea government (MSIT) (2018R1C1B5045006) and Clinical Research Institute Grant (CMCDJ-P-2020-012) funded by the Catholic University of Korea Daejeon St. Mary's Hospital. The authors also wish to acknowledge the grant funded by the Catholic Medical Center Research Foundation made in the program year of 2018.

Acknowledgments: We would like to thank the study coordinators So Yeon Kim, Young Mie Hwang, and Leeji Bae for their contributions to this study.

Conflicts of Interest: The authors declare no conflict of interest.

References

1. NCD Risk Factor Collaboration (NCD-RisC). Worldwide trends in body-mass index, underweight, overweight, and obesity from 1975 to 2016: A pooled analysis of 2416 population-based measurement studies in 128·9 million children, adolescents, and adults. *Lancet* **2017**, *390*, 2627–2642. [CrossRef]
2. Song, H.J.; Hwang, J.; Pi, S.; Ahn, S.; Heo, Y.; Park, S.; Kwon, J.W. The impact of obesity and overweight on medical expenditures and disease incidence in Korea from 2002 to 2013. *PLoS ONE* **2018**, *13*, e0197057. [CrossRef] [PubMed]
3. Specchia, M.L.; Veneziano, M.A.; Cadeddu, C.; Ferriero, A.M.; Mancuso, A.; Ianuale, C.; Parente, P.; Capri, S.; Ricciardi, W. Economic impact of adult obesity on health systems: A systematic review. *Eur. J. Public Health* **2015**, *25*, 255–262. [CrossRef] [PubMed]
4. Roberto, C.A.; Swinburn, B.; Hawkes, C.; Huang, T.T.; Costa, S.A.; Ashe, M.; Zwicker, L.; Cawley, J.H.; Brownell, K.D. Patchy progress on obesity prevention: Emerging examples, entrenched barriers, and new thinking. *Lancet* **2015**, *385*, 2400–2409. [CrossRef]
5. Murphy, N.; Cross, A.J.; Abubakar, M.; Jenab, M.; Aleksandrova, K.; Boutron-Ruault, M.C.; Dossus, L.; Racine, A.; Kuhn, T.; Katzke, V.A.; et al. A Nested Case-Control Study of Metabolically Defined Body Size Phenotypes and Risk of Colorectal Cancer in the European Prospective Investigation into Cancer and Nutrition (EPIC). *PLoS Med.* **2016**, *13*, e1001988. [CrossRef]
6. Meigs, J.B.; Wilson, P.W.; Fox, C.S.; Vasan, R.S.; Nathan, D.M.; Sullivan, L.M.; D'Agostino, R.B. Body mass index, metabolic syndrome, and risk of type 2 diabetes or cardiovascular disease. *J. Clin. Endocrinol. Metab.* **2006**, *91*, 2906–2912. [CrossRef]
7. Lu, Y.; Hajifathalian, K.; Ezzati, M.; Woodward, M.; Rimm, E.B.; Danaei, G. Metabolic mediators of the effects of body-mass index, overweight, and obesity on coronary heart disease and stroke: A pooled analysis of 97 prospective cohorts with 1.8 million participants. *Lancet* **2014**, *383*, 970–983.
8. Yun, H.R.; Kim, H.; Park, J.T.; Chang, T.I.; Yoo, T.H.; Kang, S.W.; Choi, K.H.; Sung, S.; Kim, S.W.; Lee, J.; et al. Obesity, Metabolic Abnormality, and Progression of CKD. *Am. J. Kidney Dis.* **2018**, *72*, 400–410. [CrossRef]
9. Panwar, B.; Hanks, L.J.; Tanner, R.M.; Muntner, P.; Kramer, H.; McClellan, W.M.; Warnock, D.G.; Judd, S.E.; Gutierrez, O.M. Obesity, metabolic health, and the risk of end-stage renal disease. *Kidney Int.* **2015**, *87*, 1216–1222. [CrossRef]
10. Okabayashi, Y.; Tsuboi, N.; Sasaki, T.; Haruhara, K.; Kanzaki, G.; Koike, K.; Miyazaki, Y.; Kawamura, T.; Ogura, M.; Yokoo, T. Glomerulopathy Associated with Moderate Obesity. *Kidney Int. Rep.* **2016**, *1*, 250–255. [CrossRef]
11. Goumenos, D.S.; Kawar, B.; El Nahas, M.; Conti, S.; Wagner, B.; Spyropoulos, C.; Vlachojannis, J.G.; Benigni, A.; Kalfarentzos, F. Early histological changes in the kidney of people with morbid obesity. *Nephrol. Dial. Transplant.* **2009**, *24*, 3732–3738. [CrossRef]
12. Kato, S.; Nazneen, A.; Nakashima, Y.; Razzaque, M.S.; Nishino, T.; Furusu, A.; Yorioka, N.; Taguchi, T. Pathological influence of obesity on renal structural changes in chronic kidney disease. *Clin. Exp. Nephrol.* **2009**, *13*, 332–340. [CrossRef] [PubMed]

13. Kambham, N.; Markowitz, G.S.; Valeri, A.M.; Lin, J.; D'Agati, V.D. Obesity-related glomerulopathy: An emerging epidemic. *Kidney Int.* **2001**, *59*, 1498–1509. [CrossRef] [PubMed]
14. Chen, H.M.; Li, S.J.; Chen, H.P.; Wang, Q.W.; Li, L.S.; Liu, Z.H. Obesity-related glomerulopathy in China: A case series of 90 patients. *Am. J. Kidney Dis.* **2008**, *52*, 58–65. [CrossRef] [PubMed]
15. Praga, M.; Hernandez, E.; Morales, E.; Campos, A.P.; Valero, M.A.; Martinez, M.A.; Leon, M. Clinical features and long-term outcome of obesity-associated focal segmental glomerulosclerosis. *Nephrol. Dial. Transplant.* **2001**, *16*, 1790–1798. [CrossRef] [PubMed]
16. Bonnet, F.; Deprele, C.; Sassolas, A.; Moulin, P.; Alamartine, E.; Berthezene, F.; Berthoux, F. Excessive body weight as a new independent risk factor for clinical and pathological progression in primary IgA nephritis. *Am. J. Kidney Dis.* **2001**, *37*, 720–727. [CrossRef]
17. Kataoka, H.; Ohara, M.; Shibui, K.; Sato, M.; Suzuki, T.; Amemiya, N.; Watanabe, Y.; Honda, K.; Mochizuki, T.; Nitta, K. Overweight and obesity accelerate the progression of IgA nephropathy: Prognostic utility of a combination of BMI and histopathological parameters. *Clin. Exp. Nephrol.* **2012**, *16*, 706–712. [CrossRef]
18. Berthoux, F.; Mariat, C.; Maillard, N. Overweight/obesity revisited as a predictive risk factor in primary IgA nephropathy. *Nephrol. Dial. Transplant.* **2013**, *28* (Suppl. 4), 160–166. [CrossRef]
19. Shimamoto, M.; Ohsawa, I.; Suzuki, H.; Hisada, A.; Nagamachi, S.; Honda, D.; Inoshita, H.; Shimizu, Y.; Horikoshi, S.; Tomino, Y. Impact of Body Mass Index on Progression of IgA Nephropathy Among Japanese Patients. *J. Clin. Lab. Anal.* **2015**, *29*, 353–360. [CrossRef]
20. Nagaraju, S.P.; Rangaswamy, D.; Mareddy, A.S.; Prasad, S.; Kaza, S.; Shenoy, S.; Saraf, K.; Attur, R.P.; Parthasarathy, R.; Kosuru, S.; et al. Impact of body mass index on progression of primary immunoglobulin a nephropathy. *Saudi J. Kidney Dis. Transpl.* **2018**, *29*, 318–325. [CrossRef]
21. Ouyang, Y.; Xie, J.; Yang, M.; Zhang, X.; Ren, H.; Wang, W.; Chen, N. Underweight Is an Independent Risk Factor for Renal Function Deterioration in Patients with IgA Nephropathy. *PLoS ONE* **2016**, *11*, e0162044. [CrossRef] [PubMed]
22. Wu, C.; Wang, A.Y.; Li, G.; Wang, L. Association of high body mass index with development of interstitial fibrosis in patients with IgA nephropathy. *BMC Nephrol.* **2018**, *19*, 381. [CrossRef] [PubMed]
23. Pan, W.H.; Yeh, W.T. How to define obesity? Evidence-based multiple action points for public awareness, screening, and treatment: An extension of Asian-Pacific recommendations. *Asia Pac. J. Clin. Nutr.* **2008**, *17*, 370–374. [PubMed]
24. James, P.T.; Leach, R.; Kalamara, E.; Shayeghi, M. The worldwide obesity epidemic. *Obes. Res.* **2001**, *9* (Suppl. 4), 228s–233s. [CrossRef] [PubMed]
25. Nam, G.E.; Park, H.S. Perspective on Diagnostic Criteria for Obesity and Abdominal Obesity in Korean Adults. *J. Obes. Metab. Syndr.* **2018**, *27*, 134–142. [CrossRef]
26. Levey, A.S.; Stevens, L.A.; Schmid, C.H.; Zhang, Y.L.; Castro, A.F., 3rd; Feldman, H.I.; Kusek, J.W.; Eggers, P.; Van Lente, F.; Greene, T.; et al. A new equation to estimate glomerular filtration rate. *Ann. Intern. Med.* **2009**, *150*, 604–612. [CrossRef]
27. Cattran, D.C.; Coppo, R.; Cook, H.T.; Feehally, J.; Roberts, I.S.; Troyanov, S.; Alpers, C.E.; Amore, A.; Barratt, J.; Berthoux, F.; et al. The Oxford classification of IgA nephropathy: Rationale, clinicopathological correlations, and classification. *Kidney Int.* **2009**, *76*, 534–545. [CrossRef]
28. Sinniah, R. IgA mesangial nephropathy: Berger's disease. *Am. J. Nephrol.* **1985**, *5*, 73–83. [CrossRef]
29. Tanaka, M.; Yamada, S.; Iwasaki, Y.; Sugishita, T.; Yonemoto, S.; Tsukamoto, T.; Fukui, S.; Takasu, K.; Muso, E. Impact of obesity on IgA nephropathy: Comparative ultrastructural study between obese and non-obese patients. *Nephron. Clin. Pract.* **2009**, *112*, c71–c78. [CrossRef]
30. Wolf, G.; Hamann, A.; Han, D.C.; Helmchen, U.; Thaiss, F.; Ziyadeh, F.N.; Stahl, R.A. Leptin stimulates proliferation and TGF-beta expression in renal glomerular endothelial cells: Potential role in glomerulosclerosis. *Kidney Int.* **1999**, *56*, 860–872. [CrossRef]
31. D'Agati, V.D.; Chagnac, A.; de Vries, A.P.; Levi, M.; Porrini, E.; Herman-Edelstein, M.; Praga, M. Obesity-related glomerulopathy: Clinical and pathologic characteristics and pathogenesis. *Nat. Rev. Nephrol.* **2016**, *12*, 453–471. [CrossRef] [PubMed]
32. Fogo, A.B. Mesangial matrix modulation and glomerulosclerosis. *Exp. Nephrol.* **1999**, *7*, 147–159. [CrossRef] [PubMed]
33. Serra, A.; Romero, R.; Lopez, D.; Navarro, M.; Esteve, A.; Perez, N.; Alastrue, A.; Ariza, A. Renal injury in the extremely obese patients with normal renal function. *Kidney Int.* **2008**, *73*, 947–955. [CrossRef] [PubMed]

34. Wlazlo, N.; van Greevenbroek, M.M.J.; Ferreira, I.; Jansen, E.J.H.M.; Feskens, E.J.M.; van der Kallen, C.J.H.; Schalkwijk, C.G.; Bravenboer, B.; Stehouwer, C.D.A. Low-grade inflammation and insulin resistance independently explain substantial parts of the association between body fat and serum C3: The CODAM study. *Metabolism* **2012**, *61*, 1787–1796. [CrossRef]
35. Gabrielsson, B.G.; Johansson, J.M.; Lonn, M.; Jernas, M.; Olbers, T.; Peltonen, M.; Larsson, I.; Lonn, L.; Sjostrom, L.; Carlsson, B.; et al. High expression of complement components in omental adipose tissue in obese men. *Obes. Res.* **2003**, *11*, 699–708. [CrossRef]
36. Al Haj Ahmad, R.M.; Al-Domi, H.A. Complement 3 serum levels as a pro-inflammatory biomarker for insulin resistance in obesity. *Diabetes Metab. Syndr.* **2017**, *11* (Suppl. 1), S229–S232. [CrossRef]
37. Karkhaneh, M.; Qorbani, M.; Mohajeri-Tehrani, M.R.; Hoseini, S. Association of serum complement C3 with metabolic syndrome components in normal weight obese women. *J. Diabetes Metab. Disord.* **2017**, *16*, 49. [CrossRef]
38. Ohsawa, I.; Inoshita, H.; Ishii, M.; Kusaba, G.; Sato, N.; Mano, S.; Onda, K.; Gohda, T.; Horikoshi, S.; Ohi, H.; et al. Metabolic impact on serum levels of complement component 3 in Japanese patients. *J. Clin. Lab. Anal.* **2010**, *24*, 113–118. [CrossRef]
39. Engstrom, G.; Hedblad, B.; Janzon, L.; Lindgarde, F. Weight gain in relation to plasma levels of complement factor 3: Results from a population-based cohort study. *Diabetologia* **2005**, *48*, 2525–2531. [CrossRef]
40. Zhu, B.; Zhu, C.F.; Lin, Y.; Perkovic, V.; Li, X.F.; Yang, R.; Tang, X.L.; Zhu, X.L.; Cheng, X.X.; Li, Q.; et al. Clinical characteristics of IgA nephropathy associated with low complement 4 levels. *Ren. Fail.* **2015**, *37*, 424–432. [CrossRef]
41. Nakagawa, H.; Suzuki, S.; Haneda, M.; Gejyo, F.; Kikkawa, R. Significance of glomerular deposition of C3c and C3d in IgA nephropathy. *Am. J. Nephrol.* **2000**, *20*, 122–128. [CrossRef] [PubMed]
42. Kim, S.J.; Koo, H.M.; Lim, B.J.; Oh, H.J.; Yoo, D.E.; Shin, D.H.; Lee, M.J.; Doh, F.M.; Park, J.T.; Yoo, T.H.; et al. Decreased circulating C3 levels and mesangial C3 deposition predict renal outcome in patients with IgA nephropathy. *PLoS ONE* **2012**, *7*, e40495. [CrossRef] [PubMed]
43. Park, S.; Kim, H.W.; Park, J.T.; Chang, T.I.; Kang, E.W.; Ryu, D.R.; Yoo, T.H.; Chin, H.J.; Jeong, H.J.; Kang, S.W.; et al. Relationship between complement deposition and the Oxford classification score and their combined effects on renal outcome in immunoglobulin A nephropathy. *Nephrol. Dial. Transplant.* **2019**. [CrossRef] [PubMed]
44. Wang, L.; Zhang, Y.; Chen, S.; Chen, J.; Zhuang, Y.; Chen, J. Association of metabolic syndrome and IgA nephropathy. *J. Clin. Pathol.* **2010**, *63*, 697–701. [CrossRef]
45. Park, S.; Lee, S.; Kim, Y.; Lee, Y.; Kang, M.W.; Han, K.; Lee, H.; Lee, J.P.; Joo, K.W.; Lim, C.S.; et al. Reduced risk for chronic kidney disease after recovery from metabolic syndrome: A nationwide population-based study. *Kidney Res. Clin. Pract.* **2020**, *39*, 180–191. [CrossRef] [PubMed]

© 2020 by the authors. Licensee MDPI, Basel, Switzerland. This article is an open access article distributed under the terms and conditions of the Creative Commons Attribution (CC BY) license (http://creativecommons.org/licenses/by/4.0/).

Review

History of IgA Nephropathy Mouse Models

Batoul Wehbi [1], Virginie Pascal [1], Lina Zawil [1], Michel Cogné [2] and Jean-Claude Aldigier [1,*]

[1] Immunology Department, UMR CNRS 7276 INSERM 1262, Limoges University, 87032 Limoges, France; batoulwehbi@gmail.com (B.W.); virginie.pascal@unilim.fr (V.P.); lina.zawil@unilim.fr (L.Z.)
[2] Immunology Department, EFS Bretagne, INSERM 1236, Rennes 1 University, 35000 Rennes, France; michel.cogne@unilim.fr
* Correspondence: jean-claude.aldigier@unilim.fr

Abstract: IgA nephropathy (IgAN) is the most common primary glomerulonephritis in the world. It was first described in 1968 by Jean Berger and Nicole Hinglais as the presence of intercapillary deposits of IgA. Despite this simple description, patients with IgAN may present very broad clinical features ranging from the isolated presence of IgA in the mesangium without clinical or biological manifestations to rapidly progressive kidney failure. These features are associated with a variety of histological lesions, from the discrete thickening of the mesangial matrix to diffuse cell proliferation. Immunofluorescence on IgAN kidney specimens shows the isolated presence of IgA or its inconsistent association with IgG and complement components. This clinical heterogeneity of IgAN clearly echoes its complex and multifactorial pathophysiology in humans, inviting further analyses of its various aspects through the use of experimental models. Small-animal models of IgAN provide the most pertinent strategies for studying the multifactorial aspects of IgAN pathogenesis and progression. Although only primates have the IgA1 subclass, several murine models have been developed in which various aspects of immune responses are deregulated and which are useful in the understanding of IgAN physiopathology as well as in the assessment of IgAN therapeutic approaches. In this manuscript, we review all murine IgAN models developed since 1968 and discuss their remarkable contribution to understanding the disease.

Keywords: IgA nephropathy; IgA; kidney mesangium; mouse model

1. IgAN Epidemiology

The true prevalence of IgAN cannot be exactly determined. IgA deposits on the kidney are indeed frequent in asymptomatic patients and were reported in 16.1% of a population of kidney donors in Japan [1]. However, the overt disease can evolve to a rapidly progressive glomerulopathy (Figure 1). Since the diagnosis of IgAN requires a kidney biopsy, available data only refer to cases recorded after this procedure. The prevalence of IgAN varies widely across different geographic regions and ethnic groups [2]: IgAN is most prevalent in East Asian people (with more than 40% of biopsy cases in Japan), followed by Caucasians and African individuals (respectively with about 25% and less than 5% of biopsy cases) [3]. This disparity in population distribution can be attributed to the different health screening policies as well as several genetic and environmental factors.

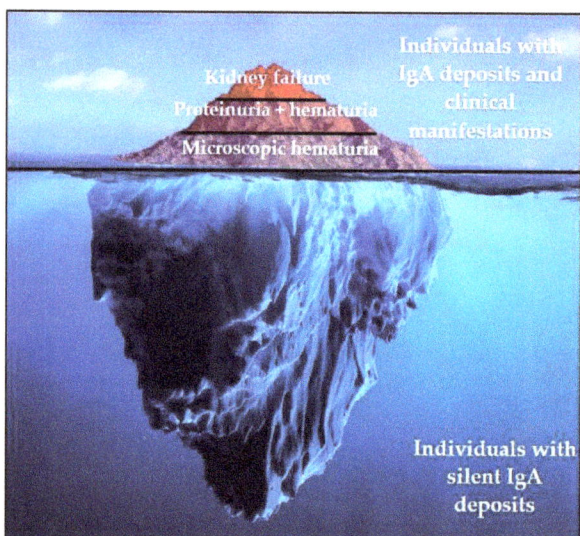

Figure 1. IgAN represent the emergent part of the IgA deposition iceberg with a heterogeneity underscoring the multifactorial pathogenesis of the disease.

2. IgAN: Clinical and Histopathological Presentation

There is significant heterogeneity in the clinical manifestations of IgAN since even healthy subjects with no clinical signs of IgAN may have mesangial deposits. By contrast, for those patients developing glomerulopathy with proteinuria and/or hematuria, one-third of the cases will progress to end stage renal disease (ESRD) [4]. High blood pressure may also be an indicative sign of IgAN; it is always present as soon as kidney failure begins. In patients presenting such features, renal biopsy is the only method to confirm diagnosis. The anatomo-pathological study of renal biopsy specimens reveals mesangial lesions: mesangial matrix expansion and hypercellularity sometimes associated with a mesangial cell proliferation with possible endo- or extra-capillary proliferation or even significant glomerular inflammation and crescent formation. Other lesions can also be identified: segmental sclerosis, tubular atrophy, and interstitial fibrosis [5]. The analysis of these different lesions makes it possible to establish the Oxford predictive score for disease progression [6]. Immunofluorescence on biopsies reveals the presence of more or less diffuse granular or filamentous IgA deposits in the form of "dead trees" or "nail strokes" [5]. The presence of lambda and kappa light chain deposits has been reported [7]. IgA deposits most often co-localize with C3, sometimes with IgG and IgM [3]. Moreover, the presence of deposits at the level of single glomeruli is sufficient to make the diagnosis [5].

3. Enigmatic Functions of IgA

IgA antibodies (Ab) are exceptionally abundant at mucosal surfaces; more than 80% of mammalian Ab secreting plasma cells reside in the gut and secrete IgA. Notably, with the exception of germ-free animals or germ-free mucosal tissues, these antibodies arise prominently during homeostasis in the absence of overt inflammation and immunization. Consistently, the influence of super antigens expressed by bacteria present early in the intestinal flora has recently been demonstrated [8]. Despite its abundance, the in vivo specificity and dual functions of IgA still remain somehow enigmatic, although these antibodies appear as major players in the functional balance opposing tolerance and inflammation in the context of mucosal immunity and as important organizers of the microbiota composition in healthy subjects [9]. At the gut-associated lymphoid tissue (GALT) level, there are two distinct aspects of humoral immunity: first, the mechanisms of humoral homeostasis against commensal bacteria seem to involve the so-called "natural IgA". Their repertoires are almost germline with slightly mature variable regions [10].

These IgA share an interspecies reactivity because they are often polyreactive and partly produced by B-lymphocytes in a T-independent context. Second, during the local immune response induced by pathogens, protective high affinity IgA are produced in the mucosa-associated lymphoid tissue (MALT) germinal centers. This T-dependent response is similar to that of a general response establishing specific immunity as effective as a response generated after a systemic infection. The immune response to the presence of various commensal microorganisms constitute a homeostatic immune repertoire that echoes the variability of the microbiota which evolves according to age, environment, and diet and which is accompanied by an increase in the IgA affinity, whether T-dependent or not. This repertoire is not limited to controlling the commensal microbiota, it is also the source of protective immunity against pathogens [8,10]. Abnormalities in the microbiota following a modification in the environment or an alteration of the immune response and therefore of the repertoire can promote the development of an immunopathological process; IgAN could be such an example.

4. IgAN: A Multifactorial Disease

IgAN is a mysterious disease. The heterogeneity of the clinical features and prognosis variability between patients explain why IgAN pathophysiology remains poorly understood despite the remarkable achieved advances. It is known that IgAN is not a primary (intrinsic) renal defect. The recurrence of IgA deposits on a normal kidney transplanted into a patient with IgAN or, on the contrary, the disappearance of deposits on kidneys from donors with IgA deposits accidentally transplanted into individuals without IgAN are two arguments supporting the extra-renal origin of the disease [11]. Currently, all studies show that IgAN is a multifactorial disease involving the intervention of many actors including genetic factors, aberrant IgA glycosylation, environmental factors, as well as dysregulation of the immune system [11]. The hypothesis of a change in the mucosa-kidney axis during IgAN is also highlighted [12,13]. In this context, a recent study reported the beneficial effect of tonsillectomy in patients with IgAN [14].

5. Genetic Factors

Over time, the idea of a genetic component in IgAN has been raised. This is especially evident with the wide disparity of IgAN incidence by ethnicity and geographic region [2]. Most IgAN cases are sporadic, with familial forms reaching no more than 5% of total cases [3]. About 100 Genome Wide Association Studies (GWAS) have already been conducted in IgAN patients as well as healthy individuals. The results highlight the polymorphism of certain genes involved in the immune response as well as protein glycosylation mechanisms [15–18]. GWAS on the ddY model identified four susceptibility loci linked to the early onset disease phenotype; these loci seem to be located on murine chromosome 10 in a region syntenic to human IGAN1, a candidate gene of familial IgAN [19].

6. Aberrant IgA Glycosylation

IgA glycosylation plays important roles in protein conformation, stability, transport, and clearance from the circulation [20]. The hinge region of IgA1 contains three to five O-linked glycans, however murine IgA has N- but not O-glycans. Under-galactosylated IgA has an increased capacity for self-aggregation and binding to mesangial cells. The nephritogenic potential of hypogalactosylated IgA was first studied in 1990 and it was shown that circulating IgA in IgAN patients is abnormally glycosylated [21]. Subsequent studies detected circulating galactose-deficient IgA1 (Gd-IgA) in IgAN patients [22,23]. In addition, immortalized plasma cells from IgAN patients not only produce polymeric and hypoglycosylated IgA characterized by the exposure of GalNac residues of the hinge region but also induce antiglycan IgG or IgA creating an immune complex disease. Some of these circulating complexes deposit in glomeruli and thereby activating mesangial cells and inducing renal injury through cellular proliferation and overproduction of extracellular matrix components [24]. It is worthy to note, however, that several observations showed that a glycosylation defect of IgA is not the sole cause and is not a prerequisite for IgA deposition. Plasma levels of Gd-IgA varied greatly between IgAN patients with diverse clinical manifestations [25]. High Gd-IgA concentrations were detected in asymptomatic IgAN patients [26] and GalNAc residues linked to serine or threonine (Tn or sialylated Tn antigens) were identified on IgA1 from both IgAN patients and healthy subjects [27]. Furthermore, it has been reported that Gd-IgAs can play a protective role in preventing IgA deposition [28].

7. Environmental Factors

Environmental factors play a potential role in the pathogenesis of IgAN from IgA production to its deposition at the mesangial level. Specific pathogens such as streptococcus or staphylococcus could be implicated in IgAN pathophysiology. Mesangial deposition of IgA binding streptococcal M protein has been detected in patients with IgA nephropathy [29]. Macroscopic hematuria episodes are often concomitant with infectious events of the upper aero-digestive tract in patients with IgAN [4,15]. Moreover, the role of the microbiota has recently been highlighted. Variations in the commensal microbiota composition were also found in IgAN patients and microbiota diversity was reduced in patients with IgAN compared to healthy subjects. The amount of bacteria present in stools such as *Bactéroïdes* and *Escherichia-Shigella* is higher in patients with IgAN compared to healthy subjects unlike other bacteria such as *Bifidobacterium* and *Prevotella* 7 that are present in much lower levels [30].

Experimental studies have confirmed the implication of environmental factors. Notably, in the α1KI mouse model expressing the heavy chain of human IgA1 (hIgA1) instead of the mouse IgM, environmental antigenic challenges accelerated IgA mesangial deposition. Mice transfer from pathogen-free zone to a conventional immune stimulation zone yielded an increase in IgA polymerization levels as well as changes in the IgA glycosylation profile [31,32]. More recently, the crucial role of gut microbiota was supported by the observation that antibiotic treatment targeting the intestinal microbiota in α1KI-CD89 Tg mice decreased IgA production, proteinuria and IgA glomerular deposits [33]. Another study also showed that gluten could aggravate IgAN lesions in α1KI- CD89 Tg mice [34].

8. What Do We Learn from Experimental Models?

8.1. DNP and ddY Models

The first described IgAN experimental model was published in 1979 (Figure 2). Rifai's work showed that DNP-BSA-IgA immune complexes (IC) formed either in vitro or in vivo were able to deposit on the mesangium of injected mice. These IC only formed with polymeric but not monomeric IgA and induced functional abnormalities such as proteinuria, hematuria, and glomerulonephritis in mice [35]. Successively, other mouse models were developed using various antigen-containing IC. These studies showed that the nature of the antigen, exposure time, and quality of the immune response determined the clinical translation of IgA deposits underscoring the role of polymeric IgA [36–40].

A few years later, in 1985, the spontaneous ddY mouse model was described. ddY animals were characterized by glomerulonephritis associated with spontaneous mesangial IgA deposition co-localized with IgM, IgG, and C3 deposits. This model was also characterized by the extreme variability of disease onset and severity. Based on histologic grading in serial biopsies, ddY mice were classified in early onset, late-onset, and quiescent groups [41]. In 1997, a new mouse strain was obtained by interbreeding ddY animals with the highest serum IgA levels to assess a possible correlation between serum IgA levels and IgAN development. Although IgA production was enhanced, HIGA (High IgA ddY) mice revealed that the severity of glomerular injuries was not associated with circulating IgA levels [42]. A model of early onset IgA nephropathy called "Grouped ddY" was recently developed through selective interbreeding of mice with the early onset phenotype for more than 20 generations. Grouped ddY animals developed IgAN within 8 weeks of age with mesangial co-deposition of IgA, IgG, and C3, severe proteinuria, mesangio-proliferation, and expansion of the extracellular matrix [43]. As ddY mice had IgA molecules lacking O-glycosylation, a typical characteristic of human IgA1, aberrant mouse IgA glycosylation due to a deficiency in β1-4 galactosylation of N-glycans could have been involved in IgAN development in these mice [44]. Finally, TLR9 activation in IgAN-prone ddY mice by CpG oligodeoxynucleotides (ODNs) enhanced the overproduction of aberrantly glycosylated IgA and IgG-IgA IC, leading to immune-complex deposition and enhanced kidney injury; hematuria was not reported. This model emphasized the role of APRIL and IL-6 in producing aberrantly glycosylated IgA [45]. In conclusion, this ddY model has shown that genetic factors are predominant, IgA levels are not mandatory, APRIL and IL-6 can be implicated, and an N-glycosylation defect can be involved in the development of immune complexes.

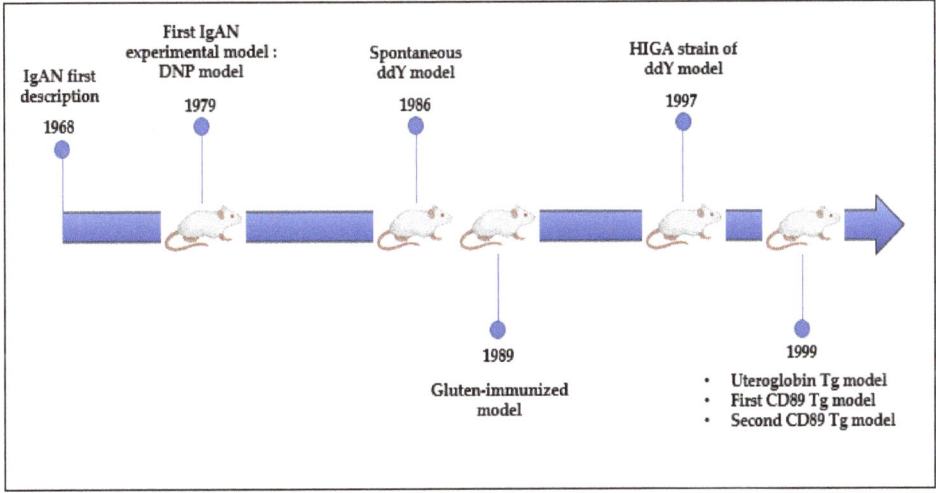

Figure 2. IgA nephropathy murine models developed since IgAN description in 1968 to 1999.

8.2. Uteroglobin Tg Model

The presence of circulating fibronectin-containing IgA complexes and their deposition in the mesangium has been reported in patients with IgAN. In 1999, Zheng et al. developed a uteroglobin-deficient mouse model. Uteroglobin, a protein known for its anti-inflammatory and immunomodulatory properties, has a strong affinity for fibronectin. In wild type mice, uteroglobin normally binds to the fibronectin heterodimer preventing its polymerization and thus the formation of IgA-fibronectin complexes. Uteroglobin-invalidated animals developed a kidney disease with microscopic hematuria associated with IgA and C3 deposits in the mesangium but neither proteinuria nor alteration of kidney function were mentioned. Circulating IgA-fibronectin complexes were also detected in uteroglobin-deficient mice. Interestingly, uteroglobin injection prevented the formation and deposition of these complexes. This study defined an essential role for uteroglobin in preventing mouse IgA nephropathy [46]. This model showed us that IgA can bind to non-antigenic proteins, for reasons possibly inherent to the IgA structure.

8.3. CD89 Tg Models

The presence of circulating soluble Fcα receptor (CD89)-IgA complexes was detected in patients with IgAN. Based on this observation, researchers have focused on the implication of IgA receptors in IgAN development. In 1999, Renato Monteiro's team developed a transgenic mouse model expressing human CD89 (no CD89 homologue exist in rodents) on macrophages and monocytes. CD89 expression was under the control of the CD11b gene promoter. Interestingly, CD89 transgenic mice having circulating CD89-IgA complexes spontaneously developed massive mesangial IgA deposition, mesangial matrix expansion, hematuria, and proteinuria [47]. In 2012, Monteiro's team crossed the α1KI model with mice expressing human CD89 on monocytes and macrophages. This double α1KI-CD89 transgenic model showed functional renal alterations with proteinuria and hematuria [48]. The role of CD89 remained controversial; a second CD89 transgenic model was generated in 2016 by knocking-in the human CD89-encoding gene under the control of the mouse CD14 gene promoter. This transgenic mouse did not show any IgA deposition or glomerular infiltration, nor have any deposits of IgA-CD89 complexes due to increased liver clearance through Kupffer cells [49]. Another mouse model expressing human CD89 under the dependence of its own promoter and regulators was also developed [50]. In our laboratory, we used this CD89 model mimicking the receptor expression seen in humans with CD89 expression restricted to the myeloid lineage. We obtained double-mutant hα1$^{+/+}$CD89$^{+/+}$ mice by breeding this model to hIgA1-producing mice. Mouse follow-up did not show any exacerbation of glomerular lesions despite the presence of circulating IgA-CD89 immune complexes [51]. Marked discrepancies observed between these three CD89 models could be explained by a difference in their genetic constructions, promotor dependence, and expression patterns. In one case, CD89 expression was restricted to monocytes. In the second case, CD89 was expressed under the control of an authentic murine CD14 promotor on blood and tissue monocytes/macrophages, and in the third, it was mainly expressed by neutrophils, which is closer to human physiology. The CD89 role in IgAN is thus still debated.

8.4. Bcl-2 Tg Model

The human Bcl-2 transgenic mouse (NZW x C57BL/6) F1-hbcl-2 model was described in 2004 (Figure 3). Bcl-2 plays an important role in promoting cellular survival and inhibiting the action of pro-apoptotic proteins. Animals overexpressing this oncogene in B cells spontaneously develop a CD4-dependent autoimmune lupus-like syndrome characterized by IgG and IgA hyperglobulinemia in addition to glomerulonephritis that resembles human IgAN. In this model, aberrant glycosylation profiles with reduced levels of IgA galactosylation and sialylation considerably increased IgA glomerular deposition. Surprisingly, few IgG deposits were observed, which suggests that serum IgA exhibits intrinsic abnormalities that facilitated preferential mesangial deposition; IgA were hypogalactosylated and hyposialylated [52].

8.5. LIGHT Tg Model

In parallel, Wang and his collaborators tested the role of T-cell dysregulation in IgAN development by focusing on LIGHT secreted by T cells. LIGHT is the ligand of the lymphotoxin β receptor (LTβR) expressed by stromal cells whose interaction creates a local environment activating IgA-producing B cells in the intestine. LIGHT transgenic mice developed T-cell-mediated intestinal inflammation with dysregulated polymeric IgA production, transportation, and clearance. Mice produced elevated levels of polymeric IgA, anti-DNA IgG and IgA antibodies, in addition to IgA and C3 mesangial deposition accompanied by proteinuria and hematuria. Importantly, this model highlighted a direct contribution of T-cell-mediated mucosal immunity to IgAN pathogenesis [53].

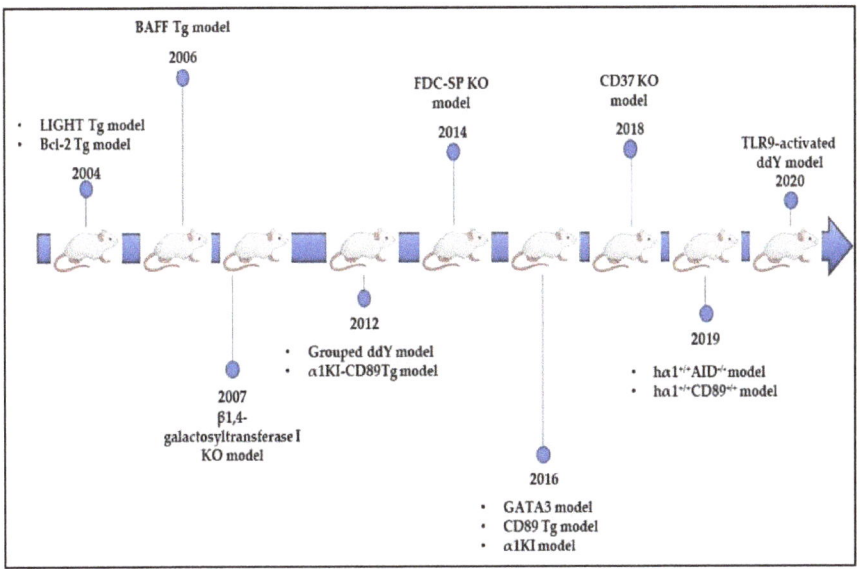

Figure 3. IgAN mouse models developed between 2004 and 2020.

8.6. BAFF and CD37 Tg Models

In 2006, another mouse model overexpressing the B-cell-activating factor (BAFF) was developed. BAFF ensures the survival of B-lymphocytes by promoting their differentiation into mature B cells and Ig class switching. Overexpression of BAFF in mice resulted in increased circulating IgA levels and mesangial deposition with glomerulonephritis. These glomerular lesions might have been most likely due to an autoimmune disorder in these mice [54]. Furthermore, this observation was most probably due to a breakdown in the barrier between mucosal and peripheral compartments [55]. Recently, it has been shown that the expression of CD37, a leukocytespecific tetraspanine, by B-lymphocytes, is significantly decreased in patients with IgAN compared to healthy subjects [56]. Tetraspanine decreases T-cell proliferation and inhibits the IgA response. In parallel, a new mouse model deficient for CD37 expression spontaneously developed IgA mesangial deposition associated with IgG and IgM deposits as well as glomerulonephritis. In contrast, CD37 × IL-6 double knockout mice showed no glomerular IgA deposition nor glomerulonephritis evoking an important role for IL-6 response in IgAN development [57]. IL-6 is not only involved in T-cell differentiation, but also promotes T-cell proliferation and activates the Th2 cytokine production. Moreover, it triggers the differentiation of Th17 cells and dampens the generation of Treg [58]. Finally, IL-6 promotes the activity of T follicular helper cells, which are strong inducers of B-cell activation [59]. Taken together, these models show that IgA deposits can be associated with or can even stand as an autoimmune syndrome.

8.7. β4GalT-I KO Model

As mouse IgA lacks the hinge region, the study of aberrant glycosylation in IgAN development seems to be complicated. In 2007, a mouse model deficient in β-1,4 galactosyltransferase (β4GalT)-I was developed. Knockout of the β4GalT-I coding gene implied the complete absence of galactosylation and sialylation in murine IgA molecules. Circulating IgA levels were significantly increased with the polymeric form predominating and mesangial deposition associated with mesangial matrix expansion [44]. In parallel, studies in our α1KI mouse model showed that IgA deposition is not necessarily associated with glycosylation anomalies [32]. Human mesangial cells express many IgA receptors:

FcαR, ASGPR, transferrin R (CD71), Fcα/μ R. Recent findings showed that tβ-1,4 galactosyltransferase 1 is a novel IgA receptor expressed on human mesangial cells and that its glomerular expression is highly increased in patients with IgA nephropathy. This receptor was shown to have an important role in both mesangial IgA clearance and the initial response to IgA deposits [60]. These studies showed that the receptors cleaning the mesangium can be saturated if the IgA deposition rate is high. This hypothesis has recently been mentioned [61].

8.8. FDC-SP KO Model

Another mouse model developed in 2014 suggested that the dysregulation of IgA production at the germinal center (GC) level led to the formation of IgA molecules prompt to deposition. Animals lacking the follicular dendritic cell secreted protein (FDC-SP) expression, a suppressive protein for IgA production secreted by FDCs, showed an increase in IgA levels in both intestinal wash and serum. This resulted from the accumulation of IgA B cells in the blood, bone marrow, Peyer's patches, and lymph nodes. IgA deposits with proteinuria were identified in 6-month-deficient mice [62]. This study showed that the regulation of IgA synthesis at the GC level could be involved in IgAN onset and progression. Abnormalities in IgA production at this level could increase their glomerular deposition ability.

8.9. $h\alpha1^{+/+}AID^{-/-}$ Model

More recently, the hypothesis of altered affinity maturation on IgA mesangial deposition was raised. The α1KI mouse model expressing the heavy chain of human IgA1 (hIgA1) in an AID-deficient background was set up [51]. In this model, it was shown that polyclonal human IgA1 are spontaneously prone to deposit on the mesangium. IgA deposition rate was affected by environmental conditions and antigen stimulation. Strict germ-free conditions delayed but did not completely prevent deposition; mice housed in these conditions had low serum IgA levels and essentially produced monomeric IgA. By contrast, mice housed in specific pathogen-free conditions had less IgA deposition than the conventional environment. However, their circulating IgA showed more galactosylation and much lower polymerization [31]. This model approached the asymptomatology of IgA deposition in 2–16% of individuals having silent IgA deposits. Using a transgenic human IgA-1 producing model lacking the DNA-editing enzyme activation induced cytidine deaminase (AID), responsible for IgA affinity maturation, we showed that IgA deposition and complement activation significantly increased and led to IgAN pathogenesis, although without significant proteinuria and hematuria. In the absence of normal antigen-driven maturation, low affinity innate-like IgA was more readily involved in IgA glomerular deposition [51]. This model thereby confirmed that IgA deposition neither depends on their polymerization degree nor on their glycosylation profile, but rather on their physical-chemical properties and their variable domain structure.

9. Conclusions

Given the wide heterogeneity of IgAN clinical features added to the multifactorial aspect of the pathology, the development of experimental models constitutes a huge challenge for researchers. Since 1979, several animal models have been developed for a better understanding of IgAN pathogenesis. Although multiple models were able to reproduce some of the IgAN characteristics, they could not cover the full spectrum of pathological manifestations observed in patients. It is evident that animal models can constitute useful tools, taking into consideration marked differences between human and mouse systems especially in IgA biosynthesis, dominant circulating forms, molecules half-life and clearance mechanisms [18]. Most importantly, murine IgA resembles human IgA2 lacking the hinge region and O-glycans which limit the utility of glycosylation aberrancy studies in mouse models. Despite these structural and immunological differences between humans and mice, experimental models developed so far have elucidated some enigmas about IgAN onset and progression.

The heterogeneity of human disease and animal models likely reflects the varying influence of genetic and environmental factors on a multitude of complex pathogenic mechanisms modulating the disease phenotype in different individuals and populations. Another explanation is that IgAN may not be a "single disease" but rather a group of distinct diseases showing a common path of mesangial IgA deposition.

Author Contributions: Conceptualization, B.W. and J.-C.A.; writing—original draft preparation, B.W.; writing—review and editing J.-C.A., M.C., L.Z. and V.P.; supervision and consultation, J.-C.A. and M.C. All authors have read and agreed to the published version of the manuscript.

Funding: This review was funded by grants from Région Nouvelle-Aquitaine (appel d'offre 2017); Chaire d'Immuno-pathologie des Maladies Rénales, Limoges University and Association Limousine pour l'Utilisation du Rein Artificiel à Domicile.

Conflicts of Interest: The authors declare no conflict of interest.

References

1. Suzuki, K.; Honda, K.; Tanabe, K.; Toma, H.; Nihei, H.; Yamagushi, Y. Incidence of Latent Mesangial IgA Deposition in Renal Allograft Donors in Japan. *Kidney Int.* **2003**, *63*, 2286–2294. [CrossRef] [PubMed]
2. Cheung, C.K.; Barratt, J. Is IgA Nephropathy a Single Disease. In *Pathogenesis and Treatment in IgA Nephropathy*; Springer: Tokyo, Japan, 2016; pp. 3–17. ISBN 978-4-431-55587-2.
3. Mestecky, J.; Raska, M.; Julian, B.A.; Gharavi, A.G.; Renfrow, M.B.; Moldoveanu, Z.; Novak, L.; Matousovic, K.; Novak, J. IgA Nephropathy: Molecular Mechanisms of the Disease. *Annu. Rev. Pathol. Mech. Dis.* **2013**, *8*, 217–240. [CrossRef]
4. Wyatt, R.J.; Julian, B.A. IgA Nephropathy. *N. Engl. J. Med.* **2013**, *368*, 2402–2414. [CrossRef]
5. Noel, L.-H. *Atlas de Pathologie Rénale*; FLAMMARION MEDECINE-SCIENCE Edition; LAVOISIER MSP: Paris, France, 2008.
6. Roberts, I.S.; Cook, H.T.; Troyanov, S.; Alpers, C.E.; Amore, A.; Barratt, J.; Berthoux, F.; Bonsib, S.; Bruijn, J.A.; Cattran, D.C. The Oxford Classification of IgA Nephropathy: Pathology Definitions, Correlations, and Reproducibility. *Kidney Int.* **2009**, *76*, 546–556. [CrossRef]
7. Lai, K.-N.; Chui, S.-H.; Lai, F.M.-M.; Lam, C.W. Predominant Synthesis of IgA with Lambda Light Chain in IgA Nephropathy. *Kidney Int.* **1988**, *33*, 584–589. [CrossRef] [PubMed]
8. Bunker, J.J.; Drees, C.; Watson, A.R.; Plunkett, C.H.; Nagler, C.R.; Schneewind, O.; Eren, A.M.; Bendelac, A. B Cell Superantigens in the Human Intestinal Microbiota. *Sci. Transl. Med.* **2019**, *11*, 507. [CrossRef]
9. Pascal, V.; Hiblot, M.; Wehbi, B.; Aldigier, J.-C.; Cogné, M. Homéostasie de la réponse IgA et microbiote. *Med. Sci.* **2021**, *37*, 35–40. [CrossRef]
10. Bunker, J.J.; Bendelac, A. IgA Responses to Microbiota. *Immunity* **2018**, *49*, 211–224. [CrossRef] [PubMed]
11. Knoppova, B.; Reily, C.; Maillard, N.; Rizk, D.V.; Moldoveanu, Z.; Mestecky, J.; Raska, M.; Renfrow, M.B.; Julian, B.A.; Novak, J. The Origin and Activities of IgA1-Containing Immune Complexes in IgA Nephropathy. *Front. Immunol.* **2016**, *7*. [CrossRef]
12. Floege, J.; Feehally, J. The Mucosa–Kidney Axis in IgA Nephropathy. *Nat. Rev. Nephrol.* **2016**, *12*, 147–156. [CrossRef]
13. Zhang, Y.; Zhang, H. Insights into the Role of Mucosal Immunity in IgA Nephropathy. *Clin. J. Am. Soc. Nephrol.* **2018**, CJN.04370418. [CrossRef]
14. Liu, L.; Wang, L.; Jiang, Y.; Yao, L.; Dong, L.; Li, Z.; Li, X. Tonsillectomy for IgA Nephropathy: A Meta-Analysis. *Am. J. Kidney Dis.* **2015**, *65*, 80–87. [CrossRef]
15. Kiryluk, K.; Novak, J.; Gharavi, A.G. The Genetics and Immunobiology of IgA Nephropathy. *J. Clin. Investig.* **2014**, *124*, 2325–2332. [CrossRef]
16. Kiryluk, K.; Novak, J.; Gharavi, A.G. Pathogenesis of Immunoglobulin A Nephropathy: Recent Insight from Genetic Studies. *Annu. Rev. Med.* **2013**, *64*, 339–356. [CrossRef] [PubMed]
17. Li, M.; Wang, L.; Shi, D.-C.; Foo, J.-N.; Zhong, Z.; Khor, C.-C.; Lanzani, C.; Citterio, L.; Salvi, E.; Yin, P.-R.; et al. Genome-Wide Meta-Analysis Identifies Three Novel Susceptibility Loci and Reveals Ethnic Heterogeneity of Genetic Susceptibility for IgA Nephropathy. *J. Am. Soc. Nephrol.* **2020**, *31*, 2949–2963. [CrossRef] [PubMed]
18. Wang, Y.-N.; Zhou, X.-J.; Chen, P.; Yu, G.-Z.; Zhang, X.; Hou, P.; Liu, L.-J.; Shi, S.-F.; Lv, J.-C.; Zhang, H. Interaction between *G ALNT12* and *C1GALT1* Associates with Galactose-Deficient IgA1 and IgA Nephropathy. *J. Am. Soc. Nephrol.* **2021**, *32*, 545–552. [CrossRef]
19. Suzuki, H.; Suzuki, Y.; Yamanaka, T.; Hirose, S.; Nishimura, H.; Toei, J.; Horikoshi, S.; Tomino, Y. Genome-Wide Scan in a Novel IgA Nephropathy Model Identifies a Susceptibility Locus on Murine Chromosome 10, in a Region Syntenic to Human *IGAN1* on Chromosome 6q22–23. *J. Am. Soc. Nephrol.* **2005**, *16*, 1289–1299. [CrossRef]
20. Rifai, A.; Fadden, K.; Morrison, S.L.; Chintalacharuvu, K.R. The N-Glycans Determine the Differential Blood Clearance and Hepatic Uptake of Human Immunoglobulin (Ig)A1 and Iga2 Isotypes. *J. Exp. Med.* **2000**, *191*, 2171–2182. [CrossRef] [PubMed]

21. Andre, P.M.; Le Pogamp, P.; Chevet, D. Impairment of Jacalin Binding to Serum IgA in IgA Nephropathy. *J. Clin. Lab. Anal.* **1990**, *4*, 115–119. [CrossRef]
22. Moldoveanu, Z.; Wyatt, R.J.; Lee, J.Y.; Tomana, M. Patients with IgA Nephropathy Have Increased Serum Galactose-Deficient IgA1 Levels. *Kidney Int.* **2007**, *71*, 1148–1154. [CrossRef]
23. Shimozato, S.; Hiki, Y.; Odani, H.; Takahashi, K.; Yamamoto, K.; Sugiyama, S. Serum Under-Galactosylated IgA1 Is Increased in Japanese Patients with IgA Nephropathy. *Nephrol. Dial. Transplant.* **2008**, *23*, 1931–1939. [CrossRef]
24. Suzuki, H.; Moldoveanu, Z.; Hall, S.; Brown, R.; Vu, H.L.; Novak, L.; Julian, B.A.; Tomana, M.; Wyatt, R.J.; Edberg, J.C.; et al. IgA1-Secreting Cell Lines from Patients with IgA Nephropathy Produce Aberrantly Glycosylated IgA1. *J. Clin. Investig.* **2008**. [CrossRef] [PubMed]
25. Yanagawa, H.; Suzuki, H.; Suzuki, Y.; Kiryluk, K.; Gharavi, A.G.; Matsuoka, K.; Makita, Y.; Julian, B.A.; Novak, J.; Tomino, Y. A Panel of Serum Biomarkers Differentiates IgA Nephropathy from Other Renal Diseases. *PLoS ONE* **2014**, *9*, e98081. [CrossRef]
26. Gharavi, A.G.; Moldoveanu, Z.; Wyatt, R.J.; Barker, C.V.; Woodford, S.Y.; Lifton, R.P.; Mestecky, J.; Novak, J.; Julian, B.A. Aberrant IgA1 Glycosylation Is Inherited in Familial and Sporadic IgA Nephropathy. *J. Am. Soc. Nephrol.* **2008**, *19*, 1008–1014. [CrossRef] [PubMed]
27. Lehoux, S.; Mi, R.; Aryal, R.P.; Wang, Y.; Schjoldager, K.T.-B.G.; Clausen, H.; van Die, I.; Han, Y.; Chapman, A.B.; Cummings, R.D.; et al. Identification of Distinct Glycoforms of IgA1 in Plasma from Patients with Immunoglobulin A (IgA) Nephropathy and Healthy Individuals. *Mol. Cell. Proteom.* **2014**, *13*, 3097–3113. [CrossRef] [PubMed]
28. Hiki, Y.; Takahashi, K.; Shimozato, S.; Odani, H.; Yamamoto, K.; Tomita, M.; Hasegawa, M.; Murakami, K.; Nabeshima, K.; Nakai, S.; et al. Protective Role of Anti-Synthetic Hinge Peptide Antibody for Glomerular Deposition of Hypoglycosylated IgA1. *Clin. Exp. Nephrol.* **2008**, *12*, 20–27. [CrossRef]
29. Schmitt, R.; Carlsson, F.; Mörgelin, M.; Tati, R.; Lindahl, G.; Karpman, D. Tissue Deposits of IgA-Binding Streptococcal M Proteins in IgA Nephropathy and Henoch-Schönlein Purpura. *Am. J. Pathol.* **2010**, *176*, 608–618. [CrossRef]
30. Zhong, Z.; Tan, J.; Tan, L.; Tang, Y.; Qiu, Z.; Pei, G.; Qin, W. Modifications of Gut Microbiota Are Associated with the Severity of IgA Nephropathy in the Chinese Population. *Int. Immunopharmacol.* **2020**, *89*, 107085. [CrossRef]
31. Duchez, S.; Amin, R.; Cogne, N.; Delpy, L.; Sirac, C.; Pascal, V.; Corthesy, B.; Cogne, M. Premature Replacement of with Immunoglobulin Chains Impairs Lymphopoiesis and Mucosal Homing but Promotes Plasma Cell Maturation. *Proc. Natl. Acad. Sci. USA* **2010**, *107*, 3064–3069. [CrossRef]
32. Oruc, Z.; Oblet, C.; Boumediene, A.; Druilhe, A.; Pascal, V.; Le Rumeur, E.; Cuvillier, A.; El Hamel, C.; Lecardeur, S.; Leanderson, T.; et al. IgA Structure Variations Associate with Immune Stimulations and IgA Mesangial Deposition. *J. Am. Soc. Nephrol.* **2016**. [CrossRef]
33. Chemouny, J.M.; Gleeson, P.J.; Abbad, L.; Lauriero, G.; Boedec, E.; Le Roux, K.; Monot, C.; Bredel, M.; Bex-Coudrat, J.; Sannier, A.; et al. Modulation of the Microbiota by Oral Antibiotics Treats Immunoglobulin A Nephropathy in Humanized Mice. *Nephrol. Dial. Transplant.* **2018**. [CrossRef]
34. Papista, C.; Lechner, S.; Mkaddem, S.B. Gluten Exacerbates IgA Nephropathy in Humanizedmice through Gliadin–CD89 Interaction. *Kidney Int.* **2015**, *88*, 276–285. [CrossRef]
35. Rifai, A. Complement Activation in Experimental IgA Nephropathy: An Antigen-Mediated Process. *Kidney Int.* **1987**, *32*, 838–844. [CrossRef]
36. Coppo, R.; Roccatello, D.; Amore, A.; Quattrocchio, G.; Molino, A.; Gianoglio, B.; Amoroso, A.; Bajardi, P.; Piccoli, G. Effects of a Gluten-Free Diet in Primary IgA Nephropathy. *Clin. Nephrol.* **1990**, *33*, 72–86. [PubMed]
37. Yagame, M.; Tomino, Y.; Eguchi, K.; Miura, M. Levels of Circulating IgA Immune Complexes after Gluten-Rich Diet in Patients with IgA Nephropathy. *Nephron* **1988**, *49*, 104–106. [CrossRef] [PubMed]
38. Coppo, R.; Mazzucco, G.; Martina, G.; Roccatello, D. Gluten-Induced Experimental IgA Glomerulopathy. *Lab. Investig.* **1989**, *60*, 499–506.
39. Petska, J.; Moorman, M.; Warner, R. Dysregulation of IgA Production and IgA Nephropathy Induced by the Trichothecene Vomitoxin. *Food Chem. Toxicol.* **1989**, *27*, 361–368.
40. Chintalacharuvu, S.R.; Nagy, N.U.; Sigmund, N.; Nedrud, J.G.; Amm, M.L.; Emancipator, S.N. T Cell Cytokines Determine the Severity of Experimental IgA Nephropathy by Regulating IgA Glycosylation. *Clin. Exp. Immunol.* **2001**, *126*, 326–333. [CrossRef]
41. Imai, H.; Nakamoto, Y.; Asakura, K. Spontaneous Glomerular IgA Deposition in DdY Mice: An Animal Model of IgA Nephritis. *Kidney Int.* **1985**, *27*, 756–761. [CrossRef]
42. Muso, E.; Yoshida, H.; Takeuchi, E.; Yashiro, M.; Matsushima, H.; Oyama, A.; Suyama, K.; Kawamura, T.; Kamata, T.; Miyawaki, S.; et al. Enhanced Production of Glomerular Extracellular Matrix in a New Mouse Strain of High Serum IgA DdY Mice. *Kidney Int.* **1996**, *50*, 1946–1957. [CrossRef]
43. Okazaki, K.; Suzuki, Y.; Otsuji, M.; Suzuki, H.; Kihara, M.; Kajiyama, T.; Hashimoto, A.; Nishimura, H.; Brown, R.; Hall, S.; et al. Development of a Model of Early-Onset IgA Nephropathy. *J. Am. Soc. Nephrol.* **2012**, *23*, 1364–1374. [CrossRef]
44. Nishie, T.; Miyaishi, O.; Azuma, H.; Kameyama, A.; Naruse, C.; Hashimoto, N.; Yokoyama, H.; Narimatsu, H.; Wada, T.; Asano, M. Development of Immunoglobulin A Nephropathy- Like Disease in β-1,4-Galactosyltransferase-I-Deficient Mice. *Am. J. Pathol.* **2007**, *170*, 447–456. [CrossRef] [PubMed]
45. Makita, Y.; Suzuki, H.; Kano, T.; Takahata, A.; Julian, B.A.; Novak, J.; Suzuki, Y. TLR9 Activation Induces Aberrant IgA Glycosylation via APRIL-and IL-6–Mediated Pathways in IgA Nephropathy. *Kidney Int.* **2020**, *97*, 340–349. [CrossRef] [PubMed]

46. Zheng, F.; Kundu, G.C.; Zhang, Z.; Ward, J.; DeMayo, F.; Mukherjee, A.B. Uteroglobin Is Essential in Preventing Immunoglobulin A Nephropathy in Mice. *Nat. Med.* **1999**, *5*, 1018. [CrossRef] [PubMed]
47. Launay, P.; Grossetete, B.; Arcos-Fajardo, M.; Gaudin, E.; Torres, S.P.; Beaudoin, L.; Patey-Mariaud de Serre, N. Fca Receptor (CD89) Mediates the Development of Immunoglobulin A (IgA) Nephropathy (Berger's Disease): Evidence for Pathogenic Soluble Receptor–IgA Complexes in Patients and CD89 Transgenic Mice. *J. Exp. Med.* **2000**, *191*, 1999–2010. [CrossRef]
48. Berthelot, L.; Papista, C.; Maciel, T.T.; Biarnes-Pelicot, M.; Tissandie, E.; Wang, P.H.M.; Tamouza, H.; Jamin, A.; Bex-Coudrat, J.; Gestin, A.; et al. Transglutaminase Is Essential for IgA Nephropathy Development Acting through IgA Receptors. *J. Exp. Med.* **2012**, *209*, 793–806. [CrossRef]
49. Xu, L.; Li, B.; Huang, M.; Xie, K.; Li, D.; Li, Y.; Gu, H.; Fang, J. Critical Role of Kupffer Cell CD89 Expression in Experimental IgA Nephropathy. *PLoS ONE* **2016**, *11*, e0159426. [CrossRef]
50. Van Egmond, M.; van Vuuren, A.H.; Morton, H.C.; van Spriel, A.B.; Shen, L.; Hofhuis, F.M.A.; Saito, T.; Mayadas, T.N.; Verbeek, J.S.; van de Winkel, J.G. Human Immunoglobulin A Receptor (FcaRI, CD89) Function in Transgenic Mice Requires Both FcR g Chain and CR3 (CD11b/CD18). *Blood* **1999**, *93*, 4387–4394. [CrossRef]
51. Wehbi, B.; Oblet, C.; Boyer, F.; Huard, A.; Druilhe, A.; Paraf, F.; Cogné, E.; Moreau, J.; El Makhour, Y.; Badran, B.; et al. Mesangial Deposition Can Strongly Involve Innate-Like IgA Molecules Lacking Affinity Maturation. *J. Am. Soc. Nephrol.* **2019**, *30*, 1238–1249. [CrossRef]
52. Marquina, R.; Díez, M.A.; López-Hoyos, M.; Buelta, L.; Kuroki, A.; Kikuchi, S.; Villegas, J.; Pihlgren, M.; Siegrist, C.-A.; Arias, M.; et al. Inhibition of B Cell Death Causes the Development of an IgA Nephropathy in (New Zealand White × C57BL/6)F $_1$-Bcl-2 Transgenic Mice. *J. Immunol.* **2004**, *172*, 7177–7185. [CrossRef]
53. Wang, J.; Anders, R.A.; Wu, Q.; Peng, D.; Cho, J.H.; Sun, Y.; Karaliukas, R.; Kang, H.-S.; Turner, J.R.; Fu, Y.-X. Dysregulated LIGHT Expression on T Cells Mediates Intestinal Inflammation and Contributes to IgA Nephropathy. *J. Clin. Investig.* **2004**, *113*, 826–835. [CrossRef]
54. McCarthy, D.D.; Chiu, S.; Gao, Y.; Summers-deLuca, L.E.; Gommerman, J.L. BAFF Induces a Hyper-IgA Syndrome in the Intestinal Lamina Propria Concomitant with IgA Deposition in the Kidney Independent of LIGHT. *Cell. Immunol.* **2006**, *241*, 85–94. [CrossRef]
55. McCarthy, D.D.; Kujawa, J.; Wilson, C.; Papandile, A.; Poreci, U.; Porfilio, E.A.; Ward, L.; Lawson, M.A.E.; Macpherson, A.J.; McCoy, K.D.; et al. Mice Overexpressing BAFF Develop a Commensal Flora–Dependent, IgA-Associated Nephropathy. *J. Clin. Investig.* **2011**, *121*, 3991–4002. [CrossRef] [PubMed]
56. Rops, A.L.; Figdor, C.G.; van der Schaaf, A.; Tamboer, W.P.; Bakker, M.A.; Berden, J.H.; Dijkman, H.B.P.M.; Steenbergen, E.J.; van der Vlag, J.; van Spriel, A.B. The Tetraspanin CD37 Protects Against Glomerular IgA Deposition and Renal Pathology. *Am. J. Pathol.* **2010**, *176*, 2188–2197. [CrossRef] [PubMed]
57. Rops, A.L.; Jansen, E.; van der Schaaf, A.; Pieterse, E.; Rother, N.; Hofstra, J.; Dijkman, H.B.; van de Logt, A.-E.; Wetzels, J.; van der Vlag, J. Interleukin-6 Is Essential for Glomerular Immunoglobulin A Deposition and the Development of Renal Pathology in Cd37-Deficient Mice. *Kidney Int.* **2018**, *93*, 1356–1366. [CrossRef]
58. Bettelli, E.; Carrier, Y.; Gao, W.; Korn, T.; Strom, T.B.; Oukka, M.; Weiner, H.L.; Kuchroo, V.K. Reciprocal Developmental Pathways for the Generation of Pathogenic Effector TH17 and Regulatory T Cells. *Nature* **2006**, *441*, 235–238. [CrossRef]
59. Linterman, M.A.; Vinuesa, C.G. Signals That Influence T Follicular Helper Cell Differentiation and Function. *Semin. Immunopathol.* **2010**, *32*, 183–196. [CrossRef] [PubMed]
60. Molyneux, K.; Wimbury, D.; Pawluczyk, I.; Muto, M.; Bhachu, J.; Mertens, P.R.; Feehally, J.; Barratt, J. B1,4-Galactosyltransferase 1 Is a Novel Receptor for IgA in Human Mesangial Cells. *Kidney Int.* **2017**, *92*, 1458–1468. [CrossRef]
61. Xie, X.; Liu, P.; Gao, L.; Zhang, X.; Lan, P.; Bijol, V.; Lv, J.; Zhang, H.; Jin, J. Renal Deposition and Clearance of Recombinant Poly-IGA Complexes in a Model of IGA Nephropathy. *J. Pathol.* **2021**. [CrossRef]
62. Hou, S.; Landego, I.; Jayachandran, N.; Miller, A.; Gibson, I.W.; Ambrose, C.; Marshall, A.J. Follicular Dendritic Cell Secreted Protein FDC-SP Controls IgA Production. *Mucosal Immunol.* **2014**, *7*, 948–957. [CrossRef]

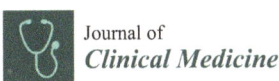

Review

New Treatment Strategies for IgA Nephropathy: Targeting Plasma Cells as the Main Source of Pathogenic Antibodies

Dita Maixnerova [1,*], Delphine El Mehdi [2], Dana V. Rizk [3], Hong Zhang [4] and Vladimir Tesar [1]

1. Department of Nephrology, First Faculty of Medicine, General University Hospital, Charles University, 128 08 Prague, Czech Republic; vladimir.tesar@lf1.cuni.cz
2. MorphoSys, MorphoSys US Inc., Boston, MA 02210, USA; delphine.elmehdi@morphosys.com
3. Division of Nephrology, University of Alabama at Birmingham, Birmingham, AL 35294, USA; drizk@uabmc.edu
4. Renal Division, Peking University First Hospital, Peking University Institute of Nephrology, Beijing 100034, China; hongzh@bjmu.edu.cn
* Correspondence: dita.dmaixnerova@vfn.cz

Abstract: Immunoglobulin A nephropathy (IgAN) is a rare autoimmune disorder and the leading cause of biopsy-reported glomerulonephritis (GN) worldwide. Disease progression is driven by the formation and deposition of immune complexes composed of galactose-deficient IgA1 (Gd-IgA1) and Gd-IgA1 autoantibodies (anti-Gd-IgA1 antibodies) in the glomeruli, where they trigger complement-mediated inflammation that can result in loss of kidney function and end-stage kidney disease (ESKD). With the risk of progression and limited treatment options, there is an unmet need for therapies that address the formation of pathogenic Gd-IgA1 antibody and anti-Gd-IgA1 antibody-containing immune complexes. New therapeutic approaches target immunological aspects of IgAN, including complement-mediated inflammation and pathogenic antibody production by inhibiting activation or promoting depletion of B cells and CD38-positive plasma cells. This article will review therapies, both approved and in development, that support the depletion of Gd-IgA1-producing cells in IgAN and have the potential to modify the course of this disease. Ultimately, we propose here a novel therapeutic approach by depleting CD38-positive plasma cells, as the source of the autoimmunity, to treat patients with IgAN.

Keywords: IgA nephropathy; galactose-deficient IgA1; plasma cells; CD38; renal pathology

1. Introduction

Immunoglobulin A nephropathy (IgAN), a rare autoimmune disorder, is the leading cause of biopsy-reported glomerulonephritis (GN) worldwide [1,2]. The global incidence of IgAN is 2.5 per 100,000, and approximately 40% of patients progress to end-stage kidney disease (ESKD) within 20 years of diagnosis [3,4]. Upon the onset of ESKD, lifelong dialysis or kidney transplantation is required and substantially increases disease burden [2]. Dialysis can decrease both physical and mental quality of life due to fatigue and decreased ability to work, which correspond with expected social consequences and increased economic burden [5–7]. Survival rates after starting dialysis for IgAN patients are favorable (93% and 65% at 10 and 20 years, respectively) compared with those with other glomerulonephritis (64% and 32% at 10 and 20 years, respectively). This survival advantage is mostly related to the younger age of IgAN patients on dialysis; however, dialysis can increase the risk of infection and cardiovascular complications [2,8,9]. Progression to ESKD also increases mortality risk and can result in a six-year reduction in median life expectancy [10]. Transplantation occurs more frequently in people with IgAN compared with other ESKDs as patients are typically younger and have fewer comorbidities [11]. Transplantation can decrease mortality and improve quality of life, but is also associated with iatrogenic infection, disease recurrence, and risk of transplant failure [2,12,13].

Data suggest that genetic and environmental factors play a role in the pathogenesis of IgAN by triggering production of galactose-deficient IgA1 (Gd-IgA1) and, subsequently, Gd-IgA1 autoantibodies (anti-Gd-IgA1 antibodies) [1,14]. Both Gd-IgA1 and anti-Gd-IgA1 antibody production are believed to be driven by CD38$^+$ plasma cells, a cell type that contributes to autoimmune disorders by producing high quantities of autoantibodies [15–17]. Together, Gd-IgA1 and anti-Gd-IgA1 antibodies form immune complexes that accumulate in the glomerular mesangium and induce activation of the complement system leading to chronic inflammation, mesangial proliferation, glomerulosclerosis, and loss of renal function (Figure 1) [1,18–20]. Levels of Gd-IgA1, anti-Gd-IgA1 antibodies, and the resulting immune complexes are biomarkers for disease severity and progression in patients with IgAN. Estimated glomerular filtration rate (eGFR) decline and poor renal survival are associated with higher Gd-IgA1 and anti-GdIgA1 antibody levels [17,21].

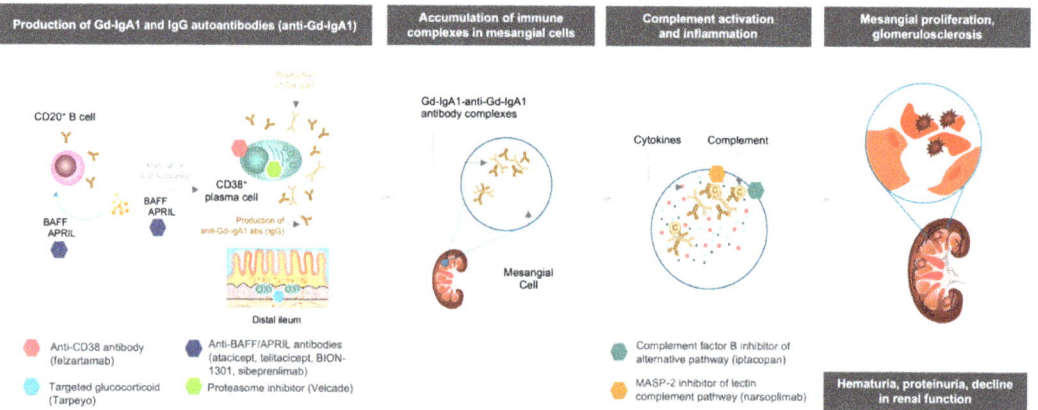

Figure 1. Immunopathogenesis of IgAN and potential therapeutic targets. Early CD20$^+$ B cells produce small amounts of antibodies (Gd-IgA1), whereas CD38$^+$ plasma cells can produce both these antibodies and high quantities of autoantibodies (anti-Gd-IgA1). The antibodies and autoantibodies form Gd-IgA1 and anti-Gd-IgA1 antibody immune complexes that can deposit and accumulate in mesangial cells. The deposition of immune complexes activates the alternative and lectin pathways of the complement system leading to chronic inflammation, which contributes to podocyte damage and, ultimately, loss of renal function that manifests in patients as hypertension, hematuria, proteinuria and reduction in glomerular filtration rate. The targets of novel therapies aim to inhibit pathogenesis by affecting the immune system at various stages of pathogenesis. Atacicept and telitacicept are recombinant fusion proteins able to bind cytokines BAFF and APRIL and interfere with B cell and plasma cell survival. BION-1301 and sibeprenlimab are monoclonal antibodies targeting the cytokine APRIL, which may reduce levels of Gd-IgA1 and IgG autoantibodies. Velcade® is a proteasome inhibitor that targets and depletes plasma cells. Felzartamab, an anti-CD38 antibody, is designed to target the highly expressed CD38 cell surface antigen on plasma cells. Tarpeyo™, a targeted-release glucocorticoid that aims at the highest concentration of Peyer's patches in the distal ileum to reduce production of Gd-IgA1. Iptacopan, a small molecule factor B inhibitor of the alternative complement pathway, acts to reduce damage caused by accumulation of immune complexes in the mesangial cells. Narsoplimab, a MASP-2 monoclonal antibody, acts as an inhibitor of the lectin complement pathway. Abs, antibodies; APRIL, a proliferation inducing ligand; BAFF, B cell activating factor; CD, cluster of differentiation; GD-IgA1, galactose-deficient immunoglobulin A1; GFR, glomerular filtration rate; MASP, mannan-binding lectin serine protease.

A differential diagnosis for IgAN is important as other conditions can present similarly but pathological mechanisms of disease and care management differ. IgA-dominant infection-associated glomerulonephritis can be challenging to distinguish from primary IgAN but imperative as immunosuppressive therapy; a standard for the latter would be contraindicated for the former. In addition, IgA vasculitis with nephritis (IgAV), previously called Henoch-Schönlein Purpura, has historically been thought of as a systemic disease on the same spectrum as IgAN. Although the two entities share some mutual steps in the pathogenesis, the signature presence of skin rash, extra-renal symptoms, and earlier age at onset indicate IgAV may require different treatment approaches and hence has been excluded from all ongoing clinical trials.

Historically, treatment of IgAN has been focused on supportive treatments that correct hypertension and proteinuria and may slow down the loss of eGFR in some patients, but most patients presenting with higher residual proteinuria still progress to ESKD. Selecting supportive care is often contingent upon balancing risks and benefits for each patient with the goal of preventing ESKD [22–24]. Renin-angiotensin system (RAS) inhibitors are often utilized to manage hypertension and slow down decreases in eGFR. There are limited risks with use of RAS inhibitors but their efficacy to prevent ESKD in high-risk patient is also limited [24,25]. An investigational dual inhibitor of the angiotensin II type 1 (AT1) and endothelin type A (ET-A) receptors, sparsentan (Travere Therapeutics, San Diego, CA, USA), may provide improved protection and reduce proteinuria levels to a greater extent than current supportive care regimens [24,26,27]. Sodium-glucose cotransporter-2 (SGLT2) inhibitor, dapagliflozin (Farxiga, AstraZeneca, Cambridge, UK) has also shown promise as a supportive treatment to decrease proteinuria and ameliorate the progression of chronic kidney disease [28,29]. Systemic corticosteroids are used to treat intermediate and high-risk patients with IgAN; however, some studies showed their limited efficacy and potentially severe toxicity [30,31].

With the risk of progression and limited treatment options, there is an unmet need for therapies that address the key mechanism of disease, which is the formation of pathogenic Gd-IgA1 containing immune complexes. In 2020, a comprehensive review was published that described therapeutic candidates that target immune components thought to contribute to disease progression [24]. Since that time, the U.S. Food and Drug Administration (FDA) granted accelerated approval for TARPEYO™ (targeted-release budesonide formulation, Calliditas Therapeutics, Stockholm, Sweden), as the first disease-specific treatment for IgAN and strengthened an ongoing discussion around targeting the primary cause of the disease, Gd-IgA1-producing cells, which are upstream of immune complex formation [32,33].

This article will review therapies, both approved and in development, that support the depletion of Gd-IgA1 and anti-Gd-IgA1 antibody-producing cells in IgAN and have the potential to modify the course of this disease (Table 1).

Table 1. Therapies in Clinical Development for Treatment of IgAN.

Agent	Target	Modality	Mechanism of Action
Atacicept	BAFF and APRIL	Fusion protein/antibody	Inhibits maturation and activation of B cells
BION-1301	APRIL	Monoclonal antibody	Inhibits maturation and activation of B cells
Felzartamab (MOR202/TJ202)	CD38	Monoclonal antibody	Depletes CD38$^+$ plasma cells
Iptacopan	Factor B	small molecule	Inhibits complement alternative pathway activation
Narsoplimab	MASP-2	Monoclonal antibody	Inhibits complement lectin pathway activation
Sibeprenlimab	APRIL	Monoclonal antibody	Inhibits maturation and activation of B cells
Tarpeyo (targeted-release budesonide)	Glucocorticoid receptors	Corticosteroid	Depletes B cells and plasma cells in the small intestine
Telitacicept	BAFF and APRIL	Fusion protein/antibody	Inhibits maturation and activation of B cells
Velcade (bortezomib)	Proteasome	Peptide	Inhibits proteasome activity in plasma cells

B cells and plasma cells both play a role in immunologic memory and play a role in autoimmune disease but regulation, location, and cell surface expression differs between these two cell types [34,35]. Plasma cells, in particular long-lived plasma cells, are capable of secreting antibodies for several years or even a lifetime. Due to their longevity, long-lived plasma cells play a crucial role in protective immunity and autoimmunity [16,34]. Plasma cells are known to be major producers of antibodies due to their expanded endoplasmic reticulum, and may represent a primary source of Gd-IgA1 and anti-Gd-IgA1 antibodies, which underlie initiation and progression of IgAN [1,16]. An increasing number of studies have revealed that Gd-IgA1 could be derived from primed plasma cells in the mucosa [36–39]. The role of plasma cells in IgAN is supported by data that show patients have significantly higher percentages of $CD38^+$ cells than healthy controls [40]. Upregulation of Toll-like receptor 9 (TLR9), higher serum levels of B cell activating factor (BAFF) and increased expression of a proliferation-inducing ligand (APRIL) have been linked to proliferation, activation, and long-term maintenance of antibody and autoantibody producing plasma cells in IgAN [41,42]. Unlike B cells, plasma cells are characterized by a high cell surface expression of CD38 and a loss of CD20 [16,34]. This is likely why anti-CD20 antibody therapeutics, such as rituximab, are able to deplete B cells but fail to eliminate plasma cells or reduce serum levels of Gd-IgA1 or anti-Gd-IgA1 antibodies [24,34,35,43,44]. A randomized controlled trial evaluating rituximab in IgAN showed no clinical benefit compared with standard therapy [44].

We propose here to explore data from approved therapies and compounds in development, as well as preliminary data on anti-CD38 antibody therapy, felzartamab, that support specific targeting of plasma cells.

2. New Strategies for the Management of IgAN

The immune system plays a multifaceted role in initiating and promoting the loss of kidney function seen in patients with IgAN [1,16,17,20]. Growing clinical data support approaches that deplete Gd-IgA1-producing cells or reduce immune complex-mediated inflammation, which hold greater promise than broad-acting immunosuppressive treatments (ISTs) that have historically demonstrated a lack of efficacy or were associated with significant toxicity.

3. Inhibition of Immune Complex-Activated Complement Activity

There is pathologic biochemical and genetic data supporting the pivotal role of the complement system in the pathogenesis and progression of IgAN that is now well established [20]. Accumulating evidence suggests that activation of both the alternative and lectin pathways, leads to glomerular inflammation and injury in IgAN [20,43,45–47]. Here, we review several complement inhibitors that are in advanced stages of clinical development.

Iptacopan (LNP023, Novartis, Basel, Switzerland) is an investigational, oral small molecule complement factor B inhibitor of the alternative pathway that is being evaluated in adults with IgAN [48,49]. Results from a Phase 2 clinical trial (NCT03373461) demonstrated a potential for effective and clinically meaningful reduction in proteinuria. The trial randomized 112 patients with IgAN into three dosing arms of iptacopan and a placebo arm. Results showed the highest dose of iptacopan (200 mg, twice daily) can reduce urine protein: creatinine ratio (UPCR) by 40% from baseline to 6 months, compared with placebo. Based on these encouraging data, the Phase 3 APPLAUSE-IgAN trial has been launched and is currently ongoing (NCT04578834) [48,50].

Similarly, narsoplimab (OMS721, Omeros, Seattle, WA, USA), an investigational humanized monoclonal antibody selectively targeting mannan-binding lectin-associated serine protease-2 (MASP-2), is a novel pro-inflammatory protein target and the effector enzyme of the lectin pathway that is being evaluated in patients with IgAN [20,51,52]. Three-year follow-up data from a Phase 2 clinical trial (NCT02682407) in 12 high-risk patients with advanced IgA nephropathy showed a median reduction in proteinuria of

64.4% and long-term improvement or sustained stabilization in eGFR when treated with narsoplimab [51,53]. A Phase 3 trial is currently ongoing (NCT03608033) [20].

Iptacopan and narsoplimab target the alternative and lectin pathways, respectively, leaving the classical complement pathway intact and able to respond to pathogens [54,55].

While complement inhibition has the potential to reduce proteinuria and slowing down eGFR loss, continued production and deposition of immune complexes in the glomeruli may require long-term treatment with complement inhibitors to prevent the progression of kidney disease.

4. Depletion of Gd-IgA1-Producing Immune Cells

New treatment strategies aim to reduce immune complex formation and subsequent inflammation by targeting sources of Gd-IgA1 and its anti-Gd-IgA1 antibody production.

4.1. Targeting Cytokines Responsible for B Cell and Plasma Cell Activation and Survival

Under normal conditions, B cells and plasma cells play an important role in producing antibodies that help defend against a multitude of infections. In autoimmune disorders, these same cells can exacerbate or contribute to the disease by producing autoantibodies [15,56]. BAFF and APRIL, cytokines from the tumor necrosis factor family, are known to mediate B cell and plasma cell function and survival [57]. BAFF and APRIL can activate the NF-kB pathway by binding to several cell surface receptors, including transmembrane activator and calcium-modulator and cyclophilin ligand interactor (TACI), which promotes plasma cell survival and can stimulate IgG antibody production [57,58]. Belimumab (Benlysta, GSK, Brentford, UK), a monoclonal antibody targeting soluble BAFF, is designed to inhibit activation of B cells and plasma cells thought to drive production of pathogenic antibodies in several autoimmune disorders [59]. Belimumab has been approved for systemic lupus erythematosus (SLE) and/or lupus nephritis, and is currently being investigated in addition to rituximab in a Phase 2 trial (NCT03949855) for primary membranous nephropathy (MN), an autoimmune kidney disease with up to 20% chance of progression to ESKD [60,61].

Increased APRIL expression has been observed in patients with IgAN and is correlated with increased expression of Gd-IgA1 antibodies [58]. Targeting APRIL has the potential to limit antibody production in autoimmune-associated plasma cells. This concept is supported by results from the first cohort of a Phase 1/2 study (NCT03945318) evaluating BION-1301 (Chinook Therapeutics, Seattle, WA, USA), an anti-APRIL monoclonal antibody, in up to 40 patients with IgAN showing sustained reduction in levels of Gd-IgA1 antibodies and proteinuria [62]. Similarly, dual targeting of both BAFF and APRIL with atacicept (Vera Therapeutics, Brisbane, CA, USA), a soluble TACI-Ig fusion protein, showed reduction in Gd-IgA1 antibody levels and proteinuria when evaluated in a Phase 2 study (NCT02808429) in 16 patients with IgAN [63]. Atacicept is being evaluated for IgAN in a Phase 2b trial (ORIGIN; NCT04716231) [64]. In addition, a Phase 2 trial with telitacicept (RemeGen, Yantai, China), a soluble TACI-Ig fusion protein, in 44 patients with IgAN also showed the proteinuria reduction (NCT04905212) [65,66]. Anti-APRIL antibody, sibeprenlimab (VIS649, Visterra/Otsuka, Cambridge, MA, USA/Tokyo, Japan), is being studied for safety and efficacy in a Phase 2 clinical trial (NCT04287985) [67,68].

These data support BAFF and APRIL inhibition as a potential treatment for IgAN; however, further studies are required to understand the broader impacts on immunogenicity when altering function of both B cells and plasma cells.

4.2. Tarpeyo, a Targeted Approach for Immune Cell Depletion in the Small Intestine

Gut-associated lymphoid tissue (GALT), including Peyer's Patches, which are thought to contain a high concentration of conventional surface IgA1-expressing primed mucosal B cells and plasma cells, may be responsible for the production of Gd-IgA1 in IgAN [69,70]. Although other studies suggest the nasopharynx-associated lymphoid tissue (NALT) or palatine tonsils may also play an important role in Gd-IgA1 production in patients with

IgAN [71,72]. Undoubtedly, reducing Gd-IgA1 levels is a promising approach for disease modification [36]. Targeted corticosteroids, such as targeted-release budesonide (Tarpeyo), have been shown to provide effective modulation and reduction in the immune cells within the gut, including long-lived plasma cells and memory B cells [32,69,73]. Tarpeyo is designed to deliver a delayed release formulation of budesonide to the distal ileum, where it locally suppresses immune cell activity, including Gd-IgA1-producing cells and reduce circulating immune complexes that cause downstream inflammation and kidney impairment [69,74,75].

In a Phase 2b study including 150 patients with IgAN and persistent proteinuria despite optimized RAS blockade (NEFIGAN; NCT01738035), Tarpeyo significantly reduced proteinuria levels and stabilized kidney function [76]. Subsequent results from the treatment period of a Phase 3 study (NefIgArd; NCT03643965) evaluating Tarpeyo in 360 patients with IgAN and persistent proteinuria despite optimized RAS blockade showed treatment with Tarpeyo reduced proteinuria by 27% and stabilized eGFR at 9 months compared with placebo, which led to its conditional accelerated approval by the FDA [77,78].

These data suggest that reducing activity of Gd-IgA1-producing immune cells, which would also reduce levels of anti-Gd-IgA1 antibodies and subsequent immune complex formation and deposition, could improve patient outcomes. However, further evidence is needed to confirm that Tarpeyo reduces Gd-IgA1-producing immune cells in Peyer's Patches.

4.3. Velcade, Plasma Cell Depletion via Proteasome Inhibition

Additional support for depletion of plasma cells has been observed with VELCADE® (bortezomib, Millennium/Takeda, Cambridge, MA, USA), a proteasome inhibitor that depletes plasma cells and is approved for treatment of MM, has also shown promise in an open-label pilot trial (NCT01103778) which enrolled 8 people with IgAN. Results showed three participants achieved complete remission (proteinuria of <300 mg/day) after treatment for 1 year, suggesting targeting plasma cells through proteasome inhibition could reduce proteinuria in patients with IgAN [79]. However, larger trials are needed to better assess safety and efficacy in patients with IgAN.

4.4. Felzartamab, Targeted CD38+ Plasma Cell Depletion

The clinical data supporting targeting of Gd-IgA1-producing immune cells in the gut showed improved outcomes for patients but not complete resolution of the disease [77]. Targeting multiple locations and types of autoantibody-producing plasma cells and thereby potentially reducing Gd-IgA1 as well as anti-Gd-IgA1 antibody levels at the same time may contribute to a more robust improvement in patient outcomes.

Felzartamab (MOR202/TJ202, MorphoSys, Planegg, Germany), a fully human immunoglobulin G1 (IgG1) monoclonal antibody designed to target the highly expressed CD38 cell surface antigen on plasma cells, is being evaluated as a potential first-in-class immunotherapy in a Phase 2a clinical trial for patients with IgAN (IGNAZ; NCT05065970) [80]. Binding of felzartamab to $CD38^+/CD20^-$ plasma cells is thought to induce cell killing through two complementary mechanisms of action (MoA) including antibody-dependent cell-mediated cytotoxicity (ADCC) via natural killer cells and antibody-dependent cell-mediated phagocytosis (ADCP) via macrophages (Figure 2) [16,81–83]. Complement-dependent cytotoxicity (CDC) is described to play a role in infusion-related reactions (IRRs), but based on in vitro testing, felzartamab does not trigger CDC or anti-drug antibodies [82,84].

Preliminary results from a Phase 1b/2a, proof-of-concept trial (M-PLACE, NCT04145440) of felzartamab in 31 patients with anti-phospholipase A2 receptor (PLA2R) antibody-positive MN showed a 46.1% reduction in pathogenic anti-PLA2R autoantibody levels after 1 week in 89% (24/27) of patients with evaluable results. The reduction was sustained, and most patients showed a further increase in reduction over time (12-week treatment). These results support successful and sustained depletion of $CD38^+$ plasma cells with felzartamab [85]. Although further trials are required to collect safety data and address any concerns about therapies that modulate the immune system, the safety profile of felzartamab in the M-PLACE trial was found to be consistent with the proposed MoA, and treatment-emergent adverse events were manageable in patients with MN [85]. Treatment-emergent adverse events (TEAEs) occurred in 26/31 patients and were mostly mild or moderate in severity and the majority resolved. A total of 5 patients experienced treatment-emergent serious adverse events, 2 of which were related to felzartamab (type-I hypersensitivity and grade 3 IRR), and no events resulted in death [86].

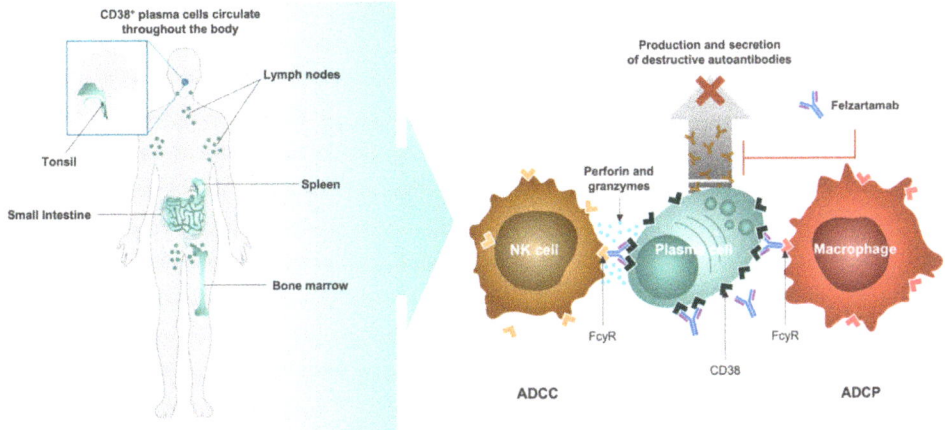

Figure 2. Proposed mechanism of action of felzartamab (MOR202/TJ202) for depleting antibody and auto-antibody-producing CD38$^+$ plasma cells. ADCC, antibody-dependent cell-mediated cytotoxicity; ADCP, antibody-dependent cell mediated phagocytosis; CD, cluster of differentiation; FcγR, Fc-gamma receptor; NK, natural killer.

Anti-CD38 activity has also been established for felzartamab in multiple myeloma (MM) clinical trials. In a Phase 1/2a clinical trial (NCT01421186) evaluating felzartamab in 91 adults with relapsed/refractory (r/r) MM, felzartamab reduced M-protein levels, supporting systemic depletion of CD38$^+$ plasma cells [82,87]. Limited downregulation of CD38 on MM cells was also observed in patients treated with felzartamab, indicating potential for sustained efficacy [88].

Taken together, the preliminary efficacy and safety data on felzartamab in MN and the proof-of-concept results in r/r MM provide further support for clinical development of anti-CD38 antibody therapies in IgAN and highlight their potential application in other plasma cell-driven autoimmune diseases.

As with any immunomodulatory therapies, there is an increased risk of infection due to downregulation of the natural immune defenses. With therapeutics such as complement inhibitors, there is a potential for disrupting the innate immune system, which is one of the first immunologic responses to pathogenic bacteria [89]. The complement pathway, however, does have redundancies within the three main pathways—classical, lectin and alternative—that allow for therapeutic targeting of this pathway while mitigating risk of infection [54,55]. When depleting B cells with general immunosuppression therapies, such as systemic glucocorticoids, there is potential to disrupt the adaptive immune system, which is responsible for clearing bacteria, viruses, fungi, and parasites [90]. Taking a more targeted approach, as is the case with several of the therapies in development, could reduce the risk of infection and potentially improve the risk/benefit profile in patients treated for IgAN.

5. Conclusions

IgAN is an autoimmune disease with a disease burden that greatly disrupts patients' lives and increases their risk for chronic kidney disease and, ultimately, ESKD. Safe and effective disease-modifying agents that target the source of the disease are greatly needed for this patient population. As the scientific community has learned more about the immunopathology of this disease, new approaches are being investigated that may slow or stop disease progression by targeting the underlying disease triggers.

Preliminary data evaluating complement inhibitors in IgAN, which act downstream of plasma cells and immune complex formation, indicate their potential to improve kidney function by reducing levels of chronic inflammation that contribute to disease progression. This approach, however, is aimed at preventing or ameliorating damage but cannot suppress the ongoing production of pathogenic autoantibodies.

Targeting B cell and plasma cell activators BAFF and APRIL have emerged as a promising approach for reducing Gd-IgA1 antibody and autoantibody production. Early clinical studies evaluating both BION-1301, atacicept, and telitacicept have shown that targeting APRIL and BAFF may reduce antibody levels and proteinuria.

An alternative approach is to target the tissues and cell types most associated with production of disease-causing antibodies (Gd-IgA1). This approach was recently validated through approval of targeted release budesonide (Tarpeyo). The clinical data on Tarpeyo showed substantial benefit for patients with IgAN over current standard of care, indicating the potential of a therapy that can interrupt immunopathogenesis by reducing mucosal production of Gd-IgA1. Tarpeyo is designed to act locally on immune cells in the small intestine, potentially missing other sources of Gd-IgA1-producing cells throughout the body, including NALT and tonsils. As plasma cells are found in mucosa throughout the body, specifically targeting all plasma cells may provide even more robust reduction in circulating pathogenic antibodies and immune complexes by removing the main source of autoantigen and/or autoantibody production in all lymphoid tissues [36–39]. Furthermore, targeting CD38 selectively targets plasma cells and allows for continued immune protection by CD38 negative B cells. The anti-CD38 antibody therapy, felzartamab, has shown successful depletion of plasma cells in the autoimmune-driven nephropathy MN and hematologic cancers, such as MM. An anti-CD38 approach may also have great potential for treatment of patients with IgAN.

Altogether, these data support development of strategies that deplete plasma cells, which aim to stop generation of Gd-IgA1 and anti-Gd-IgA1 antibodies and potentially reduce immune complex deposition, inflammation, and tissue damage, thereby preserving kidney function in patients with IgAN. However, modulating the immune system comes with an increased risk of infection and more clinical data is needed to understand the long-term effects of treatment with these novel immunotherapies.

Author Contributions: Conceptualization, D.M., D.E.M., D.V.R., H.Z. and V.T.; resources, D.M., D.V.R., H.Z. and V.T.; writing—original draft preparation, D.E.M.; writing—review and editing, D.M., D.V.R., H.Z. and V.T.; visualization, D.M., D.E.M. and V.T.; supervision, D.M. and V.T.; funding acquisition, D.E.M. All authors have read and agreed to the published version of the manuscript.

Funding: Dita Maixnerova and Vladimir Tesar are supported by: Cooperatio 207034 Internal disciplines, MH CZ-DRO-VFN64165, General University Hospital in Prague, Czech Republic. The APC was funded by MorphoSys AG.

Conflicts of Interest: D.M. has served as principal investigator for MorphoSys AG clinical trials. D.E.M. is a full-time employee of MorphoSys AG. D.V.R. reports research funding from Reata Pharmaceuticals, Travere Therapeutics (Retrophin), Achillion Pharmaceuticals, Pfizer, Calliditas Therapeutics (Pharmalinks), Otsuka Pharmaceuticals (Visterra); has served as a consultant for Novartis, George Clinical, Otsuka Pharmaceuticals (Visterra), Calliditas Therapeutics (Pharmalinks), Angion Biomedica, Catalyst Biosciences; and has ownership in Reliant Glycosciences LLC. H.Z. has served as a consultant for Janssen, Novartis, Omeros, Calliditas Therapeutics, and Chinook Therapeutics. V.T. has served as a consultant for Calliditas, Novartis, Omeros, Otsuka, Pfizer and Travere and as principal investigator for MorphoSys AG clinical trials. The APC funders had a role in in the writing of the manuscript and in the decision to publish the review.

References

1. Rodrigues, J.C.; Haas, M.; Reich, H.N. IgA Nephropathy. *Clin. J. Am. Soc. Nephrol.* **2017**, *12*, 677–686. [CrossRef] [PubMed]
2. Lai, K.N.; Tang, S.C.W.; Schena, F.P.; Novak, J.; Tomino, Y.; Fogo, A.B.; Glassock, R.J. IgA Nephropathy. *Nat. Rev. Dis. Prim.* **2016**, *2*, 16001. [CrossRef] [PubMed]
3. McGrogan, A.; Franssen, C.F.M.; de Vries, C.S. The Incidence of Primary Glomerulonephritis Worldwide: A Systematic Review of the Literature. *Nephrol. Dial. Transplant.* **2011**, *26*, 414–430. [CrossRef] [PubMed]
4. Schena, F.P.; Nistor, I. Epidemiology of IgA Nephropathy: A Global Perspective. *Semin. Nephrol.* **2018**, *38*, 435–442. [CrossRef]
5. Hakim, R.M.; Saha, S. Dialysis Frequency versus Dialysis Time, That Is the Question. *Kidney Int.* **2014**, *85*, 1024–1029. [CrossRef]
6. Tattersall, J.; Martin-Malo, A.; Pedrini, L.; Basci, A.; Canaud, B.; Fouque, D.; Haage, P.; Konner, K.; Kooman, J.; Pizzarelli, F.; et al. EBPG Guideline on Dialysis Strategies. *Nephrol. Dial. Transplant.* **2007**, *22* (Suppl. S2), ii5–ii21. [CrossRef]
7. Dąbrowska-Bender, M.; Dykowska, G.; Żuk, W.; Milewska, M.; Staniszewska, A. The Impact on Quality of Life of Dialysis Patients with Renal Insufficiency. *Patient Prefer. Adherence* **2018**, *12*, 577–583. [CrossRef]
8. Foley, R.N.; Parfrey, P.S.; Sarnak, M.J. Clinical Epidemiology of Cardiovascular Disease in Chronic Renal Disease. *Am. J. Kidney Dis.* **1998**, *32*, S112–S119. [CrossRef]
9. Komatsu, H.; Kikuchi, M.; Nakagawa, H.; Fukuda, A.; Iwakiri, T.; Toida, T.; Sato, Y.; Kitamura, K.; Fujimoto, S. Long-Term Survival of Patients with IgA Nephropathy after Dialysis Therapy. *Kidney Blood Press. Res.* **2013**, *37*, 649–656. [CrossRef]
10. Jarrick, S.; Lundberg, S.; Welander, A.; Carrero, J.-J.; Höijer, J.; Bottai, M.; Ludvigsson, J.F. Mortality in IgA Nephropathy: A Nationwide Population-Based Cohort Study. *J. Am. Soc. Nephrol.* **2019**, *30*, 866–876. [CrossRef]
11. Wyld, M.L.; Chadban, S.J. Recurrent IgA Nephropathy After Kidney Transplantation. *Transplantation* **2016**, *100*, 1827–1832. [CrossRef] [PubMed]
12. Moroni, G.; Gallelli, B.; Quaglini, S.; Leoni, A.; Banfi, G.; Passerini, P.; Montagnino, G.; Messa, P. Long-Term Outcome of Renal Transplantation in Patients with Idiopathic Membranous Glomerulonephritis (MN). *Nephrol. Dial. Transplant.* **2010**, *25*, 3408–3415. [CrossRef] [PubMed]
13. Maixnerova, D.; Hruba, P.; Neprasova, M.; Bednarova, K.; Slatinska, J.; Suchanek, M.; Kollar, M.; Novak, J.; Tesar, V.; Viklicky, O. Outcome of 313 Czech Patients With IgA Nephropathy After Renal Transplantation. *Front. Immunol.* **2021**, *12*, 726215. [CrossRef] [PubMed]
14. Knoppova, B.; Reily, C.; Maillard, N.; Rizk, D.V.; Moldoveanu, Z.; Mestecky, J.; Raska, M.; Renfrow, M.B.; Julian, B.A.; Novak, J. The Origin and Activities of IgA1-Containing Immune Complexes in IgA Nephropathy. *Front. Immunol.* **2016**, *7*, 117. [CrossRef] [PubMed]
15. Halliley, J.L.; Tipton, C.M.; Liesveld, J.; Rosenberg, A.F.; Darce, J.; Gregoretti, I.V.; Popova, L.; Kaminiski, D.; Fucile, C.F.; Albizua, I.; et al. Long-Lived Plasma Cells Are Contained within the CD19(-)CD38(Hi)CD138(+) Subset in Human Bone Marrow. *Immunity* **2015**, *43*, 132–145. [CrossRef]
16. Khodadadi, L.; Cheng, Q.; Radbruch, A.; Hiepe, F. The Maintenance of Memory Plasma Cells. *Front. Immunol.* **2019**, *10*, 721. [CrossRef]
17. Suzuki, H. Biomarkers for IgA Nephropathy on the Basis of Multi-Hit Pathogenesis. *Clin. Exp. Nephrol.* **2019**, *23*, 26–31. [CrossRef]
18. Lai, K.N. Pathogenesis of IgA Nephropathy. *Nat. Rev. Nephrol.* **2012**, *8*, 275–283. [CrossRef]
19. Suzuki, H.; Kiryluk, K.; Novak, J.; Moldoveanu, Z.; Herr, A.B.; Renfrow, M.B.; Wyatt, R.J.; Scolari, F.; Mestecky, J.; Gharavi, A.G.; et al. The Pathophysiology of IgA Nephropathy. *J. Am. Soc. Nephrol.* **2011**, *22*, 1795–1803. [CrossRef]
20. Rizk, D.V.; Maillard, N.; Julian, B.A.; Knoppova, B.; Green, T.J.; Novak, J.; Wyatt, R.J. The Emerging Role of Complement Proteins as a Target for Therapy of IgA Nephropathy. *Front. Immunol.* **2019**, *10*, 504. [CrossRef]
21. Maixnerova, D.; Ling, C.; Hall, S.; Reily, C.; Brown, R.; Neprasova, M.; Suchanek, M.; Honsova, E.; Zima, T.; Novak, J.; et al. Galactose-Deficient IgA1 and the Corresponding IgG Autoantibodies Predict IgA Nephropathy Progression. *PLoS ONE* **2019**, *14*, e0212254. [CrossRef]
22. Rovin, B.H.; Adler, S.G.; Barratt, J.; Bridoux, F.; Burdge, K.A.; Chan, T.M.; Cook, H.T.; Fervenza, F.C.; Gibson, K.L.; Glassock, R.J.; et al. Executive Summary of the KDIGO 2021 Guideline for the Management of Glomerular Diseases. *Kidney Int.* **2021**, *100*, 753–779. [CrossRef] [PubMed]
23. Huang, L.; Guo, F.-L.; Zhou, J.; Zhao, Y.-J. IgA Nephropathy Factors That Predict and Accelerate Progression to End-Stage Renal Disease. *Cell Biochem. Biophys.* **2014**, *68*, 443–447. [CrossRef]
24. Maixnerova, D.; Tesar, V. Emerging Modes of Treatment of IgA Nephropathy. *Int. J. Mol. Sci.* **2020**, *21*, 9064. [CrossRef] [PubMed]
25. Bagchi, S.; Mani, K.; Swamy, A.; Barwad, A.; Singh, G.; Bhowmik, D.; Agarwal, S.K. Supportive Management of IgA Nephropathy With Renin-Angiotensin Blockade, the AIIMS Primary IgA Nephropathy Cohort (APPROACH) Study. *Kidney Int. Rep.* **2021**, *6*, 1661–1668. [CrossRef] [PubMed]
26. Travere Therapeutics, Inc. *A Randomized, Multicenter, Double-Blind, Parallel-Group, Active-Control Study of the Efficacy and Safety of Sparsentan for the Treatment of Immunoglobulin A Nephropathy*; Travere Therapeutics, Inc.: San Diego, CA, USA, 2021. Available online: https://www.clinicaltrials.gov (accessed on 28 March 2022).
27. Komers, R.; Plotkin, H. Dual Inhibition of Renin-Angiotensin-Aldosterone System and Endothelin-1 in Treatment of Chronic Kidney Disease. *Am. J. Physio.l Regul. Integr. Comp. Physiol.* **2016**, *310*, R877–R884. [CrossRef]

28. Wheeler, D.C.; Toto, R.D.; Stefánsson, B.V.; Jongs, N.; Chertow, G.M.; Greene, T.; Hou, F.F.; McMurray, J.J.V.; Pecoits-Filho, R.; Correa-Rotter, R.; et al. A Pre-Specified Analysis of the DAPA-CKD Trial Demonstrates the Effects of Dapagliflozin on Major Adverse Kidney Events in Patients with IgA Nephropathy. *Kidney Int.* **2021**, *100*, 215–224. [CrossRef]
29. Morphosys Farxiga (Dapagliflozin). [Package Insert]. 2021. Available online: https://den8dhaj6zs0e.cloudfront.net/50fd68b9-106b-4550-b5d0-12b045f8b184/0be9cb1b-3b33-41c7-bfc2-04c9f718e442/0be9cb1b-3b33-41c7-bfc2-04c9f718e442_viewable_rendition__v.pdf (accessed on 28 March 2022).
30. Rauen, T.; Wied, S.; Fitzner, C.; Eitner, F.; Sommerer, C.; Zeier, M.; Otte, B.; Panzer, U.; Budde, K.; Benck, U.; et al. After Ten Years of Follow-up, No Difference between Supportive Care plus Immunosuppression and Supportive Care Alone in IgA Nephropathy. *Kidney Int.* **2020**, *98*, 1044–1052. [CrossRef]
31. Lv, J.; Zhang, H.; Wong, M.G.; Jardine, M.J.; Hladunewich, M.; Jha, V.; Monaghan, H.; Zhao, M.; Barbour, S.; Reich, H.; et al. Effect of Oral Methylprednisolone on Clinical Outcomes in Patients With IgA Nephropathy: The TESTING Randomized Clinical Trial. *JAMA* **2017**, *318*, 432–442. [CrossRef]
32. Calliditas Therapeutics Tarpeyo (Budesonide). [Package Insert]. 2021. Available online: https://www.tarpeyo.com/prescribinginformation.pdf (accessed on 28 March 2022).
33. FDA. *FDA Approves First Drug to Decrease Urine Protein in IgA Nephropathy, a Rare Kidney Disease*; FDA: Silver Spring, MD, USA, 2021.
34. Schrezenmeier, E.; Jayne, D.; Dörner, T. Targeting B Cells and Plasma Cells in Glomerular Diseases: Translational Perspectives. *J. Am. Soc. Nephrol.* **2018**, *29*, 741–758. [CrossRef]
35. Zhang, Y.-M.; Zhang, H. Insights into the Role of Mucosal Immunity in IgA Nephropathy. *Clin. J. Am. Soc. Nephrol.* **2018**, *13*, 1584–1586. [CrossRef] [PubMed]
36. He, J.-W.; Zhou, X.-J.; Lv, J.-C.; Zhang, H. Perspectives on How Mucosal Immune Responses, Infections and Gut Microbiome Shape IgA Nephropathy and Future Therapies. *Theranostics* **2020**, *10*, 11462–11478. [CrossRef] [PubMed]
37. Tang, Y.; He, H.; Hu, P.; Xu, X. T Lymphocytes in IgA Nephropathy. *Exp. Ther. Med.* **2020**, *20*, 186–194. [CrossRef] [PubMed]
38. Meng, H.; Ohtake, H.; Ishida, A.; Ohta, N.; Kakehata, S.; Yamakawa, M. IgA Production and Tonsillar Focal Infection in IgA Nephropathy. *J. Clin. Exp. Hematop.* **2012**, *52*, 161–170. [CrossRef]
39. Chang, S.; Li, X.-K. The Role of Immune Modulation in Pathogenesis of IgA Nephropathy. *Front. Med.* **2020**, *7*, 92. [CrossRef]
40. Wang, Y.-Y.; Zhang, L.; Zhao, P.-W.; Ma, L.; Li, C.; Zou, H.-B.; Jiang, Y.-F. Functional Implications of Regulatory B Cells in Human IgA Nephropathy. *Scand. J. Immunol.* **2014**, *79*, 51–60. [CrossRef]
41. Muto, M.; Manfroi, B.; Suzuki, H.; Joh, K.; Nagai, M.; Wakai, S.; Righini, C.; Maiguma, M.; Izui, S.; Tomino, Y.; et al. Toll-Like Receptor 9 Stimulation Induces Aberrant Expression of a Proliferation-Inducing Ligand by Tonsillar Germinal Center B Cells in IgA Nephropathy. *J. Am. Soc. Nephrol.* **2017**, *28*, 1227–1238. [CrossRef]
42. Li, W.; Peng, X.; Liu, Y.; Liu, H.; Liu, F.; He, L.; Liu, Y.; Zhang, F.; Guo, C.; Chen, G.; et al. TLR9 and BAFF: Their Expression in Patients with IgA Nephropathy. *Mol. Med. Rep.* **2014**, *10*, 1469–1474. [CrossRef]
43. Selvaskandan, H.; Cheung, C.K.; Muto, M.; Barratt, J. New Strategies and Perspectives on Managing IgA Nephropathy. *Clin. Exp. Nephrol.* **2019**, *23*, 577–588. [CrossRef]
44. Lafayette, R.A.; Canetta, P.A.; Rovin, B.H.; Appel, G.B.; Novak, J.; Nath, K.A.; Sethi, S.; Tumlin, J.A.; Mehta, K.; Hogan, M.; et al. A Randomized, Controlled Trial of Rituximab in IgA Nephropathy with Proteinuria and Renal Dysfunction. *J. Am. Soc. Nephrol.* **2017**, *28*, 1306–1313. [CrossRef]
45. Coppo, R.; Peruzzi, L.; Loiacono, E.; Bergallo, M.; Krutova, A.; Russo, M.L.; Cocchi, E.; Amore, A.; Lundberg, S.; Maixnerova, D.; et al. Defective Gene Expression of the Membrane Complement Inhibitor CD46 in Patients with Progressive Immunoglobulin A Nephropathy. *Nephrol. Dial. Transplant.* **2019**, *34*, 587–596. [CrossRef] [PubMed]
46. Zhu, L.; Zhai, Y.-L.; Wang, F.-M.; Hou, P.; Lv, J.-C.; Xu, D.-M.; Shi, S.-F.; Liu, L.-J.; Yu, F.; Zhao, M.-H.; et al. Variants in Complement Factor H and Complement Factor H-Related Protein Genes, CFHR3 and CFHR1, Affect Complement Activation in IgA Nephropathy. *J. Am. Soc. Nephrol.* **2015**, *26*, 1195–1204. [CrossRef] [PubMed]
47. Jennette, J.C. The Immunohistology of IgA Nephropathy. *Am. J. Kidney Dis.* **1988**, *12*, 348–352. [CrossRef]
48. Barratt, J. Interim Analysis of a Phase 2 Dose Ranging Study to Investigate the Effect and Safety of Iptacopan in Primary IGA Nephropathy. Available online: https://era-edta.conference2web.com/#!resources/interim-analysis-of-a-phase-2-dose-ranging-study-to-investigate-the-efficacy-and-safety-of-iptacopan-in-primary-iga-nephropathy-20ec3f83-fd34-441e-8745-44587bda74da (accessed on 15 March 2022).
49. Novartis Announces Iptacopan Met Phase II Study Primary Endpoint in Rare Kidney Disease IgA Nephropathy (IgAN). Available online: https://www.novartis.com/news/media-releases/novartis-announces-iptacopan-met-phase-ii-study-primary-endpoint-rare-kidney-disease-iga-nephropathy-igan (accessed on 15 March 2022).
50. Barratt, J.; Rovin, B.; Zhang, H.; Kashihara, N.; Maes, B.; Rizk, D.; Trimarchi, H.; Sprangers, B.; Meier, M.; Kollins, D.; et al. Pos-546 Efficacy and Safety of Iptacopan in Iga Nephropathy: Results of a Randomized Double-Blind Placebo-Controlled Phase 2 Study at 6 Months. *Kidney Int. Rep.* **2022**, *7*, S236. [CrossRef]
51. Lafayette, R.A.; Carroll, K.; Barratt, J. Long-Term Phase 2 Efficacy of the MASP-2 Inhibitor Narsoplimab for Treatment of Severe IgA Nephropathy. In Proceedings of the ASN Kidney Week 2021, San Diego, CA, USA, 4–7 November 2021.
52. Lafayette, R.A.; Rovin, B.H.; Reich, H.N.; Tumlin, J.A.; Floege, J.; Barratt, J. Safety, Tolerability and Efficacy of Narsoplimab, a Novel MASP-2 Inhibitor for the Treatment of IgA Nephropathy. *Kidney Int. Rep.* **2020**, *5*, 2032–2041. [CrossRef]

53. Wire, B. Omeros Announces Results From Nearly Three-Year Follow-Up of Patients in Phase 2 IgA Nephropathy Trial. Available online: https://www.benzinga.com/node/23920855 (accessed on 15 March 2022).
54. Schubart, A.; Anderson, K.; Mainolfi, N.; Sellner, H.; Ehara, T.; Adams, C.M.; Mac Sweeney, A.; Liao, S.-M.; Crowley, M.; Littlewood-Evans, A.; et al. Small-Molecule Factor B Inhibitor for the Treatment of Complement-Mediated Diseases. *Proc. Natl. Acad. Sci. USA* **2019**, *116*, 7926–7931. [CrossRef]
55. Rambaldi, A.; Gritti, G.; Micò, M.C.; Frigeni, M.; Borleri, G.; Salvi, A.; Landi, F.; Pavoni, C.; Sonzogni, A.; Gianatti, A.; et al. Endothelial Injury and Thrombotic Microangiopathy in COVID-19: Treatment with the Lectin-Pathway Inhibitor Narsoplimab. *Immunobiology* **2020**, *225*, 152001. [CrossRef]
56. Piedra-Quintero, Z.L.; Wilson, Z.; Nava, P.; Guerau-de-Arellano, M. CD38: An Immunomodulatory Molecule in Inflammation and Autoimmunity. *Front. Immunol.* **2020**, *11*, 597959. [CrossRef]
57. Samy, E.; Wax, S.; Huard, B.; Hess, H.; Schneider, P. Targeting BAFF and APRIL in Systemic Lupus Erythematosus and Other Antibody-Associated Diseases. *Int. Rev. Immunol.* **2017**, *36*, 3–19. [CrossRef]
58. Zhai, Y.-L.; Zhu, L.; Shi, S.-F.; Liu, L.-J.; Lv, J.-C.; Zhang, H. Increased APRIL Expression Induces IgA1 Aberrant Glycosylation in IgA Nephropathy. *Medicine* **2016**, *95*, e3099. [CrossRef]
59. Struemper, H.; Kurtinecz, M.; Edwards, L.; Freimuth, W.W.; Roth, D.A.; Stohl, W. Reductions in Circulating B Cell Subsets and Immunoglobulin G Levels with Long-Term Belimumab Treatment in Patients with SLE. *Lupus Sci. Med.* **2022**, *9*, e000499. [CrossRef] [PubMed]
60. Couser, W.G. Primary Membranous Nephropathy. *Clin. J. Am. Soc. Nephrol.* **2017**, *12*, 983–997. [CrossRef] [PubMed]
61. National Institute of Allergy and Infectious Diseases (NIAID). *NCT03949855: Efficacy of Belimumab and Rituximab Compared to Rituximab Alone for the Treatment of Primary Membranous Nephropathy (ITN080AI)*; National Institute of Allergy and Infectious Diseases (NIAID): Rockville, MD, USA, 2021. Available online: https://www.clinicaltrials.gov (accessed on 28 March 2022).
62. Barratt, J.; Hour, B.T.; Schwartz, B.S.; Sorensen, B.; Roy, S.E.; Stromatt, C.L.; MacDonald, M.; Endsley, A.N.; Lo, J.; Glicklich, A.; et al. Pharmacodynamic and Clinical Responses to BION-1301 in Patients with IgA Nephropathy: Initial Results of a Ph1/2 Trial. In Proceedings of the ASN Kidney Week 2021, San Diego, CA, USA, 4–7 November 2021.
63. Barratt, J.; Tumlin, J.A.; Suzuki, Y.; Kao, A.; Aydemir, A.; Zima, Y.; Appel, G.B. 24-Week Interim Analysis of a Randomized, Double-Blind, Placebo-Controlled Phase 2 Study of Atacicept in Patients with IgA Nephropathy and Persistent Proteinuria. In Proceedings of the ASN Kidney Week 2020, Denver, CO, USA, 20–25 October 2020.
64. Vera Therapeutics, Inc. *NCT04716231: A Phase IIb Randomized, Double-Blinded, Placebo-Controlled, Dose-Ranging Study to Evaluate the Efficacy and Safety of Atacicept in Subjects With IgA Nephropathy (IGAN)*; Vera Therapeutics, Inc.: South San Francisco, CA, USA, 2022. Available online: https://www.clinicaltrials.gov (accessed on 28 March 2022).
65. Lv, J.; Liu, L.-J.; Hao, C.-M.; Li, G.; Fu, P.; Xing, G.; Zheng, H.; Chen, N.; Caili, W.; Luo, P.; et al. A Phase 2, Randomized, Double-Blind, Placebo-Controlled Trial of Telitacicept in Patients with IgA Nephropathy and Persistent Proteinuria. In Proceedings of the ASN Kidney Week 2021, San Diego, CA, USA, 4–7 November 2021.
66. RemeGen Co. Ltd. *NCT04905212: A Phase 2, Randomized, Double-Blind, Multicenter Study of Telitacicept for Injection (RC18) in Subjects With IgA Nephropathy*; RemeGen Co., Ltd.: Yantai, China, 2022. Available online: https://www.clinicaltrials.gov (accessed on 28 March 2022).
67. Mathur, M.; Barratt, J.; Suzuki, Y.; Engler, F.; Pasetti, M.F.; Yarbrough, J.; Sloan, S.; Oldach, D. Safety, Tolerability, Pharmacokinetics, and Pharmacodynamics of VIS649 (Sibeprenlimab), an APRIL-Neutralizing IgG2 Monoclonal Antibody, in Healthy Volunteers. *Kidney Int. Rep.* **2022**, *7*, 993–1003. [CrossRef]
68. Visterra NCT04287985: Safety and Efficacy Study of VIS649 for IgA Nephropathy—Full Text View—ClinicalTrials.Gov. Available online: https://www.clinicaltrials.gov/ct2/show/NCT04287985?term=nct04287985&draw=2&rank=1 (accessed on 22 March 2022).
69. Barratt, J.; Rovin, B.H.; Cattran, D.; Floege, J.; Lafayette, R.; Tesar, V.; Trimarchi, H.; Zhang, H.; NefIgArd Study Steering Committee. Why Target the Gut to Treat IgA Nephropathy? *Kidney Int. Rep.* **2020**, *5*, 1620–1624. [CrossRef]
70. Macpherson, A.J.; McCoy, K.D.; Johansen, F.-E.; Brandtzaeg, P. The Immune Geography of IgA Induction and Function. *Mucosal Immunol.* **2008**, *1*, 11–22. [CrossRef]
71. Kano, T.; Suzuki, H.; Makita, Y.; Fukao, Y.; Suzuki, Y. Nasal-Associated Lymphoid Tissue Is the Major Induction Site for Nephritogenic IgA in Murine IgA Nephropathy. *Kidney Int.* **2021**, *100*, 364–376. [CrossRef]
72. Nakata, J.; Suzuki, Y.; Suzuki, H.; Sato, D.; Kano, T.; Yanagawa, H.; Matsuzaki, K.; Horikoshi, S.; Novak, J.; Tomino, Y. Changes in Nephritogenic Serum Galactose-Deficient IgA1 in IgA Nephropathy Following Tonsillectomy and Steroid Therapy. *PLoS ONE* **2014**, *9*, e89707. [CrossRef]
73. Lanzillotta, M.; Della-Torre, E.; Milani, R.; Bozzolo, E.; Bozzalla-Cassione, E.; Rovati, L.; Arcidiacono, P.G.; Partelli, S.; Falconi, M.; Ciceri, F.; et al. Increase of Circulating Memory B Cells after Glucocorticoid-Induced Remission Identifies Patients at Risk of IgG4-Related Disease Relapse. *Arthritis Res. Ther.* **2018**, *20*, 222. [CrossRef]
74. Floege, J. Mucosal Corticosteroid Therapy of IgA Nephropathy. *Kidney Int.* **2017**, *92*, 278–280. [CrossRef]
75. Coppo, R.; Mariat, C. Systemic Corticosteroids and Mucosal-Associated Lymphoid Tissue-Targeted Therapy in Immunoglobulin A Nephropathy: Insight from the NEFIGAN Study. *Nephrol. Dial. Transplant.* **2020**, *35*, 1291–1294. [CrossRef]
76. Fellström, B.C.; Barratt, J.; Cook, H.; Coppo, R.; Feehally, J.; de Fijter, J.W.; Floege, J.; Hetzel, G.; Jardine, A.G.; Locatelli, F.; et al. Targeted-Release Budesonide versus Placebo in Patients with IgA Nephropathy (NEFIGAN): A Double-Blind, Randomised, Placebo-Controlled Phase 2b Trial. *Lancet* **2017**, *389*, 2117–2127. [CrossRef]

77. Barratt, J.; Stone, A.; Kristensen, J. POS-830 NEFECON for the Treatment of IgA Nephropathy in Patients at Risk of Progressing to End-Stage Renal Disease: The NEFIgArd Phase 3 Trial Results. *Kidney Int. Rep.* **2021**, *6*, S361. [CrossRef]
78. Calliditas Therapeutics AB. *NCT03643965: A Randomized, Double-Blind, Placebo Controlled Study to Evaluate Efficacy and Safety of Nefecon in Patients With Primary IgA (Immunoglobulin A) Nephropathy at Risk of Progressing to End-Stage Renal Disease (NefIgArd)*; Calliditas Therapeutics AB: Stockholm, Sweden, 2021. Available online: https://www.clinicaltrials.gov (accessed on 28 March 2022).
79. Hartono, C.; Chung, M.; Perlman, A.S.; Chevalier, J.M.; Serur, D.; Seshan, S.V.; Muthukumar, T. Bortezomib for Reduction of Proteinuria in IgA Nephropathy. *Kidney Int. Rep.* **2018**, *3*, 861–866. [CrossRef] [PubMed]
80. MorphoSys AG. *NCT05065970: A Double Blind, Randomized, Placebo-Controlled, Multicenter Phase IIa, Clinical Trial to Assess Efficacy and Safety of the Human Anti-CD38 Antibody Felzartamab in IgA Nephropathy*; MorphoSys AG: Planegg, Germany, 2021. Available online: https://www.clinicaltrials.gov (accessed on 28 March 2022).
81. Boxhammer, R.; Weirather, J.; Steidl, S.; Endell, J. MOR202, a Human Anti-CD38 Monoclonal Antibody, Mediates Potent Tumoricidal Activity In Vivo and Shows Synergistic Efficacy in Combination with Different Antineoplastic Compounds. *Blood* **2015**, *126*, 3015. [CrossRef]
82. Raab, M.S.; Engelhardt, M.; Blank, A.; Goldschmidt, H.; Agis, H.; Blau, I.W.; Einsele, H.; Ferstl, B.; Schub, N.; Röllig, C.; et al. MOR202, a Novel Anti-CD38 Monoclonal Antibody, in Patients with Relapsed or Refractory Multiple Myeloma: A First-in-Human, Multicentre, Phase 1-2a Trial. *Lancet Haematol.* **2020**, *7*, e381–e394. [CrossRef]
83. Endell, J.; Boxhammer, R.; Wurzenberger, C.; Ness, D.; Steidl, S. The Activity of MOR202, a Fully Human Anti-CD38 Antibody, Is Complemented by ADCP and Is Synergistically Enhanced by Lenalidomide in Vitro and in Vivo. *Blood* **2012**, *120*, 4018. [CrossRef]
84. Tawara, T.; Hasegawa, K.; Sugiura, Y.; Harada, K.; Miura, T.; Hayashi, S.; Tahara, T.; Ishikawa, M.; Yoshida, H.; Kubo, K.; et al. Complement Activation Plays a Key Role in Antibody-Induced Infusion Toxicity in Monkeys and Rats. *J. Immunol.* **2008**, *180*, 2294–2298. [CrossRef]
85. Rovin, B.H.; Adler, S.G.; Hoxha, E.; Sprangers, B.; Stahl, R.; Wetzels, J.F.; Schwamb, B.; Boxhammer, R.; Nguyen, Q.; Haertle, S.; et al. Felzartamab in Patients with Anti-Phospholipase A2 Receptor Autoantibody Positive (Anti-PLA2R+) Membranous Nephropathy (MN): Interim Results from the M-PLACE Study. In Proceedings of the ASN Kidney Week 2021, San Diego, CA, USA, 4–7 November 2021.
86. Rovin, B.; Adler, S.G.; Hoxha, E.; Sprangers, B.; Stahl, R.; Wetzels, J.F.; Jauch-Lembach, J.; Griese, J.; Boxhammer, R.; Xu, L.; et al. Felzartamab in Patients with Anti-Phospholipase A2 Receptor Autoantibody-Positive (Anti-PLA2R Ab+) Membranous Nephropathy (MN): Preliminary Results from the M-PLACE Study. In Proceedings of the National Kidney Foundation Spring Clinical Meetings, Boston, MA, USA, 6–10 April 2022.
87. Liyasova, M.; McDonald, Z.; Taylor, P.; Gorospe, K.; Xu, X.; Yao, C.; Liu, Q.; Yang, L.; Atenafu, E.G.; Piza, G.; et al. A Personalized Mass Spectrometry-Based Assay to Monitor M-Protein in Patients with Multiple Myeloma (EasyM). *Clin. Cancer Res.* **2021**, *27*, 5028–5037. [CrossRef]
88. Raab, M.S.; Chatterjee, M.; Goldschmidt, H.; Agis, H.; Blau, I.; Einsele, H.; Engelhardt, M.; Ferstl, B.; Gramatzki, M.; Röllig, C.; et al. A Phase I/IIa Study of the CD38 Antibody MOR202 Alone and in Combination with Pomalidomide or Lenalidomide in Patients with Relapsed or Refractory Multiple Myeloma. *Blood* **2016**, *128*, 1152. [CrossRef]
89. Heesterbeek, D.A.C.; Angelier, M.L.; Harrison, R.A.; Rooijakkers, S.H.M. Complement and Bacterial Infections: From Molecular Mechanisms to Therapeutic Applications. *J. Innate Immun.* **2018**, *10*, 455–464. [CrossRef]
90. Johnson, A.; Lewis, J.; Raff, M.; Roberts, K.; Walter, P. *Molecular Biology of the Cell*, 4th ed.; Alberts, B., Ed.; Garland Science: New York, NY, USA, 2002; ISBN 978-0-8153-3218-3.

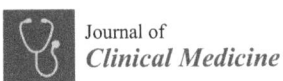

Review

An Update on the Current State of Management and Clinical Trials for IgA Nephropathy

Chee Kay Cheung [1,2], Arun Rajasekaran [3], Jonathan Barratt [1,2,†] and Dana V. Rizk [3,*,†]

1. Department of Cardiovascular Sciences, University of Leicester, Leicester LE1 7RH, UK; ckc15@le.ac.uk (C.K.C.); jb81@le.ac.uk (J.B.)
2. John Walls Renal Unit, University Hospitals of Leicester NHS Trust, Leicester LE5 4PW, UK
3. Division of Nephrology, Department of Medicine, University of Alabama at Birmingham, ZRB 614, 1720 2nd Avenue South, Birmingham, AL 35294, USA; arajasekaran@uabmc.edu
* Correspondence: drizk@uabmc.edu
† Both authors contributed equally to this work.

Abstract: IgA nephropathy remains the most common primary glomerular disease worldwide. It affects children and adults of all ages, and is a leading cause of end-stage kidney disease, making it a considerable public health issue in many countries. Despite being initially described over 50 years ago, there are still no disease specific treatments, with current management for most patients being focused on lifestyle measures and renin-angiotensin-aldosterone system blockade. However, significant advances in the understanding of its pathogenesis have been made particularly over the past decade, leading to great interest in developing new therapeutic strategies, and a significant rise in the number of interventional clinical trials being performed. In this review, we will summarise the current state of management of IgAN, and then describe major areas of interest where new therapies are at their most advanced stages of development, that include the gut mucosal immune system, B cell signalling, the complement system and non-immune modulators. Finally, we describe clinical trials that are taking place in each area and explore future directions for translational research.

Keywords: IgA; IgA nephropathy; clinical trials

1. Introduction

IgA nephropathy (IgAN) remains the most common primary glomerular disease in the world. It often affects younger adults, and in approximately 30% of patients it progresses to end-stage kidney disease (ESKD) within 20 years of diagnosis, placing a considerable burden on individuals, carers and healthcare systems globally. To date there is no approved disease-specific treatment available. The role of corticosteroids in the management of IgAN is uncertain, and there has been no consistent evidence to support the use of other existing immunosuppressive agents. Over the past few decades, significant advances have been made in understanding the complex pathogenesis that underlies IgAN. This has driven an explosion of interest in developing new therapeutic strategies for this condition, and several global phase II and phase III clinical trials are currently underway. In this review, we will focus on current treatment guidelines and new therapies for IgAN that range from being in the initial stages of development to the late phases of clinical trials.

2. Current Treatment Strategies

Despite advances in the understanding of the underlying pathogenic mechanisms in IgAN, there are currently no approved treatments that can specifically alter the production of galactose-deficient IgA1 (Gd-IgA1) nor its corresponding autoantibody that are central to the disease process, IgA1-immune complex formation, or their deposition within the glomerular mesangium.

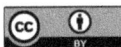

Long-term registry data have shown that patients with IgAN who have preserved kidney function, non-visible haematuria and minimal proteinuria <0.5 g/day are at low risk of progressive kidney disease, and do not require disease-specific treatment [1]. However, these patients should be followed up at least annually, so that any worsening of proteinuria, development of chronic kidney disease (CKD) or hypertension can be detected and managed appropriately.

The primary focus of management for those who have proteinuria above this threshold should be on optimized goal-directed supportive care. This includes renin-angiotensin-aldosterone system (RAAS) blockade, with either an angiotensin-converting enzyme inhibitor (ACEi) or angiotensin II receptor blocker (ARB), but not both, to the maximum tolerated amount, and addressing overall cardiovascular risk, including strict blood pressure control (to a recommended target of <130/80 mm Hg for those with proteinuria > 0.3 g/day and <125/75 mm Hg when proteinuria is >1 g/day) [2], dietary sodium reduction, smoking cessation if appropriate, weight control, and exercise. The Supportive versus immunosuppressive Therapy for the treatment of Progressive IgA Nephropathy (STOP-IgAN) trial has provided robust evidence to support this approach [3]. All participants in this trial underwent a 6-month run-in period, where an intensive program of supportive care was provided utilizing the measures outlined above. A key finding was that around one-third of participants, originally thought by their treating nephrologist to be suitable for treatment of their disease with immunosuppression, were no longer eligible to continue in the trial after this period, as proteinuria had fallen to below the set criteria to proceed.

A substantial proportion of patients will have persistent proteinuria of >1 g/day despite these measures, and observational data have demonstrated that these patients are at high risk of progressive kidney disease and ESKD. Reducing proteinuria to below this threshold is also associated with improved renal outcomes [4]. Long-term follow-up data from the STOP-IgAN trial have shown that IgAN still has a poor prognosis in those with persistent proteinuria, even with optimized supportive care, with almost half of the participants reaching the composite of death, ESKD, or decline in estimated glomerular filtration rate (eGFR) of over 40% over a median time interval of 7.4 years [5]. In the next sections, we will discuss potential additional treatments to supportive care.

3. Systemic Corticosteroid Treatment

Corticosteroids have long been used in the management of IgAN, due to their anti-inflammatory and immunosuppressive effects, but their role is controversial. Many of the clinical trials that have supported their use were conducted at a time when the concept of optimized supportive care was not well established, meaning that trial participants were not consistently treated to strict blood pressure targets and the use of RAAS inhibitors was variable. In addition, data regarding adverse events were often not systematically collected.

In an early randomized controlled trial by Pozzi et al., treatment with corticosteroids resulted in significantly reduced proteinuria and prevented progression to ESKD over a 10-year follow-up period [6]. The treatment regimen included pulsed IV methylprednisolone at induction, and at months 2 and 4, with alternate day oral prednisolone for 6 months. This would be expected to be associated with significant toxicity, yet only one significant adverse event of steroid-induced diabetes mellitus was recorded. In keeping with standard of care at the time, RAAS blockade use was low and the achieved blood pressure was higher than current treatment targets. Subsequent studies by Manno et al. and Lv et al. also reported a beneficial effect from a 6-month course of corticosteroids in high-risk patients, defined by having proteinuria > 1 g/day [7,8]. However, temporary discontinuation of RAAS blockade was mandated before re-introduction at baseline in both trials, and it is possible that a number of included patients would have responded to optimized RAAS blockade and supportive care alone.

Two recent RCTs have addressed these points, the STOP-IgAN and the Therapeutic Evaluation of Steroids in IgA Nephropathy Global (TESTING) studies, by including a run-in period where supportive care could be optimized. STOP-IgAN, conducted in Germany, compared intensive supportive care to immunosuppressive therapy (corticosteroids if estimated glomerular filtration rate (eGFR) was ≥ 60 mL/min/1.73m^2, or cyclophosphamide followed by azathioprine with prednisolone if eGFR was between 30–59 mL/min/1.73m^2) in patients at high risk of progressive kidney disease [3]. Although a reduction in proteinuria was observed in the immunosuppressed group compared to supportive care alone, there was no difference in eGFR decline between the groups, and more episodes of infection (with one fatal pneumonia) and other adverse events, including malignancy, impaired glucose tolerance and weight gain, occurred in those receiving immunosuppression. In a follow-up study, no significant difference in renal outcomes was observed between the immunosuppressed and supportive care groups at a median of 7.4 years follow-up [5]. The TESTING trial, conducted mainly in centers in China, of oral methylprednisolone vs. placebo in IgAN patients at high risk of progression was stopped early due to an excess of serious adverse events in the methylprednisolone group, including one fatal case of *Pneumocystis jirovecii*, although interestingly, there was a significant reduction in those reaching the composite renal outcome (40% reduction in eGFR, ESKD, or death due to renal failure) in this group [9]. Important differences between these two RCTs have been discussed in detail previously [10].

Currently, the risk-benefit ratio for corticosteroids in the treatment of IgAN remains uncertain, and significant questions remain regarding their optimum dose and duration, and patient selection. The TESTING low-dose study will assess whether a lower dose of methylprednisolone together with *Pneumocystis jirovecii* prophylaxis can be beneficial while avoiding the rate of serious adverse events observed in the earlier trial, and this is due to be reported in 2023 (ClinicalTrials.gov Identifier: NCT01560052). It should also be noted that corticosteroids are typically pursued as part of treatment in the rare circumstances where IgAN is associated with nephrotic syndrome, or with rapidly progressive glomerulonephritis. Both scenarios have been excluded from clinical trials addressing the benefit of steroids in the treatment of IgAN.

Forthcoming Kidney Disease: Improving Global Outcomes (KDIGO) guidelines emphasize that although patients with IgAN who have proteinuria >1 g/day despite 90 days of optimized supportive care can be considered for corticosteroid therapy, their clinical benefit is not established, and that it is much preferred that such patients be offered an opportunity to take part in a therapeutic clinical trial.

4. Clinical Trial Design in IgAN

There has been a welcomed increase in the number of clinical trials being performed in IgAN over the past decade. However, a number of difficulties are inherent to studying this disease. Firstly, it should be recognized that IgAN may not be a single disease, but instead may represent a common histological endpoint towards which distinct pathogenic mechanisms may contribute [11]. Its clinical presentation and rate of progression is highly variable between individuals, with evidence that these factors vary according to geographical location and ethnicity. The implication of this is that findings from trials conducted in certain populations may not be applicable to others. Secondly, in most cases, IgAN is a slowly progressive disease, where the traditional renal endpoints of death, dialysis, or doubling of serum creatinine may take many years to occur. This has previously meant that clinical trials have been prohibitively expensive and difficult to conduct, especially as IgAN is a rare disease. Incorporation of a 'pre-' and 'post-treatment' kidney biopsy in clinical trials can yield significant mechanistic insights into a certain drug's effectiveness, although this is an invasive procedure that is associated with a small risk of complications, and would not be accepted by all participants. Recent data have demonstrated that proteinuria reduction and the rate of change/slope of eGFR decline are accurate surrogate endpoints for these renal outcomes [12,13]. Trial-level analysis of 13 controlled trials in IgAN by a Kidney Health Initiative workgroup demonstrated an association between proteinuria reduction and effects on a composite of time to doubling of serum creatinine, ESKD or death, that was independent of the therapeutic intervention used [13]. These endpoints have recently been approved by the US Food and Drug Administration (FDA) for use in clinical trials in IgAN, generating further interest in drug development in this field.

In the following sections, we will describe the systems in IgAN that are affected, with a view to discussing interventional treatment strategies targeting these areas.

5. The Gut Mucosal Immune system and IgAN

There is an increasing recognition of the role of the gut-associated lymphoid tissue (GALT), particularly the Peyer's patches, in the generation of the pathogenic Gd-IgA1 molecules [14–17]. Gd-IgA1 enters the systemic circulation either via direct passage and/or displacement of GALT-derived B cells to systemic sites, including the bone marrow, secondary to an error in the homing mechanism, and eventually leads to secretion of mucosal-type Gd-IgA1 into the bloodstream (Figure 1) [18]. A novel, oral, targeted-release formulation (TRF) of the glucocorticoid, budesonide (NEFECON®) was designed to deliver the drug to the distal ileum where the highest concentration of mucosal Peyer's patches reside to reduce Gd-IgA1 release into the circulation [19–21] (Table 1). An exploratory phase IIa trial of TRF-budesonide in 16 IgAN patients revealed a statistically significant reduction in proteinuria and was also well tolerated [22]. Subsequently, the Targeted-Release Budesonide Versus Placebo in Patients with IgAN (NEFIGAN) trial compared TRF-budesonide (n = 100) with placebo (n = 50) in a phase IIb randomized, controlled, double-blind clinical trial [21]. Enrolled IgAN patients had persistent proteinuria, defined by a urine protein-to-creatinine ratio (UPCR) > 0.5 g/g or proteinuria or at least 0.75 g/day, despite optimal RAAS blockade. The study consisted of a 6-month run-in, 9-month treatment phase, and 3 months of follow-up. Two doses of TRF-budesonide (16 mg/day; 8 mg/day) were compared to placebo. The baseline proteinuria was 1.2 g/day (interquartile range: 0.9–2 g/day), and the baseline eGFR was 78 ± 5 mL/min/1.73m^2. The study achieved its primary end point of mean change in proteinuria with a UPCR reduction by an average of 24.4% (-0.212 g/g) in the combined treatment arms versus an increase by 2.7% ($+0.024$ g/g) in the placebo arm (geometric least-square mean change in UPCR vs. placebo 0.74; 95% CI 0.59-0.94; p = 0.006). Importantly, this effect was sustained throughout the follow-up period of the investigational product. The secondary endpoint of change in eGFR was also achieved due to a decrease by 9.8% (p = 0.001) in the placebo group over the study timeframe which was somewhat surprising. No serious adverse events, including infections, were reported in the treatment group [21]. The safety profile of TRF-budesonide is proposed to be superior to high dose systemic corticosteroid therapy given its extensive first pass metabolism with <10% of budesonide entering the systemic circulation [23].

Table 1. Novel Therapies for Treatment of Primary IgA Nephropathy.

Agent	Mechanism of Action	Clinical Trial Design	Clinical Outcomes (Reported/Being Investigated)
A. Targeting the Gut Mucosal Immune System			
TRF Budesonide	Corticosteroid formulation acts on distal ileum targeting B-cells in mucosal lymphoid tissue	Randomized, double-blind, placebo-controlled Phase II clinical trial (NEFIGAN)—*completed* * NCT01738035	• Reduction in proteinuria • No change in eGFR
		Randomized, double-blind, placebo-controlled Phase III clinical trial (NefIgArd)—*recruiting* * NCT03643965	• Effect on proteinuria • Effect on eGFR
Fecal microbiota transplantation	Restoration of intestinal microecological balance	Open-Label Phase II clinical trial—*recruiting* * NCT03633864	• Effect on proteinuria

Table 1. Cont.

Agent	Mechanism of Action	Clinical Trial Design	Clinical Outcomes (Reported/Being Investigated)
		B. Targeting B-cells	
Bortezomib	Semi-selective plasma cell proteasome inhibitor	Open-label Phase IV clinical trial—*completed* * NCT01103778	• Reduction in proteinuria only in patients with T0 MEST-C score
Fostamatinib	Oral spleen tyrosine kinase inhibitor	Randomized, double-blind, placebo-controlled Phase II clinical trial—*completed* * NCT02112838	• Non-significant reduction in proteinuria • No change in eGFR
Atacicept	Blocks downstream effects of BAFF and APRIL	Randomized, double-blind, placebo-controlled Phase II clinical trial—*terminated (slow enrollment)* * NCT02808429	• Dose-dependent reduction in proteinuria • Dose-dependent reduction in immunoglobulin (particularly Gd-IgA1) levels • No change in eGFR
		Randomized, double-blind, placebo-controlled Phase II clinical trial (ORIGIN)—*not yet recruiting* * NCT04716231	• Effect on proteinuria • Effect on eGFR
Blisibimod	Selective BAFF antagonist	Randomized, double-blind, placebo-controlled Phase II/III clinical trial—*completed* * NCT02062684	• Effect on proteinuria – data analysis pending
VIS649	Monoclonal antibody against APRIL	Randomized, double-blind, placebo-controlled Phase II clinical trial (enVISion)—*recruiting* * NCT04287985	• Effect on proteinuria • Adverse events
BION-1301	Monoclonal antibody against APRIL	Open-label, non-randomized Phase II Clinical trial—*recruiting*	• Adverse events • Effect on proteinuria • Effect on eGFR
Hydroxychloroquine	Immunomodulator, inhibits mucosal and intrarenal Toll-like receptor signaling	Randomized, double-blind, placebo-controlled Phase II clinical trial—*completed* * NCT02942381	• Reduction in proteinuria • No change in eGFR
		C. Complement System Inhibitors	
Ravulizumab	Humanized monoclonal antibody against C5	Randomized, double blind, placebo-controlled Phase II clinical trial—*recruiting* * NCT04564339	• Effect on proteinuria • Effect on eGFR
Avacopan (CCX168)	C5a receptor blocker	Open-label Phase II clinical trial—*completed* * NCT02384317	• Reduction in proteinuria
Cemdisiran	Small-interfering RNA inhibits synthesis of C5	Randomized, double-blind, placebo-controlled Phase II clinical trial—*recruiting* * NCT03841448	• Effect on proteinuria

Table 1. Cont.

Pegcetacoplan (APL-2)	Peptide inhibitor of C3	Open-Label Phase II clinical trial—*active; not recruiting* * NCT03453619	• Effect on proteinuria
Iptacopan (LNP023)	Oral inhibitor of complement factor B	Randomized, double blind, placebo-controlled Phase II clinical trial—*active, not recruiting* * NCT03373461	• Effect on proteinuria
		Randomized, double blind, parallel-group, placebo-controlled Phase III clinical trial (APPLAUSE-IgAN) —*recruiting* * NCT04578834	• Effect on proteinuria • Effect on eGFR
IONIS-FB-LRx	Anti-sense inhibitor of complement factor B	Open-Label Phase II clinical trial—*recruiting* * NCT04014335	• Effect on proteinuria
Narsoplimab (OMS721)	Monoclonal antibody against MASP-2	Open-Label Phase II clinical trial—*recruiting* * NCT02682407	• Adverse events • Effect on serum and urine complement levels • Effect on proteinuria
		Randomized, double-blind, placebo-controlled Phase III clinical trial (ARTEMIS-IGAN)—*recruiting* * NCT03608033	• Effect on proteinuria
D. Non-Immune Modulators			
Sparsentan	Selective antagonist of angiotensin II receptor and endothelin A receptor	Open-label Phase II clinical trial (SPARTAN)—*recruiting* * NCT04663204	• Effect on proteinuria
		Randomized, double-blind, parallel-group, active-control Phase III clinical trial (PROTECT)—*recruiting* * NCT03762850	• Effect on proteinuria
Atrasentan	Selective antagonist of endothelin A receptor	Open-label Phase II clinical trial (AFFINITY)—*recruiting* * NCT04573920	• Effect on proteinuria
		Randomized, double-blind, placebo-controlled Phase III clinical trial (ALIGN)—*recruiting* * NCT04573478	• Effect on proteinuria
Bardoxolone methyl	Semi-synthetic triterpenoid, activator of Nrf2 pathway, inhibitor of NF-kB pathway	Non-randomized, open-label, parallel-assignment Phase II clinical trial (PHOENIX)—*completed* * NCT03366337	• Improvement in eGFR • No serious treatment related adverse events

TRF: Targeted Release Formulation; eGFR: estimated glomerular filtration rate; BAFF: B-cell Activating Factor; APRIL: A PRoliferation-Inducing Ligand; Gd-IgA1: Galactose-deficient IgA1; RNA: Ribonucleic acid; MASP-2: Mannan-binding lectin-associated serine protease-2; Nrf2: Nuclear factor erythroid 2-related factor 2; NF-kB: nuclear-factor kappa-light-chain-enhancer of activated B-cells. * shows ClinicalTrials.gov Identifier. Data from www.clinicaltrials.gov (accessed on 28 April 2021).

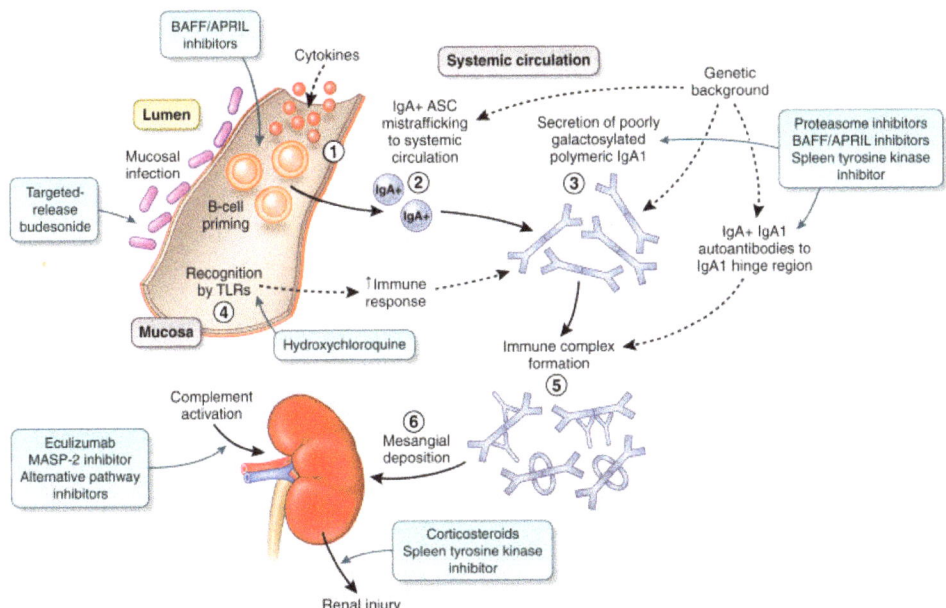

Figure 1. Proposed pathogenesis of IgAN and novel treatment strategies. (**1**) Mucosal infection primes naïve B cells to class switch to become IgA⁺ antibody secreting cells (ASCs) through T cell-dependent (cytokine mediated) and T cell-independent (Toll-like receptor (TLR) ligation) pathways. (**2**) Some IgA⁺ ASC mis-home to the systemic compartment during lymphocyte trafficking. (**3**) Displaced IgA⁺ ASCs take up residence in systemic sites and secrete normal 'mucosal-type' poorly galactosylated (galactose deficient) and polymeric IgA1 into the systemic circulation. (**4**) IgA1 secretion by displaced mucosal ASC is augmented by TLR ligation from mucosal-derived pathogen-associated molecular patterns, which have entered the systemic compartment. (**5**) IgA1 immune complexes form in the systemic circulation. Poorly galactosylated polymeric IgA1 molecules are the substrate for immune complex formation and combine with IgG and IgA autoantibodies reactive to exposed neoepitopes in the poorly galactosylated IgA1 hinge region. (**6**) IgA1 immune complexes deposit in the mesangium through a combination of mesangial trapping and increased affinity of poorly galactosylated IgA1 for extracellular matrix components. Immune complex deposition triggers a series of downstream pathways leading to glomerular injury and tubulointerstitial scarring. APRIL, a proliferation-inducing ligand; BAFF, B cell activating factor; MASP-2, mannan-binding lectin-associated serine protease-2. Reprinted from ref. [10], with permission from Elsevier.

The promising results of the NEFIGAN trial [21] led to the design of the ongoing phase III Efficacy and Safety of TRF-budesonide in Patients With Primary IgA Nephropathy (NefIgArd) study (ClinicalTrials.gov Identifier: NCT03643965). This multi-national, randomized, double-blind, placebo-controlled, phase III clinical trial aims to evaluate the efficacy, safety, and tolerability of TRF-budesonide 16 mg/day formulation in the management of patients with biopsy-proven primary IgAN at risk of progressing to end-stage kidney disease (ESKD), despite maximum tolerated RAAS blockade. Part A of the trial encompasses a 9-month treatment and a 3-month follow-up period. Part B comprises a 12-month observation period. The primary goal of Part A is to assess the effect of TRF-budesonide 16 mg/day on 24-h UPCR values over 9 months when compared to placebo. The primary objective of Part B is to assess the effect of the investigational drug on kidney function. The study aims to recruit 360 IgAN patients across 20 countries and is projected to have achieved its recruitment goal in March 2021. Interim results of the NefIgArd trial have confirmed the earlier phase IIb findings of the NEFIGAN trial [24]. The primary endpoint analysis, that included 199 patients with primary IgAN, showed a 31% mean reduction in 24-h UPCR in the TRF-budesonide 16 mg/day arm versus baseline, with placebo showing a 5% mean reduction versus baseline, resulting in a 27% mean reduction in 24-h UPCR at 9 months

(p = 0.0005) of the TRF-budesonide 16 mg/day arm versus placebo. The secondary endpoint data on eGFR showed a treatment benefit of 7% versus placebo at 9 months, reflecting stabilization in the treatment arm and a 7% decline in eGFR in the placebo arm (p = 0.0029). This reflected an absolute decline in eGFR of 4.04 mL/min/1.73m^2 in the placebo group over 9 months compared to a 0.17 mL/min/1.73m^2 eGFR decline in the treatment group. TRF-budesonide was generally well-tolerated [24].

6. Targeting B Cells

There is clear evidence that IgAN is an autoimmune disease. Production of Gd-IgA1 and glycan-specific IgG and IgA autoantibodies against Gd-IgA1 lead to the formation of IgA-containing immune complexes that deposit within the mesangium, causing subsequent effects on mesangial cells, podocytes and proximal tubular cells that drive glomerular and tubulointerstitial inflammation and fibrosis. Glycan-specific IgG autoantibodies found at increased levels in IgAN correlate with the prognosis and can be detected within mesangial deposits [25–27]. Targeting B cells in IgAN is therefore an attractive therapeutic strategy.

Effective B cell maturation and survival is dependent on BAFF (B cell activating factor) and APRIL (a proliferation inducing ligand). BAFF and APRIL bind to the tumor necrosis factor (TNF) superfamily receptors, BCMA (B cell maturation antigen), TACI (Transmembrane activator and calcium-modulating cyclophilin ligand interactor) and BAFF-R (BAFF-receptor).

There are several lines of evidence that this system plays an important role in IgAN. Transgenic mice that overexpress BAFF develop a hyper-IgA syndrome, and an IgAN-like renal phenotype [28,29]. Interestingly, this was dependent on the presence of gut commensal bacteria, presumably reflecting mucosal B cell activation. In vitro, tonsillar mononuclear cells, part of the mucosa-associated lymphoid tissue of Waldeyer's ring, from patients with IgAN exposed to the bacterial motif CpG-oligodeoxynucleotides produced increased levels of BAFF and IgA [30]. This production was blocked by the inhibition of BAFF. Levels of serum BAFF are increased in IgAN, and correlate with disease severity, as measured by renal histology (increased mesangial hypercellularity, segmental glomerulosclerosis, and tubular atrophy/interstitial fibrosis) and serum creatinine at the time of renal biopsy [31]. APRIL also plays an important role in B cell maturation and survival, and is involved in the generation of IgA-secreting plasma cells. Tonsillar APRIL and Toll-like receptor (TLR) 9 levels have been shown to be increased in IgAN, and TLR-9 stimulation increased APRIL expression by tonsillar B cells [32]. In a study of patients with IgAN, serum levels of APRIL were associated with increased Gd-IgA1 and worse clinical presentation [33]. Genome-wide associated studies have identified *TNFSF13* as a risk allele for IgAN, and this encodes for APRIL [34]. This risk variant was also associated with higher serum levels of IgA in patients with IgAN. In a recent study, APRIL inhibition reduced serum IgA and immune complex levels, and reduced glomerular IgA deposition in the ddY mouse model of IgAN [35].

There has consequently been great interest in targeting these pathways in IgAN. Blisibimod is a selective BAFF inhibitor and has been tested in a phase II trial in IgAN. Interim analysis of results suggests that subcutaneous blisibimod may reduce proteinuria in IgAN and the full results of this trial are awaited (ClinicalTrials.gov Identifier: NCT02062684). Atacicept is a fully humanized fusion protein that contains the extracellular portion of TACI and inhibits both BAFF and APRIL signaling. Preliminary results from a Phase II trial suggest a dose-dependent effect on proteinuria levels [36]. This trial was terminated early due to slow recruitment, and further studies of atacicept in IgAN are planned. Studies of other inhibitors of BAFF and APRIL in IgAN are currently ongoing, including of VIS649, a humanised IgG2 monoclonal antibody that binds to and inhibits APRIL (ClinicalTrials.gov Identifier: NCT04287985), and BION1301, a humanized IgG4 monoclonal antibody, which is also directed against APRIL (ClinicalTrials.gov Identifier: NCT03945318).

Rituximab is a chimeric murine/human monoclonal antibody that targets the CD20 antigen expressed on the surface of pre-B and mature B lymphocytes, hence leading to

B cell lysis upon binding. In contrast to targeting BAFF and APRIL, a small open label randomized controlled trial of rituximab in patients with IgAN showed no effect on proteinuria reduction, renal function, and importantly on serum levels of Gd-IgA1 and glycan-specific IgG autoantibodies, implying that peripheral B cell depletion is not an effective strategy in the management of IgAN [37]. Therefore, other B cell populations not affected by rituximab, for example plasmablasts, plasma cells, or tissue-resident B cells may play an important role in IgAN. A small open-label pilot study of the plasma cell proteasome inhibitor bortezomib demonstrated a reduction in proteinuria in eight patients with IgAN [38], and further studies of other agents are planned to examine the effects of targeting these B cell populations more specifically.

B cells express a number of TLRs, which represent an important part of the early innate immune response to invading microbial pathogens, by recognition of DAMPs (danger-associated molecular patterns) and PAMPs (pathogen-associated molecular patterns). Several TLRs, specifically -4, -9 and -10, have been implicated in the pathogenesis of IgAN [39]. Levels of TLR-4 gene expression were raised in B cells from children with IgAN and IgA vasculitis (IgAV) compared to healthy subjects [40]. Exposure to environmental antigens resulted in a higher TLR-9 gene expression and more severe renal injury in a mouse model of IgAN [41]. A small trial of hydroxychloroquine which inhibits TLR-9, and to a lesser extent TLR-7 and TLR-8, has been conducted in Chinese patients with IgAN, and was associated with a reduction in proteinuria [42]. Further larger studies in more diverse patient populations are required to see if this result can be validated.

Spleen tyrosine kinase (Syk) has a well-established role in mediating signalling from immunoreceptors, including the B cell receptor and immunoglobulin Fc receptors, and is expressed by many cell types, including B cells, myeloid cells, and renal mesangial and tubular cells. Glomerular expression of Syk has been shown to be increased in IgAN and correlates with serum creatinine levels at the time of performing a renal biopsy [43]. In vitro, pro-inflammatory cytokine release by mesangial cells in response to IgA1 from patients with IgAN is inhibited by gene silencing of Syk, or by the Syk inhibitor fostamatinib [44]. A Phase II trial of fostamatinib in IgAN (SIGN: Syk Inhibition in IgAN) was recently completed. Interim results indicated a dose-dependent reduction in proteinuria in those with urine protein excretion >1 g/day, but this did not reach statistical significance [45]. The full results from this trial are awaited.

7. Complement System Inhibitors

There is mounting clinical, biochemical, and genetic evidence regarding the pivotal role of the complement cascade in the pathogenesis, disease onset, and progression of IgAN [46–52]. Complement (C) component C3 is co-localized with glomerular IgA in >90% of biopsies with IgAN [53]. The presence of C3 distinguishes IgAN from subclinical glomerular IgA deposition. Immunohistochemical findings of C3, C4, C4d [54], properdin, mannose binding lectin (MBL) [55], and terminal complement complex (C5b-9) deposits [56] in the mesangium of IgAN biopsy samples, and the typical absence of C1q support the involvement of the alternative and lectin pathways, rather than the classical pathway [16,57–59]. Evidence of complement activation in biopsies is associated with disease activity and portends a worse renal prognosis [60–62]. C5a is a potent local inflammatory mediator, especially via its chemoattractant and neutrophilic activating properties, and its presence in the kidney correlates with histological severity and proteinuria in IgAN [63].

Serum complement levels, such as C3 and C4, are typically normal, and in some IgAN patients, even elevated [64], as are complement components C1q and C2-C9 [64–68]. Nonetheless, the utility of complement proteins in the circulation as prognostic biomarkers in IgAN is still under investigation [52,61]. The elevated serum IgA:C3 ratio is typically found in IgAN patients and is a good diagnostic marker to distinguish IgAN from other glomerular diseases [69]. Studies suggest that the serum IgA:C3 ratio can also be utilized as a prognostic marker, with higher values being associated with more severe disease histology [70] and worse clinical outcomes including proteinuria, hematuria, and elevated serum creatinine levels [71]. A Korean study involving 343 patients with IgAN showed that a decreased serum C3 level (<90 mg/dL) predicted a worse outcome, which was defined by a higher rate of doubling of serum creatinine and progression to ESKD [72]. C3 is also present in IgA1-containing circulating immune complexes of patients with IgAN [73]. In a retrospective study involving 1356 Chinese IgAN patients, serum C4 levels correlated positively with proteinuria and negatively with eGFR. Furthermore, higher serum C4 levels correlated with worse tubulointerstitial injury, global sclerosis, and crescents on kidney biopsy [74]. Serum C4 levels may be an independent risk factor for IgAN progression.

The deletion of complement factor H-related (*CFHR*) genes 1 and 3 has been identified as being protective against IgAN in genome-wide association studies [49,75,76]. Urinary excretion of complement components has also been proposed as a biomarker of the activity of IgAN. Urinary levels of Factor H and soluble C5b-9 correlated positively with proteinuria, a rise in serum creatinine levels, interstitial fibrosis, and percentage of global glomerular sclerosis, whereas urinary properdin levels were associated with only proteinuria. The urinary excretion of these biomarkers was higher in IgAN patients when compared to healthy controls [77]. Another study demonstrated increased urinary Factor H excretion in IgAN patients with more severe histologic lesions [78]. These findings have kindled a significant interest in targeting complement pathways in the management of IgAN, and ongoing clinical trials are testing several complement inhibitors using monoclonal antibodies, small molecules, and short peptides that hinder protein-complex formation and/or enzymatic reactions. However, the mechanisms linking complement activation, and subsequent levels of intact and active complement fragments, need to be further characterized to fully understand the role of the complement system in the pathogenesis, prognostic implications, and targeted therapeutics for IgAN.

Eculizumab is a humanized, recombinant, monoclonal antibody that selectively inhibits the cleavage of C5 by C5 convertase (by binding to C5 at the level of macroglobulin domain 7), thereby preventing the formation and release of the pro-inflammatory C5a and C5b components, and thereby the downstream formation of the C5b-9 membrane attack complex (MAC). Eculizumab therapy has found mixed clinical success in the management of IgAN, especially as a rescue agent in few case reports. The initial use of Eculizumab was reported from Sweden wherein a 16-year-old white male with biopsy-proven crescentic IgAN had not responded to corticosteroid and mycophenolate mofetil use, but stabilized with eculizumab treatment, although its therapeutic effects were short lived [79]. Similarly, the use of eculizumab in another 16-year-old male with crescentic IgAN resulted in transient improvement in kidney function after failure of a combination regimen consisting of corticosteroids, cyclophosphamide, and plasma exchange [80]. Eculizumab was also used as a rescue therapy in a 28-year-old male with recurrence of crescentic IgAN post kidney-transplantation but failed to salvage the allograft. It is worth mentioning that in that case, eculizumab therapy was initiated after the start of renal replacement therapy and hence it is possible that its administration was too late in the disease course [81]. Ravulizumab is a long-acting, humanized, recombinant, monoclonal antibody against C5 predicted to have similar effects to Eculizumab, that is currently being tested in a phase II clinical trial in the treatment of IgAN (ClinicalTrials.gov Identifier: NCT04564339).

C5a binds to the membrane-associated C5a receptor (C5aR) via a C-terminal C5a pentapeptide. Selectively targeting C5a offers an opportunity to dampen the local inflammation which plays a vital role in the progression of IgAN [63]. Avacopan (CCX168), a small molecule C5aR blocker, exerts its effect by binding to the C5aR surface, thereby impeding C5a binding via allosteric modulation of the C5a-binding pocket. It was evaluated in an open-label phase II trial involving seven IgAN patients (ClinicalTrials.gov Identifier: NCT02384317). At the end of 12 weeks, there was a reduction in proteinuria in six patients and UPCR decreased to <1 g/g in three patients [82]. Because avacopan does not block the downstream formation of C5b and C5b-9 MAC, as occurs with C5 inhibitors like eculizumab and ravulizumab, it has been postulated that the risk for infections with encapsulated organisms, especially belonging to the *Neisserial* species, is reduced with avacopan use. Larger studies with longer follow-up periods are warranted to confirm the efficacy of C5a inhibitors in IgAN as well as their safety.

Cemdisiran (ALN-CC5) is a synthetic, small interfering RNA (RNAi) that was designed to suppress C5 production in the liver, which can potentially limit terminal complement pathway activation and subsequent inflammation [52]. A phase II, randomized, placebo-controlled clinical trial (ClinicalTrials.gov Identifier: NCT03841448) is underway that aims to evaluate the efficacy and safety of cemdisiran in IgAN patients with persistent proteinuria >1 g/day despite optimal conservative management.

While eculizumab, ravulizumab, avacopan, and cemdisiran may be non-specific inhibitors of the distal common complement pathway, other pharmacological complement directed therapies target a specific pathway more proximally. The C3 convertase catalyzes the cleavage of C3 into C3a and C3b. This is one of the most important steps in the complement cascade and amplifies activation from the classic, alternative, and lectin pathways. The smaller, soluble C3a fragment is an anaphylatoxin that mediates inflammation. The larger subunit C3b is a highly unstable molecule and is an opsonin that covalently binds surfaces such as adjacent pathogenic cells via a reactive thioester bond, with subsequent cell phagocytosis. C3b binding can lead to C5 convertase formation by the association of C3b with C4b2a (classical and lectin complement pathways) or with C3bBb (the product of cleavage from the alternative pathway) [52,83,84]. Compstatin, a cyclic tridecapeptide; and pegcetacoplan (APL-2), a pegylated derivative of compstatin, bind to C3 and prevent its cleavage to C3a and C3b by C3 convertase [52,85]. Pegcetacoplan (APL-2) is currently being evaluated in a phase II clinical trial as a treatment option for patients with IgAN, lupus nephritis, primary membranous nephropathy or C3 glomerulopathy (ClinicalTrials.gov Identifier: NCT03453619).

The alternative complement pathway plays an important role in the essential amplification mechanism for the activation of the classical and lectin complement pathways, resulting in enhanced opsonization and generation of the terminal lytic pathway. The two proteases Factor B and Factor D play a paramount role in this tightly regulated amplification process [52,85]. Selective small-molecule reversible inhibitors of Factors B and D were developed to efficiently impede alternative complement pathway activation. Iptacopan (LNP023) is a first in class oral small molecule Factor B inhibitor. Results from a recently completed phase II clinical trial in the management of IgAN are awaited, and a phase III trial (APPLAUSE-IgAN) is currently recruiting (ClinicalTrials.gov Identifier: NCT04578834).

Mannose-binding lectin associated serine protease 2 (MASP-2) is an important component of the lectin pathway that, with MASP-1, cleaves C4 and C2 into active fragments. Thus MASP-2 triggers formation of the C3 convertase and ensuing subsequential inflammatory effects. Targeting MASP-2 inhibition can thereby curtail glomerular lectin pathway activation whilst still enabling C3 convertase to be generated via the classical and alternative pathways. Narsoplimab (OMS721) is a humanized monoclonal antibody selectively targeting MASP-2 [52,85]. In functional assays, it has shown no demonstrable effect on the classical or alternative complement pathways. In a phase II, multicenter, clinical trial, IgAN patients with proteinuria >1 g/day despite maximal tolerated RAAS blockade and baseline eGFR > 30 mL/min/1.73m^2 were enrolled into two sub-studies based on whether they were corticosteroid-dependent or -independent at baseline. Interim analysis of both groups revealed the drug was safe, well-tolerated, and decreased proteinuria with a stable eGFR [86]. Based on this preliminary data, a randomized, double-blind, placebo-controlled, phase III clinical trial (ARTEMIS-IGAN) is underway assessing the efficacy and safety of narsoplimab in IgAN patients with persistent proteinuria >1 g/day (ClinicalTrials.gov Identifier: NCT03608033). Selvaskandan et al. reported the first case of narsoplimab use in IgA vasculitis with nephritis (IgAV-N), a condition whose pathologic features are indistinguishable from those of IgAN [87–90], presenting as a rapidly progressive glomerulonephritis with crescentic features despite the use of corticosteroids in a 21-year-old female with normal baseline serum creatinine. The patient declined cyclophosphamide and was offered narsoplimab on a compassionate use basis. The patient subsequently received 12 consecutive weekly infusions of narsoplimab (4 mg/kg) which she tolerated well without any adverse events. Her kidney function stabilized, and she successfully received a deceased-donor kidney transplant within 72 h after completing the 12th infusion of narsoplimab. There was a sustained reduction in lectin pathway activity, while classical complement pathway activity and serum IgA levels remained within the normal range and were unaffected by narsoplimab therapy. Alternate complement pathway activity was not tested in this case. Interestingly, there were no significant effects on proteinuria while on narsoplimab treatment [91].

Apart from evaluating the efficacy of various inhibitors of the complement cascade, risks associated with their usage, particularly infections, need to be carefully assessed. There is a paucity of available data regarding the safety of complement therapy inhibitors. The risk of infection depends on the level of complement pathway inhibition. C5 inhibitors primarily increase the risk of *Neisseria spp.* infections given that they block the formation of C5b and C5b-9 MAC [92]. Eculizumab use considerably elevates the risk of acquiring infections with encapsulated organisms, particularly meningococcal infections (nearly 2000-fold compared to the general population). It is therefore recommended that patients considering treatment with eculizumab or ravulizumab receive meningococcal vaccination, including the serogroups A,C,Y and W-135 conjugate vaccine and serogroup B vaccine, at least 2 weeks prior to start of therapy [93]. Alternatively, if urgent treatment is needed, patients should be treated prophylactically with ciprofloxacin until the vaccination is received [94]. C3 inhibitors are more likely to confer a more expansive infectious susceptibility necessitating vaccination against several encapsulated organisms. Nonetheless, even C3 inhibitors like compstatin do not completely dampen complement-mediated immune effects against microbes given that even reticent residual complement activity confers protection [95]. Other potential safety concerns stem from the fact that certain deficiencies of the classical complement pathway escalate the risk of developing systemic lupus erythematosus, thereby raising the potential for promoting autoimmunity with complement inhibition [95].

8. Non-immune Modulators

8.1. Endothelin Receptor Antagonists

Endothelin-1 (ET-1) exerts several physiological effects in the kidneys, including the regulation of water and sodium homeostasis. ET-1 is a growth factor for mesangial cells and has been implicated in podocyte damage, proteinuria, fibrosis, and progression of chronic kidney disease (CKD) [96]. Furthermore, urinary excretion of ET-1 correlates with the severity of kidney disease [97]. The ET-1 system is complex, consisting of a converting enzyme and two active receptors: the endothelin-A receptor (ETA-R) and endothelin-B receptor (ETB-R) [98]. The activation of the ETA-R mainly located in vascular smooth muscle cells induce extremely potent vasoconstriction, cellular proliferation, endothelial dysfunction, insulin resistance, inflammation, and fibrosis. On the other hand, ETB-Rs are mainly expressed in the vascular endothelium, and induce vasodilatation via nitric oxide and prostanoid release and aid in natriuresis [98,99]. Expression of ET-1 and ETB-R, but not the ETA-R was observed in IgAN patients with high grade proteinuria providing key evidence that activation of the endothelin system in podocytes and renal tubular cells may contribute to urinary protein loss in IgAN [100]. ET-1 expression in podocytes, and polymorphisms of the ET-1 gene have been associated with IgAN disease progression, confirmed via molecular profiling studies [101,102]. A specific ET-receptor antagonist (FR 139317) was able to suppress the development of histologic lesions and proteinuria in ddY mice with IgAN [103]. Sparsentan, a dual inhibitor of the angiotensin II type 1 (AT1) receptor and ETA-R that demonstrated significant reduction in proteinuria compared to irbesartan in patients with focal segmental glomerulosclerosis (FSGS) [104] is currently being tested in the phase III PROTECT trial (ClinicalTrials.gov Identifier: NCT03762850) evaluating its long-term renoprotective potential in IgAN. Another phase III trial (ALIGN) is evaluating the effect of Atrasentan, a selective antagonist of the ETA-R, on proteinuria reduction in IgAN patients (ClinicalTrials.gov Identifier: NCT04573478).

8.2. Bardoxolone Methyl

Activation of nuclear factor erythroid 2-related factor 2 (Nrf2) and Kelch-like ECH-associated protein 1 (KEAP1) pathways by bardoxolone methyl results in the downregulation of the main proinflammatory transcription factor nuclear-factor kappa-light-chain-enhancer of activated B cells (NF-kB) and activation of certain antioxidative pathways [105]. In the IgAN cohort of phase II PHOENIX clinical study (ClinicalTrials.gov Identifier: NCT03366337), patients treated with bardoxolone experienced a temporary increase in eGFR of 8 mL/min/1.73m^2 ($n = 26$, $p < 0.0001$) at week 12 compared to baseline. Historical eGFR data were available for 23 of these patients, which demonstrated that their kidney function was declining at an average annual rate of 1.2 mL/min/1.73m^2 prior to study initiation [106]. No follow-up studies testing the benefit of bardoxolone in IgAN have been initiated so far to substantiate these preliminary results.

8.3. Sodium-Glucose Cotransporter 2 Inhibitors (SGLT2i)

SGLT2i are a novel class of medications recently introduced for the treatment of diabetes mellitus that exert their glucose lowering effect by inhibiting glucose entry into the proximal renal tubular cells through the SGLT2 co-transporter, thereby leading to enhanced glycosuria. A number of recent studies in patients with T2DM have demonstrated that SGLT2i wielded kidney protective effects independent of their antiglycemic effects [107–109]. The DAPA-CKD study enrolled 4304 CKD patients with an eGFR of 25–75 mL/min/1.73m^2 and albuminuria of 200–5000 mg/g who were randomized to receive the SGLT2i dapagliflozin either 10 mg/day or placebo. Participants had a mean age of 62 years with a mean baseline eGFR of 43.1 mL/min/1.73m^2 and a median baseline albuminuria of 949 mg/g. 68% of them had T2DM. The cause of CKD was ischemic/hypertensive nephropathy in 16%, IgAN in 6% ($n = 270$; 38 with T2DM and 232 without T2DM) and FSGS in 3%. Diagnosis had been confirmed by kidney biopsy in 20% of patients. The majority (97%) were on RAAS blockade. The trial was stopped early for overwhelming efficacy. Dapagliflozin significantly reduced the risk of the primary combined endpoint of > 50% eGFR decline, onset of ESKD or renal or cardiovascular death (HR 0.61; 95% CI 0.51–0.72; $p < 0.001$). The benefit of dapagliflozin on the primary endpoint was consistent in patients with and without T2DM (HR 0.64 (95% CI 0.52–0.79) and 0.50 (95% CI 0.35–0.72), respectively; p for interaction = 0.024). This was also observed in patients with an eGFR < 45 or $\geq$ 45 mL/min/1.73m^2 and with albuminuria $\leq$ 1000 or > 1000 mg/g, i.e., in patients with different stages of CKD and different severity of albuminuria. There were no statistically significant differences in DAPA-CKD in the primary endpoint between diabetics and non-diabetics, however, the hazard ratio was 22% lower for non-diabetics. Thus, the kidney benefit afforded by dapagliflozin was at least as large in patients with non-diabetic kidney disease (including ischemic/hypertensive nephropathy, IgAN and FSGS, among others) as in diabetic kidney disease. Dapagliflozin was also found to be safe in patients with CKD in this study [110].

A pre-specified analysis of the DAPA-CKD trial looking at the effects of dapagliflozin on major adverse kidney events in IgAN patients was recently published [111]. Of 270 participants with IgAN (254 (94%) confirmed by previous biopsy), 137 were randomized to dapagliflozin 10 mg/day and 133 to placebo and followed for a median duration of 2.1 years. Mean age was 51.2 years; 67.4% were male; 58.9% were Asian; 14.1% had T2DM; mean eGFR was 43.8 $\pm$ 12.2 mL/min/1.73 m^2; and median urinary albumin-to-creatinine ratio (UACR) was 900 mg/g. Participants had similar baseline characteristics. The primary composite outcome of $\geq$ 50% eGFR decline, onset of ESKD or renal or cardiovascular death outcome occurred in six (4%) participants on dapagliflozin and 20 (15%) on placebo (HR 0.29; 95% CI 0.12-0.73; $p = 0.005$). The absolute risk difference was −10.7% (95% CI: −17.6, −3.7). Similar results were noted for the secondary kidney-specific outcome

[HR 0.24; 95% CI 0.09–0.65; $p = 0.002$]. Five participants (4%) in the dapagliflozin group and 16 (12%) in the placebo group developed ESKD during the trial [HR 0.30; 95% CI 0.11–0.83; $p = 0.014$]. Mean rates of eGFR decline with dapagliflozin and placebo were -3.5 and -4.7 mL/min/1.73m^2/year, respectively, resulting in a between-group difference of 1.2 mL/min/1.73m^2 per year (95% CI -0.12, 2.51). Dapagliflozin reduced UACR by 26% relative to placebo (95% CI: -0.37, -14; $p < 0.001$). Additionally, blood pressures were lower in patients randomized to dapagliflozin. Adverse events leading to study drug discontinuation were similar with dapagliflozin and placebo, and there were fewer serious adverse events with dapagliflozin. There were no cases of diabetic ketoacidosis or major hypoglycemia in IgAN participants receiving dapagliflozin. While all patients in this trial had to be on a stable dose of a RAAS inhibitor for at least 4 weeks, it is unclear from the data whether RAAS blockade was maximized, and therefore it is difficult to know how much further improvement could have been achieved by the optimization of the currently available treatment before the addition of dapagliflozin [112]. The ongoing EMPA-KIDNEY trial (ClinicalTrials.gov Identifier: NCT03594110) has recruited a larger number of CKD patients and will likely shed more light on the safety of SGLT2i in IgAN patients. SGLT2i need to be further assessed, ideally in a dedicated trial where they are tested in addition to optimized supportive care but may be a promising addition to the management of nondiabetic glomerular diseases, including IgAN, treatment armamentarium.

9. Discussion

IgAN is an autoimmune disease that appears to be driven by subtle dysregulations in the adaptive and innate immune systems which we have outlined. Given its vast heterogeneity in clinical presentation and prognosis between individuals and indeed geographical locations, IgAN is unlikely to represent a single disease, but rather a common histological endpoint towards which different paths can converge. Despite being described over 50 years ago, outcomes in IgAN have remained remarkably static over the past few decades. More recently however, significant advances have been made in the understanding of the disease pathogenesis, which has driven the development of new therapeutic strategies in a number of areas that we have described in this review. It is therefore likely that new treatments will be licensed for the treatment of IgAN within the next few years. It is hoped that advances in molecular techniques will allow the capability of targeting novel therapies to an individual's disease process at its various stages, with the ultimate aim of improving outcomes for those affected by this condition.

Author Contributions: Conceptualization, J.B and D.V.R.; writing—original draft preparation, C.K.C. and A.R.; writing—review and editing, J.B. and D.V.R. All authors have read and agreed to the published version of the manuscript.

Funding: Not applicable for this publication.

Institutional Review Board Statement: Not applicable.

Informed Consent Statement: Not applicable.

Data Availability Statement: Not applicable.

Conflicts of Interest: C.K.C. has received research grants from GlaxoSmithKline and Travere Therapeutics, and personal fees from Travere Therapeutics. A.R. has no conflicts of interest to declare. J.B. has received research grants from Argenx, Calliditas Therapeutics, Chinook Therapeutics, Galapagos NV, GlaxoSmithKline, Novartis and Travere Therapeutics, and is medical/scientific advisor to Alnylam Pharmaceuticals, Argenx, Astellas Pharma, BioCryst Pharmaceuticals, Calliditas Therapeutics, Chinook Therapeutics, Dimerix, Galapagos NV, Novartis, Omeros, Travere Therapeutics, UCB, Vera Therapeutics and Visterra. D.V.R. has received grant funding from Achilion Pharmaceuticals Inc., Reata Pharmaceuticals, Calliditas Therapeutics, Travere Therapeutics, Pfizer Inc., and Morphosys Pharmaceuticals. D.V.R. has received personal fees from Visterra, Novartis and Otsuka Pharmaceuticals, and holds equity in Reliant Glycosciences LLC.

References

1. D'Amico, G. Clinical Features and Natural History in Adults with IgA Nephropathy. *Am. J. Kidney Dis.* **1988**, *12*, 353–357. [CrossRef]
2. Chapter 10: Immunoglobulin A Nephropathy. *Kidney Int. Suppl.* **2012**, *2*, 209–217. [CrossRef]
3. Rauen, T.; Eitner, F.; Fitzner, C.; Sommerer, C.; Zeier, M.; Otte, B.; Panzer, U.; Peters, H.; Benck, U.; Mertens, P.R.; et al. Intensive Supportive Care plus Immunosuppression in IgA Nephropathy. *N. Engl. J. Med.* **2015**, *373*, 2225–2236. [CrossRef]
4. Reich, H.N.; Troyanov, S.; Scholey, J.W.; Cattran, D.C. Remission of Proteinuria Improves Prognosis in IgA Nephropathy. *J. Am. Soc. Nephrol.* **2007**, *18*, 3177–3183. [CrossRef] [PubMed]
5. Rauen, T.; Wied, S.; Fitzner, F.; Eitner, F.; Sommerer, C.; Zeier, M.; Otte, B.; Panzer, U.; Budde, K.; Benck, U.; et al. After Ten Years of Follow-up, No Difference between Supportive Care plus Immunosuppression and Supportive Care Alone in IgA Nephropathy. *Kidney Int.* **2020**, *98*, 1044–1052. [CrossRef] [PubMed]
6. Pozzi, C.; Bolasco, P.G.; Fogazzi, G.; Andrulli, S.; Altieri, P.; Ponticelli, C.; Locatelli, F. Corticosteroids in IgA Nephropathy: A Randomised Controlled Trial. *Lancet* **1999**, *353*, 883–887. [CrossRef]
7. Manno, C.; Torres, D.D.; Rossini, M.; Pesce, F.; Schena, F.P. Randomized Controlled Clinical Trial of Corticosteroids plus ACE-Inhibitors with Long-Term Follow-up in Proteinuric IgA Nephropathy. *Nephrol. Dial. Transpl.* **2009**, *24*, 3694–3701. [CrossRef] [PubMed]
8. Lv, J.; Zhang, H.; Chen, Y.; Li, G.; Jiang, L.; Singh, A.K.; Wang, H. Combination Therapy of Prednisone and ACE Inhibitor Versus ACE-Inhibitor Therapy Alone in Patients with IgA Nephropathy: A Randomized Controlled Trial. *Am. J. Kidney Dis.* **2009**, *53*, 26–32. [CrossRef]
9. Lv, J.; Zhang, H.; Wong, M.G.; Jardine, M.J.; Hladunewich, M.; Jha, V.; Monaghan, H.; Zhao, M.; Barbour, S.; Reich, H.; et al. Effect of Oral Methylprednisolone on Clinical Outcomes in Patients with IgA Nephropathy: The TESTING Randomized Clinical Trial. *JAMA* **2017**, *318*, 432–442. [CrossRef]
10. Floege, J.; Barbour, S.J.; Cattran, D.C.; Hogan, J.J.; Nachman, P.H.; Tang, S.C.W.; Wetzels, J.F.M.; Cheung, M.; Wheeler, D.C.; Winkelmayer, W.C.; et al. Management and Treatment of Glomerular Diseases (Part 1): Conclusions from a Kidney Disease: Improving Global Outcomes (KDIGO) Controversies Conference. *Kidney Int.* **2019**, *95*, 268–280. [CrossRef]
11. Cheung, C.K.; Barratt, J. Is IgA nephropathy a single disease? In *Pathogenesis and Treatment in IgA Nephropathy: An. International Comparison*; Springer: Tokyo, Japan, 2016; pp. 3–17. ISBN 9784431555889.
12. Barratt, J.; Rovin, B.; Diva, U.; Mercer, A.; Komers, R. Implementing the Kidney Health Initiative Surrogate Efficacy Endpoint in Patients with IgA Nephropathy (the PROTECT Trial). *Kidney Int. Rep.* **2019**, *4*, 1633–1637. [CrossRef]
13. Thompson, A.; Carroll, K.; Inker, L.A.; Floege, J.; Perkovic, V.; Boyer-Suavet, S.; Major, R.W.; Schimpf, J.I.; Barratt, J.; Cattran, D.C.; et al. Proteinuria Reduction as a Surrogate End Point in Trials of IgA Nephropathy. *Clin. J. Am. Soc. Nephrol.* **2019**, *14*, 469–481. [CrossRef]
14. Brandtzaeg, P. The Gut as Communicator between Environment and Host: Immunological Consequences. *Eur. J. Pharmacol.* **2011**, *668*, S16–S32. [CrossRef]
15. Barratt, J.; Bailey, E.M.; Buck, K.S.; Mailley, P.; Moayyedi, P.; Feehally, J.; Turney, J.H.; Crabtree, J.E.; Allen, A.C. Exaggerated Systemic Antibody Response to Mucosal Helicobacter Pylori Infection in IgA Nephropathy. *Am. J. Kidney Dis.* **1999**, *33*, 1049–1057. [CrossRef]
16. Allen, A.C.; Harper, S.J.; Feehally, J. Galactosylation of N- and O-Linked Carbohydrate Moieties of IgA1 and IgG in IgA Nephropathy. *Clin. Exp. Immunol.* **1995**, *100*, 470–474. [CrossRef] [PubMed]
17. Smith, A.C.; Molyneux, K.; Feehally, J.; Barratt, J. O-Glycosylation of Serum IgA1 Antibodies against Mucosal and Systemic Antigens in IgA Nephropathy. *J. Am. Soc. Nephrol.* **2006**, *17*, 3520–3528. [CrossRef] [PubMed]
18. Barratt, J.; Eitner, F.; Feehally, J.; Floege, J. Immune complex formation in IgA nephropathy: A case of the 'right' antibodies in the 'wrong' place at the 'wrong' time? *Nephrol. Dial. Transplant.* **2009**, *24*, 3620–3623. [CrossRef]
19. Floege, J. Mucosal Corticosteroid Therapy of IgA Nephropathy. *Kidney Int.* **2017**, *92*, 278–280. [CrossRef]
20. Barratt, J.; Rovin, B.H.; Cattran, D.; Floege, J.; Lafayette, R.; Tesar, V.; Trimarchi, H.; Zhang, H. Why Target the Gut to Treat IgA Nephropathy? *Kidney Int. Rep.* **2020**, *5*, 1620–1624. [CrossRef]
21. Fellström, B.C.; Barratt, J.; Cook, H.; Coppo, R.; Feehally, J.; de Fijter, J.W.; Floege, J.; Hetzel, G.; Jardine, A.G.; Locatelli, F.; et al. Targeted-Release Budesonide versus Placebo in Patients with IgA Nephropathy (NEFIGAN): A Double-Blind, Randomised, Placebo-Controlled Phase 2b Trial. *Lancet* **2017**, *389*, 2117–2127. [CrossRef]
22. Smerud, H.K.; Bárány, P.; Lindström, K.; Fernström, A.; Sandell, A.; Påhlsson, P.; Fellström, B. New Treatment for IgA Nephropathy: Enteric Budesonide Targeted to the Ileocecal Region Ameliorates Proteinuria. *Nephrol. Dial. Transpl.* **2011**, *26*, 3237–3242. [CrossRef] [PubMed]
23. Edsbäcker, S.; Andersson, T. Pharmacokinetics of Budesonide (Entocort EC) Capsules for Crohn's Disease. *Clin. Pharmacokinet.* **2004**, *43*, 803–821. [CrossRef] [PubMed]
24. Barratt, J.; Stone, A.; Kristensen, J. POS-830 Nefecon for the treatment of IGa nephropathy in patients at risk of progressing to end-stage renal disease: The nefigard phase 3 trial results. *Kidney Int. Rep.* **2021**, *6*, S361. [CrossRef]
25. Moldoveanu, Z.; Wyatt, R.J.; Lee, J.Y.; Tomana, M.; Julian, B.A.; Mestecky, J.; Huang, W.-Q.; Anreddy, S.R.; Hall, S.; Hastings, M.C.; et al. Patients with IgA Nephropathy Have Increased Serum Galactose-Deficient IgA1 Levels. *Kidney Int.* **2007**, *71*, 1148–1154. [CrossRef]

26. Zhao, N.; Hou, P.; Lv, J.; Moldoveanu, Z.; Li, Y.; Kiryluk, K.; Gharavi, A.G.; Novak, J.; Zhang, H. The Level of Galactose-Deficient IgA1 in the Sera of Patients with IgA Nephropathy Is Associated with Disease Progression. *Kidney Int.* **2012**, *82*, 790–796. [CrossRef] [PubMed]
27. Rizk, D.V.; Saha, M.K.; Hall, S.; Novak, L.; Brown, R.; Huang, Z.Q.; Fatima, H.; Julian, B.A.; Novak, J. Glomerular Immunodeposits of Patients with IgA Nephropathy Are Enriched for IgG Autoantibodies Specific for Galactose-Deficient IgA1. *J. Am. Soc. Nephrol.* **2019**, *30*, 2017–2026. [CrossRef]
28. McCarthy, D.D.; Chiu, S.; Gao, Y.; Summers-deLuca, L.E.; Gommerman, J.L. BAFF Induces a Hyper-IgA Syndrome in the Intestinal Lamina Propria Concomitant with IgA Deposition in the Kidney Independent of LIGHT. *Cell Immunol.* **2006**, *241*, 85–94. [CrossRef]
29. McCarthy, D.D.; Kujawa, J.; Wilson, C.; Papandile, A.; Poreci, U.; Porfilio, E.A.; Ward, L.; Lawson, M.A.E.; Macpherson, A.J.; McCoy, K.D.; et al. Mice Overexpressing BAFF Develop a Commensal Flora-Dependent, IgA-Associated Nephropathy. *J. Clin. Investig.* **2011**, *121*, 3991–4002. [CrossRef] [PubMed]
30. Goto, T.; Bandoh, N.; Yoshizaki, T.; Nozawa, H.; Takahara, M.; Ueda, S.; Hayashi, T.; Harabuchi, Y. Increase in B-Cell-Activation Factor (BAFF) and IFN-γ Productions by Tonsillar Mononuclear Cells Stimulated with Deoxycytidyl-Deoxyguanosine Oligodeoxynucleotides (CpG-ODN) in Patients with IgA Nephropathy. *Clin. Immunol.* **2008**, *126*, 260–269. [CrossRef]
31. Xin, G.; Shi, W.; Xu, L.X.; Su, Y.; Yan, L.J.; Li, K.S. Serum BAFF Is Elevated in Patients with IgA Nephropathy and Associated with Clinical and Histopathological Features. *J. Nephrol.* **2013**, *26*, 683–690. [CrossRef]
32. Muto, M.; Manfroi, B.; Suzuki, H.; Joh, K.; Nagai, M.; Wakai, S.; Righini, C.; Maiguma, M.; Izui, S.; Tomino, Y.; et al. Toll-like Receptor 9 Stimulation Induces Aberrant Expression of a Proliferation-Inducing Ligand by Tonsillar Germinal Center B Cells in IgA Nephropathy. *J. Am. Soc. Nephrol.* **2017**, *28*, 1227–1238. [CrossRef] [PubMed]
33. Zhai, Y.L.; Zhu, L.; Shi, S.F.; Liu, L.J.; Lv, J.C.; Zhang, H. Increased April Expression Induces IgA1 Aberrant Glycosylation in IgA Nephropathy. *Medicine* **2016**, *95*. [CrossRef]
34. Kiryluk, K.; Li, Y.; Scolari, F.; Sanna-Cherchi, S.; Choi, M.; Verbitsky, M.; Fasel, D.; Lata, S.; Prakash, S.; Shapiro, S.; et al. Discovery of New Risk Loci for IgA Nephropathy Implicates Genes Involved in Immunity against Intestinal Pathogens. *Nat. Genet.* **2014**, *46*, 1187–1196. [CrossRef] [PubMed]
35. Myette, J.R.; Kano, T.; Suzuki, H.; Sloan, S.E.; Szretter, K.J.; Ramakrishnan, B.; Adari, H.; Deotale, K.D.; Engler, F.; Shriver, Z.; et al. A Proliferation Inducing Ligand (APRIL) Targeted Antibody Is a Safe and Effective Treatment of Murine IgA Nephropathy. *Kidney Int.* **2019**, *96*, 104–116. [CrossRef] [PubMed]
36. Barratt, J.; Tumlin, J.A.; Suzuki, Y.; Kao, A.; Aydemir, A.; Zima, Y.; Appel, G. MO039THE 24-week interim analysis results of a randomized, double-blind, placebo-controlled phase II study of atacicept in patients with IgA nephropathy and persistent proteinuria. *Nephrol. Dial. Transplant.* **2020**, *35*. [CrossRef]
37. Lafayette, R.A.; Canetta, P.A.; Rovin, B.H.; Appel, G.B.; Novak, J.; Nath, K.A.; Sethi, S.; Tumlin, J.A.; Mehta, K.; Hogan, M.; et al. A Randomized, Controlled Trial of Rituximab in IgA Nephropathy with Proteinuria and Renal Dysfunction. *J. Am. Soc. Nephrol.* **2017**, *28*, 1306–1313. [CrossRef] [PubMed]
38. Hartono, C.; Chung, M.; Perlman, A.S.; Chevalier, J.M.; Serur, D.; Seshan, S.V.; Muthukumar, T. Bortezomib for Reduction of Proteinuria in IgA Nephropathy. *Kidney Int. Rep.* **2018**, *3*, 861–866. [CrossRef]
39. Yeo, S.C.; Cheung, C.K.; Barratt, J. New Insights into the Pathogenesis of IgA Nephropathy. *Pediatr Nephrol* **2018**, *33*, 763–777. [CrossRef] [PubMed]
40. Donadio, M.E.; Loiacono, E.; Peruzzi, L.; Amore, A.; Camilla, R.; Chiale, F.; Vergano, L.; Boido, A.; Conrieri, M.; Bianciotto, M.; et al. Toll-like Receptors, Immunoproteasome and Regulatory T Cells in Children with Henoch-Schönlein Purpura and Primary IgA Nephropathy. *Pediatr. Nephrol.* **2014**, *29*, 1545–1551. [CrossRef] [PubMed]
41. Suzuki, H.; Suzuki, Y.; Narita, I.; Aizawa, M.; Kihara, M.; Yamanaka, T.; Kanou, T.; Tsukaguchi, H.; Novak, J.; Horikoshi, S.; et al. Toll-like Receptor 9 Affects Severity of IgA Nephropathy. *J. Am. Soc. Nephrol.* **2008**, *19*, 2384–2395. [CrossRef]
42. Liu, L.J.; Yang, Y.; Shi, S.F.; Bao, Y.F.; Yang, C.; Zhu, S.N.; Sui, G.L.; Chen, Y.Q.; Lv, J.C.; Zhang, H. Effects of Hydroxychloroquine on Proteinuria in IgA Nephropathy: A Randomized Controlled Trial. *Am. J. Kidney Dis.* **2019**, *74*, 15–22. [CrossRef]
43. McAdoo, S.P.; Bhangal, G.; Page, T.; Cook, H.T.; Pusey, C.D.; Tam, F.W.K. Correlation of Disease Activity in Proliferative Glomerulonephritis with Glomerular Spleen Tyrosine Kinase Expression. *Kidney Int.* **2015**, *88*, 52–60. [CrossRef]
44. Kim, M.J.; McDaid, J.P.; McAdoo, S.P.; Barratt, J.; Molyneux, K.; Masuda, E.S.; Pusey, C.D.; Tam, F.W.K. Spleen Tyrosine Kinase Is Important in the Production of Proinflammatory Cytokines and Cell Proliferation in Human Mesangial Cells Following Stimulation with IgA1 Isolated from IgA Nephropathy Patients. *J. Immunol.* **2012**, *189*, 3751–3758. [CrossRef] [PubMed]
45. Tam, W.K.F.; Tumlin, J.; Barratt, J.; Rovin, H.B.; Roberts, S.D.I.; Roufosse, C.; Cook, H.T.; Tong, S.; Magilavy, D.; Lafayette, R. Sun-036 Spleen Tyrosine Kinase (Syk) Inhibition In Iga Nephropathy: A Global, Phase II, Randomised Placebo-Controlled Trial Of Fostamatinib. *Kidney Int. Rep.* **2019**, *4*, S168. [CrossRef]
46. Coppo, R.; Peruzzi, L.; Loiacono, E.; Bergallo, M.; Krutova, A.; Russo, M.L.; Cocchi, E.; Amore, A.; Lundberg, S.; Maixnerova, D.; et al. Defective Gene Expression of the Membrane Complement Inhibitor CD46 in Patients with Progressive Immunoglobulin A Nephropathy. *Nephrol Dial. Transpl.* **2019**, *34*, 587–596. [CrossRef]
47. Espinosa, M.; Ortega, R.; Sánchez, M.; Segarra, A.; Salcedo, M.T.; González, F.; Camacho, R.; Valdivia, M.A.; Cabrera, R.; López, K.; et al. Association of C4d Deposition with Clinical Outcomes in IgA Nephropathy. *Clin. J. Am. Soc. Nephrol.* **2014**, *9*, 897–904. [CrossRef] [PubMed]

48. Zhu, L.; Zhai, Y.L.; Wang, F.M.; Hou, P.; Lv, J.C.; Xu, D.M.; Shi, S.F.; Liu, L.J.; Yu, F.; Zhao, M.H.; et al. Variants in Complement Factor H and Complement Factor H-Related Protein Genes, CFHR3 and CFHR1, Affect Complement Activation in IgA Nephropathy. *J. Am. Soc. Nephrol.* **2015**, *26*, 1195–1204. [CrossRef] [PubMed]
49. Xie, J.; Kiryluk, K.; Li, Y.; Mladkova, N.; Zhu, L.; Hou, P.; Ren, H.; Wang, W.; Zhang, H.; Chen, N.; et al. Fine Mapping Implicates a Deletion of CFHR1 and CFHR3 in Protection from IgA Nephropathy in Han Chinese. *J. Am. Soc. Nephrol.* **2016**, *27*, 3187–3194. [CrossRef] [PubMed]
50. Jullien, P.; Laurent, B.; Claisse, G.; Masson, I.; Dinic, M.; Thibaudin, D.; Berthoux, F.; Alamartine, E.; Mariat, C.; Maillard, N. Deletion Variants of CFHR1 and CFHR3 Associate with Mesangial Immune Deposits but Not with Progression of IgA Nephropathy. *J. Am. Soc. Nephrol.* **2018**, *29*, 661–669. [CrossRef] [PubMed]
51. Daha, M.R.; van Kooten, C. Role of Complement in IgA Nephropathy. *J. Nephrol.* **2016**, *29*, 1–4. [CrossRef] [PubMed]
52. Rizk, D.V.; Maillard, N.; Julian, B.A.; Knoppova, B.; Green, T.J.; Novak, J.; Wyatt, R.J. The Emerging Role of Complement Proteins as a Target for Therapy of IgA Nephropathy. *Front. Immunol.* **2019**, *10*, 504. [CrossRef]
53. Jennette, J.C. The Immunohistology of IgA Nephropathy. *Am. J. Kidney Dis.* **1988**, *12*, 348–352. [CrossRef]
54. Espinosa, M.; Ortega, R.; Gómez-Carrasco, J.M.; López-Rubio, F.; López-Andreu, M.; López-Oliva, M.O.; Aljama, P. Mesangial C4d Deposition: A New Prognostic Factor in IgA Nephropathy. *Nephrol. Dial. Transplant.* **2009**, *24*, 886–891. [CrossRef]
55. Roos, A.; Rastaldi, M.P.; Calvaresi, N.; Oortwijn, B.D.; Schlagwein, N.; van Gijlswijk-Janssen, D.J.; Stahl, G.L.; Matsushita, M.; Fujita, T.; van Kooten, C.; et al. Glomerular Activation of the Lectin Pathway of Complement in IgA Nephropathy Is Associated with More Severe Renal Disease. *J. Am. Soc. Nephrol.* **2006**, *17*, 1724–1734. [CrossRef]
56. Miyamoto, H.; Yoshioka, K.; Takemura, T.; Akano, N.; Maki, S. Immunohistochemical Study of the Membrane Attack Complex of Complement in IgA Nephropathy. *Virchows Arch. A Pathol. Anat. Histopathol.* **1988**, *413*, 77–86. [CrossRef]
57. Conley, M.E.; Cooper, M.D.; Michael, A.F. Selective Deposition of Immunoglobulin A1 in Immunoglobulin A Nephropathy, Anaphylactoid Purpura Nephritis, and Systemic Lupus Erythematosus. *J. Clin. Investig.* **1980**, *66*, 1432–1436. [CrossRef]
58. Hiki, Y.; Odani, H.; Takahashi, M.; Yasuda, Y.; Nishimoto, A.; Iwase, H.; Shinzato, T.; Kobayashi, Y.; Maeda, K. Mass Spectrometry Proves Under-O-Glycosylation of Glomerular IgA1 in IgA Nephropathy. *Kidney Int.* **2001**, *59*, 1077–1085. [CrossRef]
59. Wyatt, R.J.; Julian, B.A. IgA Nephropathy. *N. Engl. J. Med.* **2013**, *368*, 2402–2414. [CrossRef] [PubMed]
60. Floege, J.; Daha, M.R. IgA Nephropathy: New Insights into the Role of Complement. *Kidney Int.* **2018**, *94*, 16–18. [CrossRef] [PubMed]
61. Maillard, N.; Wyatt, R.J.; Julian, B.A.; Kiryluk, K.; Gharavi, A.; Fremeaux-Bacchi, V.; Novak, J. Current Understanding of the Role of Complement in IgA Nephropathy. *J. Am. Soc. Nephrol.* **2015**, 1–10. [CrossRef] [PubMed]
62. Wyatt, R.J.; Kanayama, Y.; Julian, B.A.; Negoro, N.; Sugimoto, S.; Hudson, E.C.; Curd, J.G. Complement Activation in IgA Nephropathy. *Kidney Int.* **1987**, *31*, 1019–1023. [CrossRef] [PubMed]
63. Liu, L.; Zhang, Y.; Duan, X.; Peng, Q.; Liu, Q.; Zhou, Y.; Quan, S.; Xing, G. C3a, C5a Renal Expression and Their Receptors Are Correlated to Severity of IgA Nephropathy. *J. Clin. Immunol.* **2014**, *34*, 224–232. [CrossRef] [PubMed]
64. Julian, B.A.; Wyatt, R.J.; McMorrow, R.G.; Galla, J.H. Serum Complement Proteins in IgA Nephropathy. *Clin. Nephrol.* **1983**, *20*, 251–258. [PubMed]
65. Clarkson, A.R.; Seymour, A.E.; Thompson, A.J.; Haynes, W.D.; Chan, Y.L.; Jackson, B. IgA Nephropathy: A Syndrome of Uniform Morphology, Diverse Clinical Features and Uncertain Prognosis. *Clin. Nephrol.* **1977**, *8*, 459–471.
66. Evans, D.J.; Williams, D.G.; Peters, D.K.; Sissons, J.G.; Boulton-Jones, J.M.; Ogg, C.S.; Cameron, J.S.; Hoffbrand, B.I. Glomerular Deposition of Properdin in Henoch-Schönlein Syndrome and Idiopathic Focal Nephritis. *Br. Med. J.* **1973**, *3*, 326–328. [CrossRef] [PubMed]
67. Gluckman, J.C.; Jacob, N.; Beaufils, H.; Baumelou, A.; Salah, H.; German, A.; Legrain, M. Clinical Significance of Circulating Immune Complexes Detection in Chronic Glomerulonephritis. *Nephron* **1978**, *22*, 138–145. [CrossRef] [PubMed]
68. Miyazaki, R.; Kuroda, M.; Akiyama, T.; Otani, I.; Tofuku, Y.; Takeda, R. Glomerular Deposition and Serum Levels of Complement Control Proteins in Patients with IgA Nephropathy. *Clin. Nephrol.* **1984**, *21*, 335–340.
69. Tomino, Y.; Suzuki, S.; Imai, H.; Saito, T.; Kawamura, T.; Yorioka, N.; Harada, T.; Yasumoto, Y.; Kida, H.; Kobayashi, Y.; et al. Measurement of Serum IgA and C3 May Predict the Diagnosis of Patients with IgA Nephropathy Prior to Renal Biopsy. *J. Clin. Lab. Anal.* **2000**, *14*, 220–223. [CrossRef]
70. Komatsu, H.; Fujimoto, S.; Hara, S.; Sato, Y.; Yamada, K.; Eto, T. Relationship between Serum IgA/C3 Ratio and Progression of IgA Nephropathy. *Intern. Med.* **2004**, *43*, 1023–1028. [CrossRef]
71. Kawasaki, Y.; Maeda, R.; Ohara, S.; Suyama, K.; Hosoya, M. Serum IgA/C3 and Glomerular C3 Staining Predict Severity of IgA Nephropathy. *Pediatr. Int.* **2018**, *60*, 162–167. [CrossRef] [PubMed]
72. Kim, S.J.; Koo, H.M.; Lim, B.J.; Oh, H.J.; Yoo, D.E.; Shin, D.H.; Lee, M.J.; Doh, F.M.; Park, J.T.; Yoo, T.H.; et al. Decreased Circulating C3 Levels and Mesangial C3 Deposition Predict Renal Outcome in Patients with IgA Nephropathy. *PLoS ONE* **2012**, *7*, e40495. [CrossRef] [PubMed]
73. Czerkinsky, C.; Koopman, W.J.; Jackson, S.; Collins, J.E.; Crago, S.S.; Schrohenloher, R.E.; Julian, B.A.; Galla, J.H.; Mestecky, J. Circulating Immune Complexes and Immunoglobulin A Rheumatoid Factor in Patients with Mesangial Immunoglobulin A Nephropathies. *J. Clin. Investig.* **1986**, *77*, 1931–1938. [CrossRef] [PubMed]
74. Bi, T.D.; Zheng, J.N.; Zhang, J.X.; Yang, L.S.; Liu, N.; Yao, L.; Liu, L.L. Serum Complement C4 Is an Important Prognostic Factor for IgA Nephropathy: A Retrospective Study. *BMC Nephrol.* **2019**, *20*, 244. [CrossRef]

75. Gharavi, A.G.; Kiryluk, K.; Choi, M.; Li, Y.; Hou, P.; Xie, J.; Sanna-Cherchi, S.; Men, C.J.; Julian, B.A.; Wyatt, R.J.; et al. Genome-Wide Association Study Identifies Susceptibility Loci for IgA Nephropathy. *Nat. Genet.* **2011**, *43*, 321–327. [CrossRef] [PubMed]
76. Kiryluk, K.; Li, Y.; Sanna-Cherchi, S.; Rohanizadegan, M.; Suzuki, H.; Eitner, F.; Snyder, H.J.; Choi, M.; Hou, P.; Scolari, F.; et al. Geographic Differences in Genetic Susceptibility to IgA Nephropathy: GWAS Replication Study and Geospatial Risk Analysis. *PLoS Genet.* **2012**, *8*, e1002765. [CrossRef]
77. Onda, K.; Ohsawa, I.; Ohi, H.; Tamano, M.; Mano, S.; Wakabayashi, M.; Toki, A.; Horikoshi, S.; Fujita, T.; Tomino, Y. Excretion of Complement Proteins and Its Activation Marker C5b-9 in IgA Nephropathy in Relation to Renal Function. *BMC Nephrol.* **2011**, *12*, 64. [CrossRef] [PubMed]
78. Zhang, J.J.; Jiang, L.; Liu, G.; Wang, S.X.; Zou, W.Z.; Zhang, H.; Zhao, M.H. Levels of Urinary Complement Factor H in Patients with IgA Nephropathy Are Closely Associated with Disease Activity. *Scand. J. Immunol* **2009**, *69*, 457–464. [CrossRef]
79. Rosenblad, T.; Rebetz, J.; Johansson, M.; Békássy, Z.; Sartz, L.; Karpman, D. Eculizumab Treatment for Rescue of Renal Function in IgA Nephropathy. *Pediatr. Nephrol.* **2014**, *29*, 2225–2228. [CrossRef] [PubMed]
80. Ring, T.; Pedersen, B.B.; Salkus, G.; Goodship, T.H. Use of Eculizumab in Crescentic IgA Nephropathy: Proof of Principle and Conundrum? *Clin. Kidney J.* **2015**, *8*, 489–491. [CrossRef]
81. Herzog, A.L.; Wanner, C.; Amann, K.; Lopau, K. First Treatment of Relapsing Rapidly Progressive IgA Nephropathy With Eculizumab After Living Kidney Donation: A Case Report. *Transpl. Proc.* **2017**, *49*, 1574–1577. [CrossRef]
82. Bruchfeld, A.; Nachman, P.; Parikh, S.; Lafayette, R.; Potarca, A.; Diehl, J.; Lohr, L.; Miao, S.; Schall, T.; Bekker, P. TO012C5A receptor inhibitor avacopan in IgA nephropathy study. *Nephrol. Dial. Transplant.* **2017**, *32*, iii82. [CrossRef]
83. Dobó, J.; Kocsis, A.; Gál, P. Be on Target: Strategies of Targeting Alternative and Lectin Pathway Components in Complement-Mediated Diseases. *Front. Immunol.* **2018**, *9*, 1851. [CrossRef] [PubMed]
84. Merle, N.S.; Church, S.E.; Fremeaux-Bacchi, V.; Roumenina, L.T. Complement System Part I—Molecular Mechanisms of Activation and Regulation. *Front. Immunol.* **2015**, *6*, 262. [CrossRef] [PubMed]
85. Selvaskandan, H.; Cheung, C.K.; Muto, M.; Barratt, J. New Strategies and Perspectives on Managing IgA Nephropathy. *Clin. Exp. Nephrol.* **2019**, *23*, 577–588. [CrossRef] [PubMed]
86. Lafayette, R.A.; Rovin, B.H.; Reich, H.N.; Tumlin, J.A.; Floege, J.; Barratt, J. Safety, Tolerability and Efficacy of Narsoplimab, a Novel MASP-2 Inhibitor for the Treatment of IgA Nephropathy. *Kidney Int. Rep.* **2020**, *5*, 2032–2041. [CrossRef] [PubMed]
87. Allen, A.C.; Bailey, E.M.; Brenchley, P.E.; Buck, K.S.; Barratt, J.; Feehally, J. Mesangial IgA1 in IgA Nephropathy Exhibits Aberrant O-Glycosylation: Observations in Three Patients. *Kidney Int.* **2001**, *60*, 969–973. [CrossRef] [PubMed]
88. Waldo, F.B. Is Henoch-Schönlein Purpura the Systemic Form of IgA Nephropathy? *Am. J. Kidney Dis.* **1988**, *12*, 373–377. [CrossRef]
89. Novak, J.; Moldoveanu, Z.; Renfrow, M.B.; Yanagihara, T.; Suzuki, H.; Raska, M.; Hall, S.; Brown, R.; Huang, W.Q.; Goepfert, A.; et al. IgA Nephropathy and Henoch-Schoenlein Purpura Nephritis: Aberrant Glycosylation of IgA1, Formation of IgA1-Containing Immune Complexes, and Activation of Mesangial Cells. *Contrib. Nephrol.* **2007**, *157*, 134–138. [CrossRef]
90. Suzuki, H.; Moldoveanu, Z.; Julian, B.A.; Wyatt, R.J.; Novak, J. Autoantibodies Specific for Galactose-Deficient IgA1 in IgA Vasculitis With Nephritis. *Kidney Int. Rep.* **2019**, *4*, 1717–1724. [CrossRef]
91. Selvaskandan, H.; Kay Cheung, C.; Dormer, J.; Wimbury, D.; Martinez, M.; Xu, G.; Barratt, J. Inhibition of the Lectin Pathway of the Complement System as a Novel Approach in the Management of IgA Vasculitis-Associated Nephritis. *Nephron* **2020**, *144*, 453–458. [CrossRef]
92. Konar, M.; Granoff, D.M. Eculizumab Treatment and Impaired Opsonophagocytic Killing of Meningococci by Whole Blood from Immunized Adults. *Blood* **2017**, *130*, 891–899. [CrossRef]
93. Barnum, S.R. Therapeutic Inhibition of Complement: Well Worth the Risk. *Trends Pharmacol. Sci.* **2017**, *38*, 503–505. [CrossRef] [PubMed]
94. Cohn, A.C.; MacNeil, J.R.; Clark, T.A.; Ortega-Sanchez, I.R.; Briere, E.Z.; Meissner, H.C.; Baker, C.J.; Messonnier, N.E. Prevention and Control of Meningococcal Disease: Recommendations of the Advisory Committee on Immunization Practices (ACIP). *MMWR Recomm. Rep.* **2013**, *62*, 1–28.
95. Ricklin, D.; Mastellos, D.C.; Reis, E.S.; Lambris, J.D. The Renaissance of Complement Therapeutics. *Nat. Rev. Nephrol.* **2018**, *14*, 26–47. [CrossRef]
96. Simonson, M.S.; Wann, S.; Mené, P.; Dubyak, G.R.; Kester, M.; Nakazato, Y.; Sedor, J.R.; Dunn, M.J. Endothelin Stimulates Phospholipase C, Na+/H+ Exchange, c-Fos Expression, and Mitogenesis in Rat Mesangial Cells. *J. Clin. Investig.* **1989**, *83*, 708–712. [CrossRef]
97. Ohta, K.; Hirata, Y.; Shichiri, M.; Kanno, K.; Emori, T.; Tomita, K.; Marumo, F. Urinary Excretion of Endothelin-1 in Normal Subjects and Patients with Renal Disease. *Kidney Int.* **1991**, *39*, 307–311. [CrossRef]
98. Raina, R.; Chauvin, A.; Chakraborty, R.; Nair, N.; Shah, H.; Krishnappa, V.; Kusumi, K. The Role of Endothelin and Endothelin Antagonists in Chronic Kidney Disease. *Kidney Dis.* **2020**, *6*, 22–34. [CrossRef] [PubMed]
99. Kohan, D.E.; Pollock, D.M. Endothelin Antagonists for Diabetic and Non-Diabetic Chronic Kidney Disease. *Br. J. Clin. Pharmacol.* **2013**, *76*, 573–579. [CrossRef]
100. Lehrke, I.; Waldherr, R.; Ritz, E.; Wagner, J. Renal Endothelin-1 and Endothelin Receptor Type B Expression in Glomerular Diseases with Proteinuria. *J. Am. Soc. Nephrol.* **2001**, *12*, 2321–2329. [CrossRef] [PubMed]

101. Maixnerová, D.; Merta, M.; Reiterová, J.; Stekrová, J.; Rysavá, R.; Obeidová, H.; Viklický, O.; Potměsil, P.; Tesar, V. The Influence of Three Endothelin-1 Polymorphisms on the Progression of IgA Nephropathy. *Folia Biol.* **2007**, *53*, 27–32.
102. Tycová, I.; Hrubá, P.; Maixnerová, D.; Girmanová, E.; Mrázová, P.; Straňavová, L.; Zachoval, R.; Merta, M.; Slatinská, J.; Kollár, M.; et al. Molecular Profiling in IgA Nephropathy and Focal and Segmental Glomerulosclerosis. *Physiol. Res.* **2018**, *67*, 93–105. [CrossRef]
103. Nakamura, T.; Ebihara, I.; Fukui, M.; Tomino, Y.; Koide, H. Effect of a Specific Endothelin Receptor a Antagonist on Glomerulonephritis of DdY Mice with IgA Nephropathy. *Nephron* **1996**, *72*, 454–460. [CrossRef] [PubMed]
104. Trachtman, H.; Nelson, P.; Adler, S.; Campbell, K.N.; Chaudhuri, A.; Derebail, V.K.; Gambaro, G.; Gesualdo, L.; Gipson, D.S.; Hogan, J.; et al. DUET: A Phase 2 Study Evaluating the Efficacy and Safety of Sparsentan in Patients with FSGS. *J. Am. Soc. Nephrol.* **2018**, *29*, 2745–2754. [CrossRef] [PubMed]
105. Shelton, L.M.; Park, B.K.; Copple, I.M. Role of Nrf2 in Protection against Acute Kidney Injury. *Kidney Int* **2013**, *84*, 1090–1095. [CrossRef] [PubMed]
106. Pergola, P.; Appel, G.; Block, G.; Chin, M.; Goldsberry, A.; Inker, L.; Jarad, G.; Meyer, C.; Rastogi, A.; Rizk, D.; et al. FP110A phase 2 trial of the safety and efficacy of bardoxolone methyl in patients with rare chronic kidney diseases. *Nephrol. Dial. Transplant.* **2018**, *33*, i14. [CrossRef]
107. Wanner, C.; Inzucchi, S.E.; Lachin, J.M.; Fitchett, D.; von Eynatten, M.; Mattheus, M.; Johansen, O.E.; Woerle, H.J.; Broedl, U.C.; Zinman, B. Empagliflozin and Progression of Kidney Disease in Type 2 Diabetes. *N. Engl. J. Med.* **2016**, *375*, 323–334. [CrossRef]
108. Perkovic, V.; Jardine, M.J.; Neal, B.; Bompoint, S.; Heerspink, H.J.L.; Charytan, D.M.; Edwards, R.; Agarwal, R.; Bakris, G.; Bull, S.; et al. Canagliflozin and Renal Outcomes in Type 2 Diabetes and Nephropathy. *N. Engl. J. Med.* **2019**, *380*, 2295–2306. [CrossRef]
109. Neal, B.; Perkovic, V.; Mahaffey, K.W.; de Zeeuw, D.; Fulcher, G.; Erondu, N.; Shaw, W.; Law, G.; Desai, M.; Matthews, D.R. Canagliflozin and Cardiovascular and Renal Events in Type 2 Diabetes. *N. Engl. J. Med.* **2017**, *377*, 644–657. [CrossRef]
110. Heerspink, H.J.L.; Stefánsson, B.V.; Correa-Rotter, R.; Chertow, G.M.; Greene, T.; Hou, F.-F.; Mann, J.F.E.; McMurray, J.J.V.; Lindberg, M.; Rossing, P.; et al. Dapagliflozin in Patients with Chronic Kidney Disease. *N. Engl. J. Med.* **2020**, *383*, 1436–1446. [CrossRef]
111. Wheeler, D.C.; Toto, R.D.; Stefansson, B.V.; Jongs, N.; Chertow, G.M.; Greene, T.; Hou, F.F.; McMurray, J.J.V.; Pecoits-Filho, R.; Correa-Rotter, R.; et al. A Pre-Specified Analysis of the DAPA-CKD Trial Demonstrates the Effects of Dapagliflozin on Major Adverse Kidney Events in Patients with IgA Nephropathy. *Kidney Int.* **2021**. [CrossRef]
112. Barratt, J.; Floege, J. SGLT-2 Inhibition in IgA Nephropathy: The New Standard-of-Care? *Kidney Int.* **2021**. [CrossRef] [PubMed]

MDPI
St. Alban-Anlage 66
4052 Basel
Switzerland
Tel. +41 61 683 77 34
Fax +41 61 302 89 18
www.mdpi.com

Journal of Clinical Medicine Editorial Office
E-mail: jcm@mdpi.com
www.mdpi.com/journal/jcm

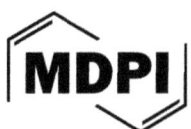

www.ingramcontent.com/pod-product-compliance
Lightning Source LLC
LaVergne TN
LVHW070715100526
838202LV00013B/1096